Eating Disorders

Eating Disorders
A Guide to Medical Care and Complications

THIRD EDITION

EDITED BY

Philip S. Mehler, MD, FACP, FAED, CEDS

Chief Medical Officer, The Eating Recovery Center
Founder and Executive Medical Director, ACUTE at Denver Health
The Glassman Professor of Medicine, University of Colorado
    School of Medicine

AND

Arnold E. Andersen, MD

Professor Emeritus, The Carver College of Medicine
Department of Psychiatry, University of Iowa
Adjunct Lecturer, Johns Hopkins Medical Institutions

JOHNS HOPKINS UNIVERSITY PRESS   BALTIMORE

Note to the Reader: This book is not meant to substitute for medical care and treatment should not be based solely on its contents. Instead, treatment must be developed in a dialogue between the individual and his or her physician. Our book has been written to help with that dialogue.

Drug dosage: The author and publisher have made reasonable efforts to determine that the selection of drugs discussed in this text conform to the practices of the general medical community. The medications described do not necessarily have specific approval by the US Food and Drug Administration for use in the diseases for which they are recommended. In view of ongoing research, changes in governmental regulation, and the constant flow of information relating to drug therapy and drug reactions, the reader is urged to check the package insert of each drug for any change in indications and dosage and for warnings and precautions. This is particularly important when the recommended agent is a new and/or infrequently used drug.

© 1999, 2010, 2017 Johns Hopkins University Press
All rights reserved. Published 2017
Printed in the United States of America on acid-free paper
9 8 7 6 5 4 3 2 1

Johns Hopkins University Press
2715 North Charles Street
Baltimore, Maryland 21218-4363
www.press.jhu.edu

Library of Congress Cataloging-in-Publication Data
Names: Mehler, Philip S., author. | Andersen, Arnold E., author.
Title: Eating disorders : a guide to medical care and complications / Philip S. Mehler and Arnold E. Andersen.
Description: Third edition. | Baltimore : Johns Hopkins University Press, [2017] | Includes bibliographical references and index.
Identifiers: LCCN 2017034510| ISBN 9781421423425 (hardcover : alk. paper) | ISBN 1421423421 (hardcover : alk. paper) | ISBN 9781421423432 (pbk. : alk. paper) | ISBN 142142343X (pbk. : alk. paper) | ISBN 9781421423449 (electronic) | ISBN 1421423448 (electronic)
Subjects: | MESH: Feeding and Eating Disorders—therapy | Feeding and Eating Disorders—complications
Classification: LCC RC552.E18 | NLM WM 175 | DDC 616.85/26—dc23
LC record available at https://lccn.loc.gov/2017034510

A catalog record for this book is available from the British Library.

Special discounts are available for bulk purchases of this book. For more information, please contact Special Sales at 410-516-6936 or specialsales@press.jhu.edu.

Johns Hopkins University Press uses environmentally friendly book materials, including recycled text paper that is composed of at least 30 percent post-consumer waste, whenever possible.

To my wife, Leah, and Avi, Ilana, and Benji and their families, for their devotion and love, and to the memory of my late parents, Irving and Bernice Mehler, for their unfailing efforts and invaluable guidance

—Philip S. Mehler

To Helen, my wife, and Allan, Karl, and Ellie, for their loving patience and encouragement

—Arnold E. Andersen

Contents

Preface

This third edition was prompted by both the repeat success of the second edition and the ongoing explosive increase in medical information available for the care of persons with eating disorders. As with previous editions, the intended audience for this new edition is primarily clinicians with direct patient care responsibility for treating eating disorders, but it also extends to include a host of other devoted professionals who are involved in the detection of eating disorders and the treatment of these patients, including teachers and various types of mental health professionals, along with the families whose loved ones are struggling with the potential ravages of these diseases. However, overall, we emphasize the role of eating disorder clinicians and primary care clinicians.

Our overarching goal is to promote excellence in medical care with requisite detail, while attempting to minimize excessive obscure medical terminology. This has been achieved by being directive, albeit selective, based on our expansive and long clinical practice in both internal medicine and psychiatry, and supported by current and updated references from the relevant medical literature. Our collective experience in this field exceeds 75 years at all levels of care. Whenever possible, our immutable tenet is to predicate our writings on an evidence-based approach, tempered by hands-on, practical methods of treatment and reasonable explanation, knowing that the vicissitudes of patient care and individual circumstance also factor in the calculus of medical and psychiatric care. We truly remain convinced that this approach will continue to be most useful for our readers and offer substantial benefit.

The approach of each chapter is to identify common questions to be answered and to offer a clinical case or two with highlights pertinent to the subject. We strive to describe the background for understanding the nature of the medical psychiatric issue, to offer an approach to diagnosis and treatment, and, finally, to recommend selected up-to-date and pertinent references. The full literature is so voluminous at present, and will continue to expand, that winnowing pertinent references is crucial. All chapters in the third edition have been at least partially written by myself or Dr. Andersen, making a close working relationship between an iconic and highly experienced psychiatrist and a widely published internist to achieve a pragmatic and feasible method for fully updating this edition. For this edition, we also reached out to include a select number of devoted and highly experienced clinicians who are viewed as national thought leaders in this field of endeavor. Their work has been closely edited by us for content, accuracy, and utility.

Besides our commitment to substantially update the knowledge presented in this third edition, we have also opted to make some significant changes, mostly driven by new and emerging evidence in this field. Thus, the chapter on the multidisciplinary approach is completely rewritten by a well-respected and highly experienced cadre of eating disorder clinicians. The discussion of osteoporosis is much expanded to comprehensively address this vitally important subject matter. The cardiology chapter is very different from that in the previous edition in deference to rapidly emerging evidence related to cardiovascular complications. The information on diabetes has been culled out into its own chapter and completely written anew in recognition of the increased knowledge about the care of the patient who has diabetes and an eating disorder and the increasingly recognized entity of diabulimia. Lastly, the chapter on ethics is completely revised in the light of new legal opportunities that have become available in the past seven years that greatly affect care. As a result of these efforts, this new edition is much lengthier than the previous ones.

Growing and learning always go together as a medium to advocate for the protection of our patients and their families who have grown to trust our advice. We have aimed to emphasize and strive to provide a practical treatment approach with tools, references, and resources to define a process we believe will enhance patient outcomes in your clinics, practices, and health care systems. Clinicians play a vital, trusted, and influential role in providing needed care and counsel to these vulnerable patients. The time to demand excellence in their care is now. The heterogeneity of eating disorders adds to the inherent complexity of this patient population. Diagnosis and medical treatment must be cognizant of the confluence of multiple interacting body systems. Therefore, while trying to avoid being pedantic, we advocate for humility with a modicum of informed confidence to accomplish excellent patient care.

Tributes should be plentiful, but I am limited by space. Many patients, clinicians, and mentors have helped inform our practice and writings over our combined eight decades of involvement in this field. Ralph Emerson wrote, "The only way to have a friend is to be one." We have many friends in our network of eating disorder professionals, for whom we are ever grateful. They are helping to flip the script toward better care by their devoted efforts directed at the seeds of unhealthy eating, which are sown in all facets of life. Specifically, however, we want to acknowledge the ongoing support of the Johns Hopkins University Press and our editor, Jackie Wehmueller, who constantly guided and encouraged our work while demanding unrelenting excellence.

In addition, I would be remiss if I did not offer my personal and sincere gratitude to my coeditor, Dr. Arnold Andersen, an iconic, beloved, and highly respected colleague, who has long been a mentor to multitudes and an irrefutable leader in this field for four decades. His wealth of experience, measured approach, and wisdom made this third edition a reality. In addition, I want to express my appreciation to Dr. Ken Weiner for his unfailing support and friendship since he introduced me to the eating disorder field 30 years ago. Also, many thanks to Dr. Margherita Mascolo, Medical Director of ACUTE, and her devoted team. Since I founded this medical stabilization unit, I have greatly benefited from the amazing medical lessons ACUTE's patients have taught me, as well as from the patients and dedicated staff at the Eating Recovery Center. Finally, I would like to acknowledge the unfailing and superb help of my long-time assistant, Ms. Adrianna Padgett, as well as Ms. Bobbi West-Stemple.

Philip S. Mehler, MD, FACP, FAED, CEDS

Eating Disorders

1

Diagnosis and Treatment of the Eating Disorders Spectrum in Primary Care Medicine

Arnold E. Andersen, MD

Common Questions

What are eating disorders? Why are they a public health concern?

How do eating disorders present to physicians, psychologists, teachers, coaches, and others?

What risk factors increase the probability of developing an eating disorder?

How are eating disorders diagnosed? How have *DSM*-5 and ICD-10 changed diagnosis?

How does a transdiagnostic approach compare with *DSM*-5 and ICD-10?

Why are eating disorders best understood as a spectrum disorder?

Is a simple screening instrument available?

How do subgroups of the eating disorders spectrum (EDOS) differ from each other?

What are the most common comorbid psychiatric disorders accompanying eating disorders?

What is the natural history and development of eating disorders over time?

What about overlooked groups: how are males, older women, minorities, and people with intellectual disabilities affected?

How serious are eating disorders? What are the causes of death?

What are the key principles of treatment? What role do medications play?

When should a primary care clinician refer a patient rather than carry out treatment?

What are the criteria for hospitalization?
What role does genetics play?
Is prevention possible?
How can the burden on caregivers be alleviated?

Case 1

A.H., a 25-year-old female, was referred by her local psychiatrist for treatment of severe anorexia nervosa, complicated by a fractured humerus. She had developed body image distress and perception of fatness starting at age 13. She had been slightly chubby and was teased by her peers, especially about her "thunder thighs." She restricted food and lost weight from 151 pounds at 5 feet 4 inches (body mass index [BMI] of 26) to 84.9 pounds (BMI 14.6) at admission. In addition to eating fewer than 500 calories a day, she ran 6–8 miles a day and lifted weights. She limited herself to no more than 5 grams of fat a day and became vegetarian, not a family tradition. She developed fearfulness about "dangerous foods," such as cheese.

A.H. stated: "I felt cold all the time. My skin was dry. My hair started to fall out and my nails were brittle." Menses stopped at age 19. She was preoccupied with thoughts of food, weight, and shape for "80% to 90% of the day." She experienced a severe fear of becoming fat, even as her weight plummeted. Her mood became fragile, often tearful. Family "walked on eggshells" to avoid displeasing her and provoking irritability. Her temperament was that of a self-critical, perfectionistic young woman for whom expression of emotions was a foreign experience.

Three previous residential treatments resulted in only temporary improvement, followed by relapse into her anorexic pattern of behavior and thinking. No binges or purges developed. Shortly before admission, she fell on an icy sidewalk and fractured her humerus. Bone mineral density by dual-energy X-ray absorptiometry (DEXA) scan for L1–L4 was 0.675 g/cm^3, T = −3.4. Left hip bone density was 0.674 g/cm^3, T = −2.2. Hemoglobin of 5.4 required four transfusions. Labs showed hyponatremia of 126 mEq/L. Calcium was low, but potassium and phosphorus were within normal limits. EKG showed bradycardia of 45. Her displaced fracture was treated surgically with a rod, followed by physical therapy. A.H. had never abused alcohol or street drugs. Her two previous relationships had ended poorly, and she had a sense of distrust about future relationships.

During the inpatient portion of comprehensive treatment, A.H. restored her weight to 85% of her goal weight of 122–126 pounds. She accomplished the remainder of her weight restoration in partial hospital (day hospital, 5 days a week), achieving 100% of her goal weight. Her morbid fear of fatness diminished, and she developed an acceptance of a healthy weight and body image, learning cognitive behavioral skills in group, individual, and family therapy to challenge her overvalued beliefs. Her mood became euthymic and stable. No psychotropic medications were needed. She made considerable progress in catching up with normal development during a year of relapse prevention outpatient therapy after discharge.

Figure 1.1 shows severe starvation in a woman with anorexia nervosa.

Case 2

G.M. was an 18-year-old male who had reached a weight of 205 pounds at 6 feet tall. He was teased by his classmates and was advised by his coach to take off weight. He gradually cut down food intake to the point of having only an orange a day plus a health shake, and he lost almost 60 pounds over 3 months. He developed the superior mesenteric artery syndrome, becoming nauseated and vomiting after meals. His primary care physician recognized the compressive effect of a full stomach on the superior mesenteric artery, caused by the absence of the abdominal fat pad, which had been severely diminished by self-starvation. G.M. was promptly treated in the hospital, and though he minimized his desire for drastic weight loss, no other cause for his nausea and vomiting was found. He fully restored his weight and went on to maintain himself in a healthy range with full relief of abdominal symptoms. He was diagnosed with a probable eating disorder and associated depressive symptomatology, as well as the superior mesenteric artery syndrome.

Figure. 1.2 shows a young man starved from anorexia nervosa. See chapter 13 for an extended discussion.

Background

In the nineteenth century, tuberculosis and syphilis were called "great pretenders," presenting to clinicians in many disguised forms. In a similar manner, eating disorders in the twenty-first century appear in a variety of disguises before physicians and other health professionals.

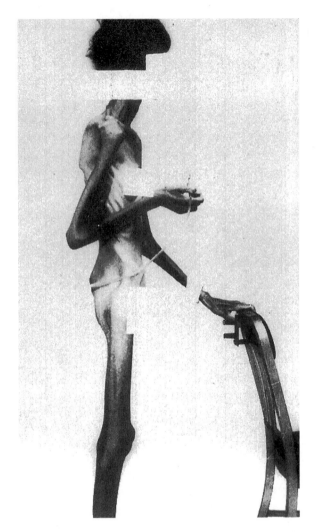

Figure 1.1. A typical very ill woman with anorexia nervosa. Note the extreme emaciation and lack of soft tissue.

They are underdiagnosed and overlooked. See table 1.1 for typical ways in which eating disorders present to primary care physicians.

Eating disorders constitute a public health concern with a greater prevalence than childhood diabetes or schizophrenia. They carry the highest probability of death among all psychiatric disorders, resulting in 6–12 times the expected mortality for females 12–25 years old (Arcelus et al.,

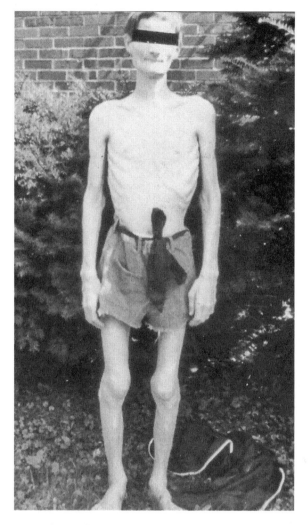

Figure 1.2. A typical very ill man with anorexia nervosa. Reproduced with permission of the patient.

2011; Fichter and Quadflieg, 2016). Even when subclinical by formal diagnostic criteria, these disorders impose a significant burden on the normal development of a healthy identity in young people entrained in their symptomatology. Preoccupation with weight, shape, and body image results in functional psychosocial impairment during the adolescence of a large percentage of young women and significant numbers of young men.

Table 1.1. Typical ways in which eating disorders present to primary care physicians

- Physician notes unexplained decreased weight; preoccupation with dieting or body shape; abnormal laboratory signs; failure to increase weight proportional to height in preteen or teenaged patient; or unexplained amenorrhea in menstruating patient.
- Parent or significant other expresses concerns about child/partner being preoccupied with weight or having unexplained weight loss; unexplained loss of periods in daughter; signs of vomiting without medical illness; excessive use of bathroom or shower after meals; signs of binge eating / disappearance of food; relentless workouts.
- Referral by coach, teacher, or psychologist for evaluation of possible eating disorder.
- Presentation of patient *complaints* seemingly compatible with disorders of specific organ systems: thyroid (hyperactive, weight loss), malabsorption (diarrhea), other GI disorders (reflux, ulcers, lactose intolerance, stomach pain, bloating), cancer (weight loss, loss of appetite in older patients), parasites (unexplained weight loss), dermatologic (loss of hair), dental (multiple new caries, loss of enamel). *Rule in* eating disorders before *ruling out* medical causes of eating disorder symptoms.
- Positive answers to routine behavioral surveys, written or in person, for presence of an eating disorder; e.g., (modified) SCOFF (mSCOFF) questionnaire.
- Routine history and examination of a patient in high-risk sports or interest group, or with gay orientation.

Eating disorders are, at their core, disorders of eating behavior that develop to deal with problems in a variety of areas of life, including self-esteem, emotional regulation, fears of growing up, and relationship conflicts, developing from an overvaluation of the benefits of slimness or shape change as methods to deal with these issues. They have almost nothing to do with food, just as fear of riding in elevators has little to do with the actual risk of elevators. They serve as strategies, as pseudo-solutions, to deal with a variety of distressed emotions and personal conflicts, especially a sense of lack of adequate control and effectiveness in life situations.

Our society promotes the belief that weight loss and shape change are ways to improve low self-esteem, to become respected and envied by others, and to feel effective, conferring the belief that an individual is in control of life's challenges and promising to be a means of warding off criticism, external or internal. While often discussed as separate disorders, anorexia nervosa, bulimia nervosa, and binge-eating disorder are all part of one overarching, larger disorder of eating dysregulation driven by cognitive distortions—specifically, a shared overvalued belief in the benefits of thinness, usually combined with an excessive fear of fatness, and often associated with distortion in body perception (Andersen and Yager, 2009). It may be helpful to conceptualize a novel term used for other disorders, such as autism disorders: the *eating disorders spectrum* (EDOS). These disorders occur on a *spectrum of severity*, changing in severity of symptoms over time in response to life events and therapeutic interventions. They also evolve on a *spectrum of migration* between different subgroups, having porous boundaries between these subgroups. As autism has recently come to be understood as a spectrum disorder, so eating disorders are best understood as a spectrum disorder.

Not everyone is equally vulnerable to developing an illness on the eating disorders spectrum. Table 1.2 summarizes some of the risk factors predisposing to the development of an eating disorder (Gonçalves, Machado, and Martins, 2014; Hilbert et al., 2014; Machado et al., 2014; Meier et al., 2015; Steinhausen et al., 2015). The greater the number of risk factors present, the more intense these factors, and the more likely these factors are to be present during vulnerable windows in development, the higher is the likelihood of developing an eating disorder. Risk factors are therefore *probabilistic*, not deterministic. They are *culture-bound*, occurring primarily in industrialized cultures that value thinness and have sufficient availability of food so that being overweight is a realistic possibility. Anorexia as a goal in societies experiencing widespread starvation is rare, except in the governing or wealthy classes of developing countries that have adopted westernized body images.

Incidentally, throughout this chapter, the term *patient*, meaning a person who suffers, is used in preference to *client*, which is a term focused on an economic relationship.

Epidemiology

The probability of accurately and validly identifying the incidence and prevalence of disorder X depends on (1) how an investigator defines disorder X, (2) in what populations disorder X is sought, and (3) the methods of diagnosis used. So it is with eating disorders. Changes in the diagnostic

Table 1.2. Risk factors that increase the probability of developing an eating disorder

Risk factor	Comments
Gender	More females than males, but not as large a discrepancy as commonly believed (10:1 in clinical referrals, 2–3:1 in community sample), meaning males are underdiagnosed.
Age	Persons in teens and early 20s most likely, with peaks at ages 13–14 and 17–18; cases noted from 7 to 77 years old.
Geography	Highest incidence in westernized societies and upper socioeconomic classes in developing countries.
Personality (typical, though not required, features)	Anorexia nervosa: sensitive, perfectionist, persevering, self-critical features of temperament, persevering.
	Bulimia nervosa: impulsivity, emotional intensity, mood lability, dramatic features.
	Binge-eating disorder: high harm avoidance, low self-directedness, conflict avoidant.
Family history	Increased in families with history of depressive spectrum disorder, obesity.
Heritability/genetics	Estimated 50%–70% of risk factors are heritable. Concordance in monozygotic twins 3–4 times as high as in dizygotic twins. Elevated in utero testosterone.
Interest groups	Students in strict dance schools, bodybuilders, models, wrestlers, participants in sports with high performance and appearance demands (girls gymnastics, figure skating), cross-country runners, media professionals, actors.
Sexual orientation	Increased in gay males and heterosexual females. Lesbian females may be slightly protected (controversial).
Age of onset of dieting behavior	Girls starting to worry about weight by ages 6–10; by age 14, 60%–70% trying to reduce weight.
Racial and ethnic group	Largely independent of racial and ethnic designation if westernized body ideals for thinness are adopted; increased in African American families of higher socioeconomic status.
Predisposing medical diseases	Type 1 diabetes mellitus, cystic fibrosis, medical prescription of corticosteroids or atypical antipsychotics.
Predisposing psychiatric disorders	Depressive disorders, anxiety disorders, attention deficit hyperactivity disorder, posttraumatic stress disorder, obsessive compulsive disorder.
Location	More common in urban areas than in rural.
Influence of media	Decreased self-esteem, more self-critical body image, after viewing impossible-to-achieve body size/shape ideals in media; onset of eating disorders with introduction of TV and other media, e.g., in South Sea Islands.

criteria (e.g., changes in the *Diagnostic and Statistical Manual of Mental Disorders (DSM)* from *DSM-IV* to *DSM-5*), in location of case finding (clinical admissions vs. community samples), and in method of case finding (screening instruments, clinic discharge codes, full individual diagnostic evaluations) are among the factors that contribute to differing estimates of incidence and prevalence.

Controversy remains as to whether the incidence and prevalence of eating disorders are increasing, whether the disorders are simply more accurately diagnosed, and/or whether patients are now more willing to seek help. The preponderance of evidence supports an actual increase in cases of eating disorders in westernized societies, especially bulimia nervosa and binge-eating disorders, along with improving, but still far from perfect, diagnostic criteria. The following discussion gives rough estimates of prevalence.

Anorexia nervosa may be present in 0.1%–5% of the younger population, with 0.5% being a good estimate in females 13–21 years of age. Males with full or subthreshold anorexia nervosa present to hospital clinics in, on average, a 1:10 male-to-female ratio, but more accurately are found in a 1:3 ratio in community samples. Bulimia nervosa in adolescents and young adults may be present in 0.3%–7%, with an estimate of 1.5%–2% as an approximate figure, with a ratio of 1:3 males to females. Binge-eating disorder is roughly a gender-neutral disorder, being present in 2%–3% of the vulnerable population. In selected populations such as a strict ballet school, in certain sports where appearance is important, and in weight-sensitive vocations, the prevalence of an eating disorder is much higher than the average probability for a similar age. The prevalence of subsyndromal anorexia nervosa is considerably higher than that of the full diagnostic syndrome, underlining the fact that weight loss and frequency of disordered eating in the population are *dimensional* constructs.

Diagnosis

The key concept in diagnosis of eating disorders is to *rule in* eating disorders. Avoid first attempting to *rule out* all possible medical or psychiatric causes of the presenting symptoms and signs. A delay in diagnosis may increase the severity of the eating disorder, cause iatrogenic morbidity through excessive medical testing, and make treatment more difficult. A systematic psychiatric history and mental status examination will reveal the true picture of the disorder underlying the medical presentation. For younger patients, when a patient's denial of overvalued beliefs occurs, the clinician may have to depend on the account of parents. Anorexia nervosa is a relatively "public" disorder usually presenting with obvious thinness, often in an otherwise energetic younger individual. Bulimia nervosa, however, is most commonly private, secretive, and marked by shame, and generally involves planned or impulsive exits from functions involving food. A spouse, parent, or significant other living with someone struggling with bulimia nervosa may not be aware of the condition despite years of illness.

Anorexia nervosa has been recognized for several centuries, but bulimia nervosa was given a diagnostic name as recently as 1979 (Russell). These two disorders are two sides of the same coin: they both begin with dieting to lose weight, leading in one case to sustained low weight and in the other to failure of significant weight loss but, instead, a breakthrough of hunger in the form of binge eating, followed by compensatory efforts to avoid weight gain using self-induced vomiting, laxatives, diuretics, heroic exercise, or bouts of fasting. Bulimia nervosa is in many ways a failed attempt at anorexia nervosa: a dieting effort in a person without the persevering traits of a classic anorexic, a person whose physiology and psychology do not tolerate prolonged semistarvation. The binge episodes of bulimia nervosa quickly evolve from being driven by hunger alone to being triggered by dysphoric moods and automatic habits of time and place, as well as autonomic conditioning.

Binge-eating disorder (BED) is defined by the behavior of chronic binge eating with *no* compensation for the binges—no purging and minimal dietary restriction—but with psychologic and medical distress and self-recrimination after binge eating. Binge-eating disorder is not a hedonic experience. Its definition is even more recent (Devlin, Goldfein, and Dobrow, 2003; Latner and Clyne, 2008).

Commonly there is migration between these eating disorder subtypes, most often from anorexia to bulimic symptoms, in the form of either developing binge-purge episodes while maintaining low weight (anorexia nervosa, binge-purge subtype) or restoring enough weight to no longer suffer from the medical signs of starvation (bulimia nervosa). Approximately 50% of patients with bulimia nervosa have had a past episode of anorexia nervosa, either a full or partial syndrome. Some attempts at severe weight loss quickly evolve to bulimia nervosa, while others first evolve to become the binge-purge subtype of anorexia nervosa and then, only later—weeks to years—evolve into bulimia nervosa.

Committees of specialists have continued to change the criteria for the diagnosis of eating disorder, but patients have not changed in their behaviors or mental life. Table 1.3 lists diagnostic criteria for eating disorders adapted from *DSM-5* (American Psychiatric Association, 2013), with some additions or modifications by the author. These criteria are convertible to ICD-10 (International Statistical Classification of Diseases and Related Health Problems, 10th revision) diagnoses in most cases. Fairburn and Cooper (2011) have summarized a view held by this author that "the DSM-IV scheme for classifying eating disorders is a poor reflection of clinical reality . . . DSM-5 will only partially succeed in correcting this shortcoming." With that admonition in mind, a discussion of current diagnoses by *DSM-5* follows. The most admirable contribution of *DSM-5* has been to reduce the previous greatly overused and clinically confusing diagnosis of Eating Disorders Not Otherwise Specified (in *DSM-IV*), a diagnosis not often used by experienced clinicians employing more enduring and simpler criteria. Fairburn (2008) has promoted the helpful suggestion that eating disorders are best understood by linking them through a transdiagnostic conceptualization.

The primary changes from *DSM-IV* to *DSM-5* can be summarized as follows. For anorexia nervosa, "significant" voluntary weight loss is required rather than the previous, often falsely interpreted, attainment of "less than 85%" of healthy weight (*DSM-IV*). The "less than 85%" of healthy weight was meant as an example but was most often taken to be a fixed rule. The presence of significant medical signs of underweight is now considered diagnostic, rather than, specifically, amenorrhea.

Two categories of anorexia nervosa will be commonly underdiagnosed by *DSM-5*. The first is anorexia nervosa with apparently, but falsely, "normal weight." True anorexia nervosa may occur when an individual begins dieting at a self-regulating set point that is 2 or more standard deviations above population average, is otherwise healthy and self-restricts food to a weight that would be considered within the normal weight range for many individuals, but shows signs of medical starvation. It is the "delta," or decrement, of weight change from the starting weight to the lowest weight, the degree of weight change sufficient to produce medical symptoms of

Table 1.3. Diagnostic categories and criteria for eating disorders in *DSM-5*

Anorexia Nervosa (AN)

- Substantial and medically significant voluntary *weight loss* by dieting, overexercising, laxative/diuretic abuse. Failure to gain weight appropriate to age and height.
- Duration of ≥3 months.
- Intense fear of fatness, often associated with a relentless drive for thinness.
- An overvaluation of the benefits of thinness / shape change for self-esteem.
- Frequently, body image distortion, in which the body is perceived to be larger than actual weight; denial of low weight obvious to family, friends. An egosyntonic psychopathologic symptom.
- Signs of medical starvation, especially abnormal gonadotropin hormone functioning, loss of muscle mass, skeletal appearance. Amenorrhea frequent in females, but not essential. Decreased sexual drive common in males.
- Two subtypes: (a) classic food restriction; no binge-purge; may include overexercising (AN-R); or (b) binge-purge subtype (AN-BP): significant intentional weight loss plus recurrent binge-purge behaviors with compensation.

Bulimia Nervosa (BN)

- Binge eating at least once a week (on average) for >3 months. Binges vary in amount from rapidly eaten large amounts of food in <2 hours to more subjective perception of food intake greater than internal standards allow; perception of loss of control of eating during the episode.
- Regret after binges, especially guilt or shame, fear of becoming fat, and/or medical discomfort, primarily gastric fullness.
- Inappropriate compensation for perceived overeating after binges by purging (vomiting, laxatives, diuretics), compulsive exercise, or increased fasting.
- Shared psychopathologic disturbance with anorexia nervosa of an excessive valuation of benefits of thinness for self-esteem and mood regulation.
- Two subtypes: (a) purging subtype (80%) or (b) other compensation (20%) such as fasting or excessive exercise.
- Weight in broad normal range or overweight, i.e., not weight-associated as with anorexia nervosa.

Binge-Eating Disorder (BED)

- Binge eating (average of one or more binges/week for >3 months), with a spectrum of binge severity ranging from huge caloric intake in <2 hours to subjectively distressing smaller amounts, to almost constant grazing, resulting in significant psychological distress (regret, guilt, shame) and/or medical discomfort, primarily stomach pain.
- No compensatory behaviors to minimize the unwanted consequences of the binges.
- Patients often older (30s–40s), frequently medically obese; present in about 25% of medically obese patients; equally prevalent in females and males.

Table 1.3. (*continued*)

Avoidant/Restrictive Food Intake Disorder (ARFID)

- A disturbance of feeding behavior in children or infants not explained by lack of food, cultural norms, or a diagnosed psychiatric or medical disorder that would better explain the weight loss or lack of appropriate weight gain.
- Not associated with a distorted body image or drive for thinness.
- May be manifested by lack of interest in food, abnormal rejection of food due to its sensory properties.

Source: Adapted from American Psychiatric Association, 2013, with some additions or modifications by the author.

starvation, not the final weight, that is significant for diagnosis. A patient at seemingly normal weight as judged by population average weights may well be suffering from true anorexia nervosa. This category is classified by *DSM-5* (see table 1.4) as an "atypical" eating disorder, but when the cognitive distortions of anorexia nervosa are also present, there is nothing atypical in these patients: this is simply a less common presentation of anorexia nervosa. Body weight, like body height, follows a roughly bell-shaped curve. The amount of decrease from an original weight to a final weight that produces medical signs of underweight is the critical issue, not the weight falling below population averages.

The second category of anorexia nervosa likely to be missed is sub-subclinical anorexia nervosa, characterized by a less severe continuing, voluntary restriction of food intake to achieve a socially enviable ("social X-rays") but medically symptomatic weight loss, accompanied by overvalued beliefs that preoccupy a person's life and direct her behaviors. Weight loss is dimensional, not categorical. About 8% of failures to conceive in women may be due to simply being 2 or 3 kilograms below the weight for normal gonadotropic functioning.

For bulimia nervosa, the criteria in *DSM-5* are similar to those in *DSM-IV* except for reducing the required frequency of binge episodes from two to one episode per week for 3 months. The diagnostic criteria for bulimia nervosa overlook a substantial number of sufferers because of the requirement that there be repeated ingestion of food in amounts larger than those that most *observers* would consider normal. This begs the question of how to diagnose the disorder in patients who eat amounts larger than *they* consider acceptable according to their internal goals. Even though an observer might not see what would be considered a "binge," it is a binge to the person. This may well be the case in the category of "purging disorder," still under investigation, which requires no binges—at least, no large, observable binges.

Binge-eating disorder is now an accepted diagnostic subgroup within the eating disorders spectrum, rather than a provisional category under investigation (*DSM-IV*) As in bulimia nervosa, only one binge per week for 3 months is required.

Avoidant/Restrictive Food Intake Disorder (ARFID) is introduced in *DSM-5* as a somewhat confusing cluster of criteria focusing on abnormal feeding behaviors. Disorders of *feeding behavior* are not to be confused with *eating disorders*. Although the terminology of eating and feeding behaviors might seem similar, eating disorders, by convention, require not only abnormal eating but internalization of a determined drive for thinness or shape change (and/or a morbid fear of fatness) or, in the case of binge-eating disorders, subjective psychological and usually objective medical distress after binges. Overvalued beliefs are not present in feeding disorders.

The etiology of feeding abnormalities is certainly multiple. The category of feeding disorders is a catch-all for unexplained weight loss or lack of weight gain, primarily in infants or young children. Infants and children who are below the age (using Piaget's stages of cognitive development) when they are able to internalize a drive for thinness or a fear of fatness cannot develop true eating disorders. Feeding can certainly be a problem but is not necessarily an eating disorder. Part of the confusion is that the words "*eating*" and "*feeding*" have overlapping meanings in English. With the German term for anorexia nervosa, Pubertätsmagersucht, meaning "pubertal desire for thinness," there is no confusion between eating and feeding abnormalities.

The most commonly overlooked or underdiagnosed patient populations are males, minorities, older women, and the mentally challenged. Using *DSM-IV* criteria, too many clinicians believed that males did not qualify for a diagnosis of anorexia nervosa because they obviously could not manifest amenorrhea. Diagnoses of anorexia nervosa in males were also statistically inconvenient for researchers using the male-to-female ratio for numbers of cases presenting to clinics. Males are discussed in detail in chapter 13. Recent studies have documented the high frequency of bulimia nervosa and binge-eating disorder in minority groups. Likewise, older women are increasingly found to suffer from eating disorders, disorders continued from younger years or of recent onset, even postmenopausal (Beck, Casper, and Andersen, 1996). Eating disorders in different generations within the same family are not uncommon. Finally, intellectually disabled individuals may suffer from an eating disorder (Galluci and Andersen, 2003). The intellectual level required to develop a desire for thinness includes individuals with IQs in the mildly disabled category or those within the Autistic Spectrum Disorder. The mentally challenged may achieve increased self-esteem and social acceptance from weight loss.

Table 1.4 summarizes additional *DSM-5* categories under "Other Specified Eating or Feeding Disorder," less common eating and feeding disorders undergoing continuing research. The criteria for patients simply having milder forms of illness falling short of the required formal criteria are simple and not a source of controversy, such as patients with bulimia nervosa who have fewer than one binge per week, or binge eating for less than 3 months.

Table 1.4. Other specified feeding or eating disorders *in DSM-5*

- Atypical Anorexia Nervosa: (1) Criteria for anorexia nervosa met, except final weight after dieting is within or above the "normal" range [author: not really atypical; see text]. (2) The other form of atypical anorexia nervosa is present when some but not all of the criteria for anorexia nervosa are met, e.g., duration <3 months.
- Bulimia Nervosa Syndrome (low frequency and/or limited duration): All of the criteria for BN are met except less frequent binge behaviors or duration <3 months. Not applied to "normal-abnormal" eating such as binge-purge around exam times, after drinking bouts.
- Binge-Eating Disorder (low frequency and/or limited duration): All criteria met, except binge episodes occur less than once per week, or duration <3 months.
- Purging Disorder: Repeated purging behavior in the absence of typical observer-rated binge behavior; may occur after subjective sense of eating more than amount determined by internal, pervasive, desire for low weight. May not appear excessive to observers.
- Night Eating Syndrome: Repeated episodes of overeating at night after awakening from sleep, with variable degree of alertness during eating, and variable remembrance in the morning, but usually associated with regret or confusion; not explained by medical or psychiatric disorder or most medications.

Source: Adapted from American Psychiatric Association, 2013, with some additions or modifications by the author.

The night eating syndrome is of note because of its enigmatic origin and frequent presentation to clinicians. The most common causes of repeated night eating that causes psychological and/or physical distress are (1) the presence of a true eating disorder prompted by an intense hunger due to daytime food restriction, a hunger that surfaces only when the patient spontaneously awakes to full or clouded awareness and then eats, with later regret; and (2) the use of certain sleep medications that can regularly produce night eating in an unknown percentage of people suffering from insomnia. The formal criteria exclude "most medications" as a cause of the night eating syndrome, but clinicians need to include information about sleep aids in their evaluation of night eating. These medications may be acting on predisposed individuals to a greater extent than on those without vulnerability to an eating disorder.

The "splintering" approach of listing more and more subgroups under the broad category of eating disorders, as in Other Specified Feeding or Eating Disorder, may not bear up under sustained research, given the porous boundaries between eating disorders subgroups and their transitions in severity over time. This is especially so when comparing this approach with the more robust and enduring transdiagnostic approach. The simpler, more applicable, *transdiagnostic criteria* for all eating disorders include (1) abnormal eating behaviors, typically self-starvation with or without binge eating/purging/other compensation; (2) the presence of cognitive distortions—specifically, an overvalued belief in the benefits of thinness or shape change, often associated with a phobic fear of fatness; sometimes, but not necessarily, with a distorted body image; (3) an established pattern sustained over a reasonable amount of time; (4) the presence of medical symptoms resulting from starvation, binge eating, and purging, with associated psychosocial distress (table 1.5).

Where an overvalued belief in the need for thinness or shape change is present, along with self-starvation and/or binge-purge behavior, there is almost no chance of a medical diagnosis as the primary cause, although consequential medical symptoms may be severe and numerous. Escaping the more typical pattern of onset and development of anorexia nervosa are the approximately 8% of eating disorders cases that begin *inadvertently* in a medical illness (flu, gastrointestinal disorder) or after a surgical procedure (wiring of jaws, abdominal surgery). These patients who have not previously dieted now take over the wheel of attempting additional weight

Table 1.5. Transdiagnostic features of all eating disorders

- Abnormalities of eating behavior not due to underlying medical or psychiatric diagnoses and are associated with criterion 2.
- The presence of cognitive distortions overvaluing the benefits of thinness and/ or shape change leading to dieting. Often combined with a morbid fear of fatness and body image distortion (not required).
- The presence of significant medical consequences and/or psychosocial distress. Note: Eating disorders transition from one subtype to another regularly, most often from anorexia nervosa to anorexia nervosa of the binge-purge subtype or to bulimia nervosa, but other changes in subtype also occur.
- The disorder is present for sufficient time to rule out short-term self-improving symptoms.

loss, being prompted either by a new, spontaneous, internal desire for more thinness or by positive comments by others on their new, inadvertently lowered weight.

Incidentally, there are no "bad" reasons for developing eating disorders comparable to smoking cigarettes or baking in the sun. Eating disorders always begin as strategies to deal with problems in psychosocial functioning or goals in living.

Anorexia nervosa is generally an *ego-syntonic disorder*, not considered foreign or a source of suffering by the patient, in contrast to the *ego-dystonic* nature of bulimia nervosa. Patients with bulimia nervosa or binge-eating disorder are seldom content with their disorder, being distressed by their inability to simply decrease food intake and lose weight; they most often feel shame regarding the purging behaviors, especially self-induced vomiting.

Rigid diagnostic boundaries may deprive patients who are suffering from eating disorders that do not yet meet the requirement of a duration of 3 months of symptoms, or those suffering less severe symptoms than the *DSM-5* criteria require, of appropriate diagnostic recognition and care. These patients should not be overlooked, underdiagnosed, or excluded from treatment. Milder, subsyndromal eating disorders are far more common than classic cases that meet the full criteria of either *DSM-5* or ICD-10.

ICD-10 offers some variations from *DSM-5*, but is likewise to be considered a useful if flawed guide to diagnosis for patients meeting all criteria. ICD-10 is no more to be taken as gospel than is *DSM-5* with regard to diagnosing patients presenting less classically and failing to meet all categorical or dimensional criteria. Compare with asthma, for example, which is diagnosed when there is wheezing not from a foreign body or from pulmonary edema, and so forth, independent of the severity of wheezing. One would not fail to treat a mildly asthmatic patient because the wheezing and shortness of breath were not severe. ICD-10 criteria for anorexia nervosa require either weight loss to at least 15% below expected weight or a BMI of 17.5 or less in adults, along with avoidance of high-calorie foods, a distorted body image, and, specifically, a disorder of gonadotropic endocrine functioning. It, too, would fail to diagnose patients beginning to diet at a higher than typical pre-illness weight who then go on to manifest signs of medical starvation at seemingly normal weights.

ICD-10 criteria for bulimia nervosa lack a frequency requirement for binge episodes. Like *DSM-5*, ICD-10 requires overeating episodes that appear "large" (undefined) to an observer, excluding those who simply eat externally "normal" amounts of food that exceed their internally stipulated acceptable amounts or nutritional categories of food. Under methods of compensating for binge episodes, ICD-10 helpfully includes the omission or compensatory overuse of insulin by patients with diabetes, increasingly recognized as a vulnerability in young people with type 1 insulin-dependent diabetes mellitus.

Binge-eating disorder in ICD-10 is relegated to "eating disorder, unspecified." Many health systems are moving toward requiring ICD-10 criteria for diagnosis, despite its flaws. Undoubtedly, further diagnostic adjustments by future committees will continue to produce complexity in changing diagnostic criteria that rely on a checklist rather than promoting a fundamental knowledge of eating disorders and of the limbic system's role in attempts at weight loss. Epidemiologic estimates and research studies dependent on using a particular rigid set of diagnostic criteria are also repeatedly scrambled by these diagnostic changes. *DSM-5* and ICD-10 are most useful for presenting classifications accepted by health plans for reimbursement and for research and epidemiologic studies, although these latter two require translational efforts when diagnostic criteria again change.

Table 1.6 lists the SCOFF Questionnaire's criteria, developed in London (Morgan, Reid, and Lacey, 1999). Its virtue (modified for North America by using "14 pounds" rather than the charmingly archaic "one stone") is its simplicity and documented history of high utility in identifying probable

Table 1.6. The SCOFF Questionnaire

1. Do you make yourself Sick because you feel uncomfortably full?
2. Do you worry you have lost Control over how much you eat?
3. Have you recently lost Over 14 pounds ("one stone") in a three-month period?
4. Do you believe yourself to be Fat when others say you are too thin?
5. Would you say that Food dominates your life?

Source: Adapted for American population from Morgan, Reid, and Lacey, 1999. In the original publication, item 3 reads: "One stone (14 lbs)" rather than "Over 14 pounds ('one stone')."

Note: Ask these questions of all patients 10–40 years old or in high-risk groups. Count 1 point for every yes; a score of 2 or more indicates a likely case of anorexia nervosa or bulimia nervosa.

cases of eating disorders for further, more definitive evaluation, whether anorexia nervosa or bulimia nervosa. It is helpful to have a brief but systematic set of questions for each behavioral disorder commonly seen in patients, as in the CAGE questionnaire for assessing alcohol problems. The key concept in a diagnosis of eating disorders (again) is that it is made not by ruling out all conceivable medical causation but by confidently ruling in the disorder based on a brief history and mental status examination as well as through a screening questionnaire.

Table 1.7 summarizes some clues to secretive eating disorders. These are tip-offs that should lead to a systematic history and mental status examination to ascertain whether an eating disorder, albeit often initially denied, is present.

The term *orthorexia*, occurring in the popular literature, is of uncertain clinical significance. It means an excessive, obsessional concern about eating only healthy foods. While at times it may rule a patient's life personally and socially, orthorexia has no current diagnostic criteria. However, it may be considered one hazard of a preoccupying desire for healthy eating and, when pervasive and having unhealthy consequences psychologically or interpersonally, may benefit from treatment.

Natural History

The natural history of eating disorders usually begins with months to years of a socioculturally induced preoccupation with weight talk, weight comparisons, dieting, and desire for thinness, beginning in the 6- to 10-year-old age group, with subsequent development of overvalued beliefs in the desirability of thinness, usually combined with a fear of becoming

Table 1.7. Clues to hidden/secretive eating disorders

Anorexia Nervosa

- Unexplained weight loss, especially in adolescents, or failure to gain weight proportional to height in preteens and adolescents
- Secondary amenorrhea in adolescents or preadolescents without obvious medical cause
- Membership in avocational or identity groups promoting or requiring weight loss/shape change (ballet, wrestling, modeling, female gymnastics, cross-country running, gay orientation)
- Preoccupation with need for additional weight loss or body shape change, despite obvious thinness (females) or muscularity (males)
- Frequent mirror gazing
- Frequent "weight loss talk" without a medical basis; negative comparison of self to thinner peers
- Unexplained high TSH, low T3, low LH/FSH resulting from central hypothalamic hypogonadism; feeling cold compared with peers; objective hypothermia; unexplained hair loss; development of lanugo hair (fine, downy hair on face, arms, and back)
- Unexplained hypercarotenemia

Bulimia Nervosa or Binge-Purge Form of Anorexia Nervosa

- Unexplained hypokalemia (low potassium)
- Family report of patient vomiting without medical illness; finding boxes of laxatives or diuretics; patient regularly disappears to bathroom or takes showers after meals
- Swollen or tender parotid glands
- Loss of dental enamel on lingual surface, or large number of new caries
- Gastroesophageal reflux or symptoms of esophageal erosions in young person without medical cause; hoarseness without medical cause
- Yo-yo weight pattern

Binge-Eating Disorder

- Obesity
- Continued unexplained steady weight gain or sudden rapid weight gain
- Shame or guilt in discussing eating patterns
- Hopelessness, helplessness about weight

fat. To most American women, a "normal" weight means achieving 85% or less of the population average weight. Students are encouraged by multiple sources to develop unrealistic goals of an idealized thin but fashionable body size and improbable body shape (defined by slender hips, visible abs, no "stomach," thighs that do not touch).

Nature has created young people with a dimensional variation in weight and shape. Dieting behavior most commonly (but not exclusively) begins during the pubertal years of body change (occurring at younger and younger ages) or in later adolescence, times of changes not only in body size and shape but in hormones, mood, social interactions, and family relationships. The attitudes and values learned earlier about the benefits of thinness drive the dieting behavior. A specific precipitating factor—such as comments by friends or family, especially mother, siblings, boyfriends, coaches, teachers, or peers, suggesting that a young person is overweight, is in danger of becoming overweight, or needs to change the shape of a body part—tips the incubating phase of a predisposed individual into development of an overt eating disorder. Of course, some may dip their toe in the water of thinness, attempting to lose weight, and never dive in. Or they may dive in, developing short-term eating disorder symptoms, and then get out quickly. This is especially true for self-limited binge-purge episodes during the college years. Up to 50% of 9- to 10-year-olds are already worried about becoming fat, even though far fewer are medically overweight.

There is an increasingly alarmist leapfrogging of announcements about how many children are overweight. T. Moran summarizes the nutritional state of many American children as most typically "overfed calorically, underfed nutritionally" (personal communication), the backdrop of increasing weight in the young. A lack of fitness completes the vicious circle of an increasing desire for more and more thinness in an unattainable athletic body shape, distressingly accompanied by an increase in body weight and body fat and decreased fitness. Many Northern European countries, in contrast, especially in Scandinavia, cultivate a "virtuous circle," encouraging eating a healthy, palatable lunch in schools and teaching life-time carry-over athletic skills for all students rather than only the athletically elite. Dieting is the behavioral trigger for many eating disorders, if not most.

The natural history of most eating disorders supports an ideational schematic: the combination of *precipitating factors* acts on a person vulnerable through a variety of *predisposing risk factors*, leading to onset of an eating disorder that may then be consolidated into an enduring illness by *sustaining factors*. *Therapeutic factors* have also been increasingly identified.

The sustaining factors appear to be psychosocial as well as biomedical. Comments praising weight loss are like manna from heaven for a girl or young woman who seeks approval not granted by her sensitive personality or who is in the shadow of a more extraverted sibling. Patients who have lost considerable weight will generally feel sick if made to eat large amounts of food, especially foods high in fats, confirming their beliefs that they are meant to be thin. Temporary lactose intolerance may be present. Putative changes in serotoninergic functioning as sustaining factors have been suggested but not yet fully proved as sustaining factors. There are clearly secondary serotoninergic changes. Figure 1.3 illustrates a high school student's struggle with perceptual distortion.

The classic account of men who were conscientious objectors during World War II and voluntarily agreed to lose substantial weight in order to provide information on better ways to refeed returning starved prisoners of war remains essential reading for understanding how weight loss changes thinking and behavior (Keys et al, 1950). Many of the symptoms of anorexia nervosa are symptoms of medical starvation, independent of cause. The core of eating disorders is the distorted cognitions.

Once dieting has started, a number of outcomes are possible. A frequent outcome is development of the most common eating disorder: a subsyndromal eating disorder characterized by chronic dieting, with or without binges, not fulfilling strict criteria for any diagnosable eating disorder yet a burden and a source of distress during critical developmental years. The process may then go on until, in a smaller number of these dieting individuals, an eating disorder meeting diagnostic criteria develops, either anorexia nervosa or bulimia nervosa. Binge-eating disorder tends to occur at somewhat older ages. Anorexia nervosa may present as a pure food-restricting subtype (AN-R) or as a binge and/or purge subtype (AN-BP). The first binge of bulimia nervosa is usually triggered by dieting-induced hunger, provoking binge eating and then compensatory measures to get rid of the unwanted calories due to the fear of fatness. Soon, however, the binges of bulimia nervosa generalize to become a way to deal with any distressed mood, including depression, anxiety, anger, or feeling stuck or bored. Autonomic patterning (Haedt-Matt et al., 2014) helps lock in the syndrome behaviors. Finally, both eating disorders go on to give a personal identity in which the individual cannot imagine life without either self-starving or binge-purge behavior or both. Eating disorders too often be-

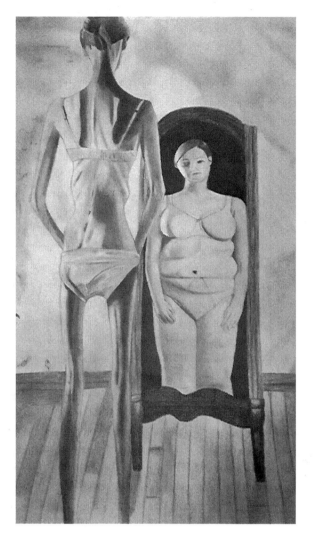

Figure 1.3. A high school student's struggle with perceptual distortion.

come an identity and a profession, which helps to explain their frequent intransigence. Although the ages for onset are most often between 11 and 22 years, a spectrum of ages of onset between 7 and 77 has been documented. Dieting should be considered a four-letter word, in contrast to a stable lifetime pattern of balanced nutritional intake.

No age, social class, or race is exempt from developing eating disorders Binge-eating disorder is now the most common eating disorder, with approximate gender neutrality. It is less obvious than the other disorders, being characterized by binge eating only (often with relentless grazing), without purging or any other compensation to avoid weight gain. It tends to present less dramatically than bulimia nervosa, generally in somewhat older patients, and may contribute to approximately 25% of cases of medical obesity. Most commonly, binge eating precedes the obesity, but it may also result from increasing weight. Binge eating and, more visibly, obesity are often dismissed by patients, families, and doctors as simply a lack of willpower.

Some males may suffer from "reverse anorexia nervosa," a syndrome also occurring in bodybuilders and weightlifters, all of whom fear they are never big enough and/or never have a low enough percentage of body fat to reveal well-defined muscles. The goal is often attainment of less than 5% body fat. A more recent term sometimes applied to this syndrome is "muscle dysmorphia," but reverse anorexia nervosa does not overlap completely with either muscle dysmorphia or body dysmorphia. Males with reverse anorexia nervosa suffer from a psychopathology that includes *megamusculophilia* (desire for large, defined muscles) and *microsomatophobia* (fear of having a too small body) (see chapter 13).

As noted earlier, a "rule out" approach to the diagnosis of eating disorders, by focusing on all possible medical causes without first appreciating the mental status changes, leads to delay in treatment and iatrogenic morbidity. Of the several thousand patients with anorexia nervosa that we have treated, in not a single case did we find that a patient having the core psychological cognitive distortions and abnormal eating behaviors had a medical disorder causing the illness. Medical illnesses by themselves do not cause patients to have a morbid fear of fatness or a relentless drive for thinness.

Comorbid Psychiatric Disorders

Once a diagnosis of an eating disorder has been made, further diagnostic work is essential. Eating disorders typically have one to four co-occurring psychiatric disorders. Comorbid psychiatric disorders may occur either before an eating disorder or as a consequence of an eating disorder. This difference is important in planning treatment (table 1.8). The presence of comorbid psychiatric disorders often makes treatment of the eating

Table 1.8. Comorbid psychiatric disorders that commonly accompany eating disorders

- Mood disorders (40%–70%): major depressive disorder, dysthymia (persistent depressive disorder), bipolar II (cycles of depression with mild highs). May have seasonal affective disorder subtype.
- Anxiety disorders: generalized anxiety disorder with or without panic.
- Obsessive-compulsive disorders (especially in anorexia nervosa)
- Alcohol and/or other substance abuse (especially in bulimia nervosa or AN-BP), especially amphetamine-type drugs.
- Personality disorders (full criteria) or vulnerable traits (<2 SD from norm).
  - Traits common in anorexia nervosa: sensitive, perfectionist, persevering, self-critical.
  - Traits common in bulimia nervosa: impulsivity, unstable moods, dramatic behaviors, emotional intensity.
  - Traits common in binge-eating disorder: high harm avoidance, low self-directedness, difficulties in emotional regulation, low self-esteem.

disorder more complex and may have a substantial influence on the outcome of treatment (Woodside and Staab, 2006).

The diagnosis of an eating disorder is virtually always an exercise in uncovering multiple diagnoses and attempting to differentiate between predisposing and consequential comorbid disorders. And, not uncommonly, and more subtly, psychiatric disorders that precede the eating disorder may simply be intensified by rather than caused by the eating disorder. In any case, unless a comorbid disorder is strongly present and interferes with treatment of the eating disorder, it makes clinical sense to fully treat the medical/weight components of the eating disorder and the cognitive distortions before treating the companion disorders. This allows clinicians to determine whether these co-occurring disorders are remitted or improved by full treatment of the eating disorder. Anorexia nervosa has a substantially increased probability of suicide (Bulik et al., 2008).

Classic food-restricting anorexia is accompanied, on average, by two additional associated psychiatric diagnoses; the binge-purge subtype of anorexia typically has four associated diagnoses; and bulimia nervosa has three (Margolis et al., 1994). Binge-eating disorder is often associated with depression and obesity. Community-based untreated cases of eating disorder may not have as high an incidence of comorbid disorders, but the majority of individuals with eating disorders who come for treatment will have some form of mood disorder, personality disorder, drug or alcohol abuse, anxiety state, or obsessive-compulsive disorder (OCD). It is important to emphasize the assessment of the comorbid syndromes because comprehensive treatment and certainly case management depend on a combined approach. Vulnerabilities of personality, whether traits or disorders, are increased in most eating disorders but are not randomly distributed. Patients with anorexia nervosa are more likely to be sensitive, persevering, self-critical, and perfectionistic, while patients with bulimia nervosa are more often (but not always) likely to be impulsive and dramatic and to have unstable moods.

Differential Diagnosis: Psychiatric and Medical

A number of psychiatric syndromes imitate anorexia nervosa, primarily in behaviors of food refusal or weight loss without the core cognitive distortions of eating disorders but with the essential psychopathology of another disorder. The guideline is to diagnose a symptom (weight loss, food refusal) by the company it keeps (low mood, delusions; see text below and table 1.9).

Major depressive illness is frequently accompanied by a weight loss of 15–20 pounds. Appetite return and weight restoration with cognitive behavioral therapy, antidepressants, or electroconvulsive therapy, and the absence of body image distortion or a morbid fear of fatness, usually confirm the correct diagnosis. Patients with obsessive-compulsive disorders or traits may be unable to eat normally because of obsessional ruminations about the nutritional content of food, making decision making about meals difficult. A choking episode may have sensitized an individual so that he or she avoids swallowing solid food of any kind, which has led to weight loss as severe as in anorexia nervosa in some patients. Paranoid states—especially paranoid schizophrenia or a delusional disorder (including delusional disorders secondary to use of substances of abuse, most commonly methamphetamine) in adolescents and young adults with narrowly focused delusions that food is poisoned—may lead to substantial weight loss but be inscrutable, as a patient's suspiciousness prevents him or her from giving the physician full awareness of the inner delusional process. Treatment with neuroleptics usually leads to increased eating and increased weight in paranoid states, as well as enabling the patient to become more candid in the mental status examination about the real reason for avoiding food.

Occasionally, medical disorders may simulate anorexia nervosa in some ways but without the crucial morbid fear of fatness and drive for thinness and without distortion of body image. For example, consider a case of Crohn's disease in a 25-year-old individual who had obsessive-compulsive personality disorder that manifested by avoidance of all solid food and limitation of caloric intake to sports drinks. This appears at first glance to be a case of anorexia nervosa. The Crohn's disease was correctly diagnosed only after a positive stool evaluation for occult blood and assessment of the absence of typical mental symptoms of anorexia nervosa. Medical assessment for reasons other than diagnosis of an eating disorder is crucial. Medical assessment is vital for understanding the consequences and complications of the disorder, as well as for decision making about the location, intensity, and methods of treatment, but not for diagnosis. Table 1.9 summarizes some common issues in the differential diagnosis of medical disorders.

Another guideline bears up in extensive, experienced clinical practice: A psychiatric disorder is not necessarily present because an extensive medical history and testing have not uncovered a medical diagnosis. Not only for eating disorders but for all psychiatric disorders, the absence of a medical diagnosis does not mean the symptoms and signs of loss of appetite, weight loss, food refusal, idiosyncratic food choices, vomiting, or abdominal pain must therefore be caused by a psychiatric disorder. Admission to

Table 1.9. Differential diagnosis of eating disorders

Psychiatric Disorders

- Major Depressive Disorder: often associated with weigh loss >15 lb
- Obsessive Compulsive Disorder: obsessional rumination about content of food
- Paranoid Delusions: fear of poisoning in food
- Behavioral Sensitization: prior choking episode

Medical Disorders

- Insulin-Dependent Diabetes Mellitus
- Cystic Fibrosis
- Medication Induced Weight Increase: corticosteroids, atypical neuroleptics

General Rule: Diagnose a symptom by the company it keeps.

an eating disorders unit with supervised refeeding and experienced nutritional prescription may benefit these idiopathic cases, regardless of the lack of diagnosis. Doctors are better at determining what disorders are not present than what the correct diagnosis is. Treatment with supervised refeeding, psychotherapy, additional efforts at a more inclusive history from the patient and from significant others, and repeated mental status examinations as weight and eating behavior improve will often reveal the true diagnosis, whether medical or psychiatric.

Vulnerabilities of personality, whether traits or disorders, are increased in all eating disorders but are not randomly distributed. As noted earlier, patients with anorexia nervosa are more likely to be sensitive, persevering, self-critical, and perfectionistic, valuing order and sameness; in contrast, patients with bulimia nervosa or the binge-purge subtype of anorexia nervosa are more likely to demonstrate impulsive, dramatic features and intense but unstable moods. For monozygotic twins, there is a 58% chance of both having an eating disorder if one is afflicted. There is no conclusion yet as to what is being transmitted for genetic vulnerability—possibly vulnerabilities in personality or mood such as a predisposition to depressive illness, persevering and sensitive personality traits, and other features that might be related to variations in the central nervous system's serotonin regulation. It has been estimated that genetic vulnerability to an eating disorder ranges from 30% to 70% (Thornton, Mazzeo, and Bulik, 2011). Case 2 (above) illustrates one of the serious medical complications than can result from rapid, severe, self-induced starvation when the diagnosis of an eating disorder is made on a probabilistic basis by comparing with other possible diagnoses.

Treatment

Primary care physicians can and should not only diagnose but also treat many early and moderate cases of eating disorders, sometimes in conjunction with colleagues in psychology, nutrition, and social work. After diagnosis and differential diagnosis, the next step is setting goals for treatment. Table 1.10 summarizes transdiagnostic treatment goals for all eating disorders.

For all patients with eating disorders, the first approach necessarily involves safety. This means correcting all severe, urgent medical disorders, distinguishing between these and self-improving signs and symptoms of

Table 1.10. Transdiagnostic treatment goals

- *Correction of all medical abnormalities*, distinguishing between (a) urgent immediate medical abnormalities, including severe hypokalemia, severe hypophosphatemia, severely decreased cardiac mass, abnormal QT interval; (b) self-improving symptoms or signs of starvation, including decreased muscle mass and strength, slow gastric emptying, slow GI transit time, bradycardia without abnormal QT interval, decreased ovarian and testicular function; (c) long-term concerns of uncertain outcome, including low bone mineral density, decreased brain mass / enlarged brain ventricles, amenorrhea despite weight restoration.

- *Fully normal individualized weight restoration*, using weight from an insurance table / pre-illness weight as an intermediate goal; full attainment of a healthy, self-regulating, individualized "set point" for weight, indicated by absence of hypothermia, normal T3, normal hunger and satiety patterns, normal gonadotropin functioning.

- *Normal eating behavior with normal dietary content* in a wide variety of social situations and emotional states. No dieting; no binge-purge behaviors.

- *Healthy thinking by challenge and change of cognitive distortions* about weight, shape, and food. "Normative cultural distress" is acceptable. Preoccupation with weight loss and/or shape change no longer dominates mental life. Self-esteem not primarily dependent on weight or shape.

- *Selective psychopharmacology and/or psychotherapy* for preexisting or persisting psychiatric disorders after normal weight and healthy thinking are restored.

- *Comfortable skills in shopping for, preparing, consuming food*, choosing clothing. Encourage life-time moderate exercise/fitness.

- *Family support and psychoeducation.*

- *Relapse prevention* through planned follow-up of a sequence of less restrictive settings, from inpatient/residential treatment or partial (day) programs to intensive outpatient or weekly outpatient treatment. Consider residential aftercare.

- *Psychodynamic goals* to include (a) return to and proceed through normal developmental trajectory where thwarted by eating disorder; (b) cultivate resilience and flexibility; (c) increase distress tolerance.

- *Gradual acquisition of stress management techniques / mindfulness.*

medical starvation, and considering strategies for other long-term medical concerns.

The methods of treatment available to a primary care physician are often low in technology, modest in cost, and yet effective, and best accomplished by a team approach. Patients with anorexia nervosa need to be restored to a full, healthy, individualized weight for multiple reasons; at a minimum, for women, a healthy weight is a weight range that leads to normal, regular menstrual cycles. The first signs of menstrual activity are not synonymous with a final healthy weight. An initial weight goal for a very starved individual, based on insurance tables or pediatric tables, should be written in pencil, not ink. A final *goal range* for each patient needs to be individualized by achievement of a cluster of signs of normality. Typically, the return of menses occurs at an average of 92% of healthy weight, meaning: don't stop there. Freedom from feeling colder than peers, increasing heart rate from a bradycardic range to a normal rate, and normalization of T3, luteinizing hormone, and estradiol (testosterone in males) are signs of being close to a healthy weight, even if menses are not yet fully restored. In females within the typical age range of menstruation, the finding of a dominant ovarian cyst on a sonogram supports the fact that the patient is close to a healthy weight range. In starved males, a dimensional increase in sexual drive and fantasies along with the metrics noted above are signs of an approach to a healthy long-term goal range. When in doubt as to whether weight restoration is adequate, follow-up treatment includes prescribing additional plateaus in weight restoration.

Treatment is not limited to achieving a weight goal. If weight is the only goal, as too often occurs when patients with anorexia nervosa are treated on general psychiatric, medical, or pediatric units, a "revolving door" with recurrent admissions often results. Weight improvement without skilled evidence-based psychotherapy is seldom effective in sustaining improvement. For substantially underweight patients, restoration of healthy weight (avoid the phrase "gaining weight"; teach "restoring weight" or "catching up to a healthy weight" for growing adolescents) is best achieved with supervised refeeding by an experienced team on a specialized unit or subunit. Evidence is mounting that the strongest predictor of long-term sustained remission of anorexia nervosa is the degree to which fully adequate weight is restored and maintained, in addition to the goal of challenging and changing cognitive distortions. It is reasonable for an experienced treatment program to safely increase weight by 2.5–3 pounds per week for females with anorexia nervosa, and 3–4 pounds for males. A kilogram per week is the minimum restoration in experienced programs. A rapid approach to weight restoration (1.98 kg/week for inpatients; 1.36 kg/week for partial-hospital patients) has been demonstrated to be safe and effective (Haynos et al., 2016; Redgrave et al., 2015).

The real core of treatment alongside weight restoration is *persuading patients to think differently* about the value of thinness, low weight, food restriction, body shape, and excessive exercise. A central treatment goal is to help patients find personalized ways other than self-starving to deal with developmental or psychosocial stresses, dysphoric moods (especially depression and anxiety), crises in family functioning, and low self-esteem.

The most validated evidence-based psychotherapeutic method for changing the driving cognitive distortions in anorexia nervosa is *cognitive behavioral therapy* (CBT) (Dalle Grave et al., 2016; Fairburn, 2008). CBT is a summary term for the method by which several goals are achieved. First, the patient receives psychoeducation on both the consequences of starvation/binge-purge behaviors and how CBT functions in goals and methods, so the patient is made *co-investigator* in understanding his or her eating disorder. The second goal is challenging and changing distorted cognitions, especially overvaluation of the benefits of thinness and excessive fear of fatness. These changes are brought about by guiding the patient in gathering evidence to support or refute the underlying cognitive distortions, which together are called "schema." Third, as a consequence of replacing cognitive distortions with healthy thinking about weight, shape, food, and exercise, the patient is guided into healthy patterns of behavior, including the capacity to eat in all social situations, shopping for and preparing food, shopping for clothing, and attending functions involving food. The physician should think of eating disorders not only as an *illness* but also as a *strategy that needs to be replaced by healthy alternatives.*

Studies of the benefits of CBT and weight restoration for patients with severe anorexia nervosa that meets diagnostic criteria lack truly randomized controlled trials, given the obvious ethical requirements of not allowing nontreated groups to further lose weight or die. Yet the evidence supporting the necessity and benefit of a combination of weight restoration and CBT for anorexia nervosa is overwhelming. Randomized controlled trials of very mildly ill patients with anorexia nervosa (such as subsyndromal anorexia without serious medical complications) might be undertaken with groups assigned to CBT plus weight restoration, CBT alone, weight restoration alone, and no treatment. Enhanced CBT has been shown to be effective for outpatients (Fairburn et al., 2013).

No medication by itself is necessary or sufficient for the treatment of anorexia nervosa, although some medications may be helpful in selected cases. For 50 years, medications to increase appetite have been prescribed by psychopharmacologically oriented physicians who act much like the carpenter for whom the whole world is a nail: prescribing based on their training limitations, patience, financial goals, or administrative/health plan bureaucracies' restrictions. Crisp (1995) and others have shown that normal appetite is returned with only a few weeks of simple, balanced nutrition. The only medication that truly works is food.

Healthy lifetime patterns of physical exercise are necessary to get patients who have engaged in driven, compulsive exercise to moderate their regimen, and for the less common "couch potatoes" to get moving. Supervised strength training is of special benefit to males with eating disorders, for whom achieving both muscle mass and muscle definition is important to their return to a more normative male role in society, with increased self-confidence and a healthy body image.

Innovative supplemental measures include directing patients to throw out the bathroom scale at home and to cover mirrors, except for enough visual reflection to check hair and make-up. Mirror gazing is nearly universal in patients with eating disorders. The figure seen in the mirror is seen through the eyes of body image distortion and seldom corresponds to objective measurements. The overall methods of treatment are summarized in table 1.11. Occasionally, compulsory treatment for anorexia nervosa may be lifesaving (Elzakkers et al., 2014).

Bulimia nervosa is a heterogeneous spectrum condition, a kind of final common pathway, variable in seriousness and in response to treatment. Bulimia nervosa treatment essentially involves working the binge episodes "out of a job." This means assessing the adaptive purposes the binges serve, beginning with identifying their triggers—a task easily accomplished for outpatients who are asked to keep a week of daily diaries on 3×5 cards, documenting time of eating, food eaten, mood, life events, and binge urges and behaviors. The three major triggers for binge episodes are (1) hunger from being underweight or restricting eating, (2) emotional distress of any kind, and (3) automatic conditioned reflexes responding to location or time of day. When any degree of underweight is present, an increase to fully normal weight is essential to decrease the intensity of hunger that continues to drive binge episodes. The psychological core of treatment in bulimia nervosa involves decreasing emotional distress,

Table 1.11. Methods of treatment for eating disorders

- *Cognitive behavioral therapy (CBT)* is the most effective evidence-based form of psychotherapy for eating disorders. CBT principles teach patients to challenge, through evidence gathering, their overvalued beliefs about the benefits of slimness / shape change. Interpersonal therapy (IPT) is slower but may be an alternative. Dialectical behavioral therapy (DBT) is also slower but may be an alternative for bulimia nervosa comorbid with borderline personality disorder. CBT is required in Great Britain as first treatment for bulimia nervosa. The preponderance of evidence supports its use in anorexia nervosa as well, but studies are harder to randomize. It is often effective in groups.
- If no experienced cognitive behavioral therapist is available, *SSRIs* (e.g., fluoxetine, sertraline, citalopram) often decrease binge-purge symptoms by 50%, but patients may have relapse if medications are discontinued or may not respond at all. Prescribe primarily for bulimia nervosa and binge-eating disorder as a supplement to CBT. SSRIs are best used if CBT is not by itself fully effective. Avoid medications to increase appetite (atypical antipsychotics, cannabinoids etc.).
- Individualized psychotherapy can *help the patient understand that the core underlying issues in treatment are not weight loss or food* but strategies to manage emotional distress, identity formation, and self-esteem, for which the eating disorder is a pseudosolution.
- *Parents and significant others should be provided with psychoeducation* about the nature of the eating disorder and companion disorders. They need empathy and coping strategies for preventing "burnout" while caring for individuals with chronic illness and for maintaining healthy family relationships without being monitors or "food police." Resolution of family functioning issues can be identified in family therapy.
- *Avoid the "revolving door" of premature discharge below healthy weight or with persisting binge eating, which is demonstrated to increase relapse and repeat admissions.*
- Family-based *outpatient treatment for adolescents with mild or moderate anorexia nervosa (preliminary support for bulimia nervosa) can be effective* using the Lock and Le Grange method. The family is empowered to act as the treatment team. Inpatient hospitalization may be avoided.
- Consider waiting until after normal weight and cognition are achieved before prescribing separate treatment for comorbid disorders. *Comorbid psychiatric diagnoses may remit or diminish with full treatment of the eating disorder.*
- If absolutely necessary, involuntary treatment has been demonstrated to improve patients' condition, without subsequent litigation.

altering habit patterns, improving distressed relationships, and developing stress management techniques.

Evidence for the effectiveness of CBT in treating bulimia nervosa is so persuasive from so many studies that it is required as the first line of treatment in Great Britain. The main problem is lack of fully trained therapists experienced in CBT. Where individual circumstances necessitate a different evidence-based approach, interpersonal psychotherapy (IPT) or dialectical behavioral therapy (DBT) have proved effective. Interpersonal psychotherapy is prescribed especially when distressed relationships appear to play a major role in the onset and maintenance of the disorder. Dialectical behavioral therapy methods have been validated especially when comorbid emotional intensity disorder ("borderline personality disorder") is part of the psychological picture.

SSRIs (selective serotonin reuptake inhibitors: fluoxetine, sertraline, citalopram) alone *may* (but do not always) decrease binge episodes and purging by about 50% within 3 months. However, symptoms tend to recur when medications are stopped, or binge-purge behaviors may break through despite medications. Antidepressants are best reserved for patients with bulimia nervosa who have not responded to CBT, IPT, or DBT after 10–12 weeks of structured treatment combining weight restoration (when necessary), interruption of binge-purge behaviors, and immersion in evidence-based psychotherapy. The exception appears to be when there is a preexisting history of depressive illness or OCD before onset of the eating disorder. Buproprion is generally contraindicated for patients with bulimia nervosa because of possible seizures. Psychopharmacology for eating disorders is summarized by Reas and Grilo (2015) and Citrome (2015).

Binge-eating disorder seldom requires inpatient treatment. It generally responds to a combination of treatment methods, but the first essential goal is to interrupt the binge eating (Wilson, 2011). Even an intelligently directed gradual weight loss plan cannot be accomplished in the presence of continued binge eating. Normalization of eating behaviors takes priority over weight loss.

Along with interrupting binge eating behavior, concurrent CBT (or, if indicated, IPT or DBT) is at the core of the treatment of binge-eating disorders. After binge eating has been substantially interrupted and CBT methods have challenged and changed cognitive distortions, only then, if body weight is associated with medical abnormalities, can safe, slow weight loss be attempted. At times, when patients with binge-eating disorder who are obese do go on to attain a goal within a BMI range of 19–25, they may suffer from mild or significant symptoms of starvation. As little as a 10% loss of weight can substantially improve the medical abnormalities associated with obesity—for example, by achieving and maintaining a BMI of about 30. The first component of weight that is lost is usually the excessive weight gained through binge eating. The next weight loss challenge often means an attack on the second source of obesity: the bedrock of genetic obesity. Where genetically predisposed obesity is present, more complex methods beyond CBT are necessary. Moderate regular exercise to increase muscle mass has a goal of decreasing body fat and increasing cardiopulmonary fitness, not weight loss. Weight loss is achieved at the dining table, while fitness is achieved by increasing physical activities. Additional supplemental goals in the comprehensive treatment of binge-eating disorder include learning assertiveness, distress tolerance, stress management, and mindfulness.

Several studies cautiously endorse the use of stimulant medications to decrease urges to overeat and to decrease binge episodes in binge-eating disorders. At most, current evidence supports a supplemental/supportive role for stimulants in binge-eating disorders. The history of the treatment of obesity is littered with the ill-advised use of stimulants to decrease hunger, generally resulting in rebound overeating.

Table 1.12 lists some of the most common reasons for referral to hospital for treatment of an eating disorder. In general, most persons with entrenched anorexia nervosa will require some form of hospitalization, either 24-hour inpatient/residential care or partial hospital (full-day treatment) care. Most patients with bulimia nervosa can generally be treated as outpatients, with exceptions for those with significant medical or psychiatric comorbidity

Le Grange et al. (2015) and Marzola et al. (2015) have pioneered and developed an intensive family treatment method that allows many adolescents (under 18 years of age) with anorexia nervosa, with a BMI exceeding 15, to be treated entirely at home—an encouraging development now supported by evidence from several studies. This method has been extended to teens with bulimia nervosa. Comprehensive treatment with insistence on attaining a healthy, fully normal, individualized weight range, whether by team-oriented inpatient treatment or family-based treatment, leads to

Table 1.12. Criteria for inpatient/residential/partial (day) hospitalization for patients with eating disorders

- Moderate to severe anorexia nervosa: some hospitalization (full or partial hospital) is required. (Exception: family-based treatment in home for teens with intact families willing to learn Locke and Le Grange methods.) Hospitalization is usually needed for *substantial or rapid* weight loss, especially weight loss below 75% of normal age-appropriate weight; sooner rather than later treatment needed if weight loss is rapid in adolescents. Also needed if mildly underweight patients with anorexia nervosa, bulimic subtype, have significant medical symptomatology (low potassium, unstable vital signs, uncontrolled insulin abuse).
- Bulimia nervosa: outpatient programs usually the best choice, except for patients with severe depression, self-harming behavior, suicide plans, or severe medical complications (hypokalemia).
- Significant psychiatric comorbidity, especially if impairing outpatient treatment progress: this includes suicidality; borderline personality disorder with self-harming; substance abuse; intrusive comorbid OCD; major depressive disorder.
- Lack of response to outpatient treatment after good effort.
- Hostile living situation or lack of experienced local therapists.
- Diagnostic uncertainty, with probable eating disorder and severe medical symptoms.
- Presence of a life-threatening situation (refusal of treatment despite severe weight loss, hypokalemia, suicidality), in which case involuntary treatment may be necessary. Involuntary treatment is as effective as voluntary treatment; generally, insight returns in about 2–3 weeks.

Note: Treatment on a unit dedicated to eating disorders, with a comprehensive, experienced team–oriented approach, is more effective than treatment on a general unit with inexperienced staff.

fewer rehospitalizations (Baran, Weltzin, and Kaye, 1995) and, in the long run, is more cost-effective (Crow and Nyman, 2004). Managed care has made ruthless inroads in length of stay for psychiatric disorders in general and eating disorders in particular. Similar refusal of adequate treatment for breast cancer or type 1 diabetes mellitus would lead to an outcry resulting in legislative action.

Hospital care is essential to achieve enduring, long-term outcomes for patients with moderate to severe anorexia nervosa and in selected cases of bulimia nervosa. Once initial safety, diagnostic assessment, and goal setting while in hospital are accomplished, planning for aftercare and relapse prevention also starts on the day of admission. With hospitalized patients under 18 years of age, treatment of the family unit as a whole after discharge

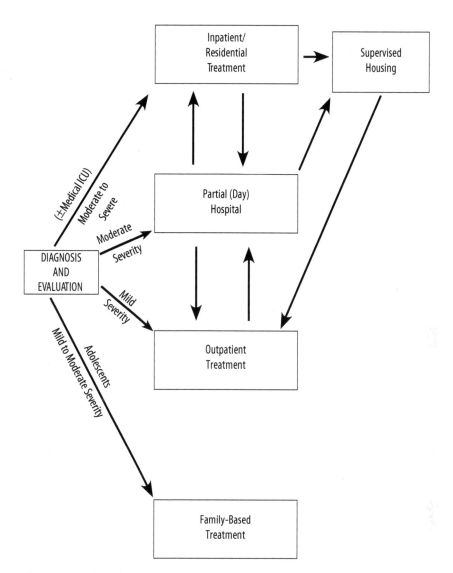

Figure 1.4. Referral to treatment levels after diagnosis.

has produced more sustained improvement and relapse prevention than treatment of the teenager alone. Figure 1.4 summarizes schematically the pathways to treatment locales on the basis of severity of illness and age.

The long-term death rate for patients with eating disorders, especially anorexia nervosa and bulimia nervosa, is the highest of all psychiatric

Table 1.13. Causes of death in eating disorders

- Anorexia nervosa: medical complications of starvation; hypokalemia in AN-BP subtype; suicide.
- Bulimia nervosa: hypokalemia causing cardiac arrhythmia; suicide.
- Binge-eating disorder: death seldom related to this eating disorder alone.

Note: Eating disorders have the highest mortality of any psychiatric disorder.

disorders. Half of deaths from anorexia nervosa are due to starvation and half to suicide. Deaths are spread out in a continuing pattern from onset of illness throughout the years of illness, rather than concentrated at one particular time. Recently, this death rate has decreased, but it is still high in most outcome studies, with death rates gradually accumulating over additional years of illness. Deaths from bulimia nervosa are most often associated with cardiovascular or metabolic consequences, as well as suicide. (table 1.13).

A few series, such as that of Strober, Freeman, and Morrell (1997), have reported no deaths in their long-term outcomes for young patients with anorexia nervosa who have been comprehensively treated. In addition, they have documented remission in more than 75% of these patients, demonstrating that full, sustained remission is achievable for anorexia nervosa. Death of patients who have bulimia nervosa or anorexia nervosa with binge-purge behaviors is generally due to arrhythmias or suicide. Death from the eating disorder is uncommon in binge-eating disorder. Bulimia nervosa and binge-eating disorder have a higher rate of spontaneous remission and high rates of remission with increasingly validated treatment methods.

The goals of treatment for all eating disorders have to be reasonable and achievable. A healthy weight range, normal patterns of eating, and healthy thinking about food, weight, and shape are achievable. Being mildly concerned about weight and shape is culturally normative and consistent with otherwise successful treatment. Rodin, Silberstein and Striegel-Moore (1985) have called this phenomenon "normative discontent," which means having a slight overconcern about achieving thinness that does not cause a disorder that meets full or subsyndromal diagnostic criteria and is not significantly preoccupying an individual's life. Giving lip service to wanting to be thinner is an almost mandatory part of the female role in western society. There is no guarantee that individuals with bulimia will be free from *urges* to binge or purge even after adequate treatment. What is completely possible is to learn to redirect binge or purge *urges* so that the individual never carries out binge or purge *behaviors* and chooses healthy alternatives instead. Urges are suggestions, not commands. Patients are on the way to wellness when they realize that the crucial issues in their lives are not food, weight, or shape, but important matters in living, relationships, mood regulation, and development.

Treatment of Comorbid Psychiatric Syndromes

The overall treatment of an eating disorder may be determined as much by comorbid psychological symptoms as by the eating disorder itself. As a general guideline, once the patient's medical status has been assessed and stabilized, treatment quickly turns, first, to the eating disorder itself: restoration of normal weight, interruption of abnormal eating behaviors, and resolution of cognitive distortions. Consideration of comorbid psychiatric syndromes comes next. Unless comorbid syndromes are severe, it is often prudent to delay their treatment until 4–8 weeks after beginning treatment for the eating disorder. The reason here is that a fair percentage of depressive symptoms, anxiety states, and obsessive-compulsive thoughts and behaviors will improve with weight restoration and normalized eating behavior alone. Initially treating both the eating disorder and comorbid syndromes often fails to recognize how many of these psychological symptoms are either secondary to or accentuated by the eating disorder.

If comorbid psychiatric syndromes are not improved after treatment of the eating disorder itself, the following approaches may be useful.

1. *Depressive disorders:* Any SSRI (fluoxetine, sertraline, or citalopram) is effective. We recommend starting with one-half the usual minimum maintenance dose for 1 or 2 weeks, then increasing to the typical starting dosage for 6 weeks; for example, beginning with 10 mg of fluoxetine, then increasing gradually to 40–60 mg of fluoxetine. Typical ranges of other SSRIs are 50–150 mg of sertraline and 20–40 mg of citalopram, beginning with lower doses. Where a seasonal worsening of depression is evident in the lower-light months of fall and winter (not uncommon), the addition of bright light therapy (10,000 lux for one-half hour at 18–22 inches each morning) will add incremental benefit. Occasionally, a mood stabilizer is helpful for bipolar II disorders. CBT has the additional virtue of being effective

not only for eating disorders but for many mild to moderate depressive illnesses. First-generation antidepressants such as nortriptyline may produce QT prolongation. As noted above, buproprion is generally contraindicated because of the report of seizures in patients with bulimia. In retrospect, the seizures leading to a delay in introducing buproprion to the market may well have resulted from unrecognized electrolyte abnormalities; nonetheless, buproprion should be used cautiously.

2. *Anxiety disorders:* Panic disorder responds to the same treatments as depressive illness—SSRIs plus CBT—with additional psychoeducation about the nature of panic symptoms. Generalized anxiety is less responsive to medication but does improve, though more slowly, with CBT, behavioral relaxation techniques, stress management teaching, and sometimes short-term benzodiazepines for individuals without substance abuse histories. Binge eating episodes are often used to self-treat intolerable anxiety. When the need to self-medicate anxiety by binge eating is diminished by CBT, with or without antidepressants, binge episodes decrease more rapidly.

3. *Obsessive-compulsive disorder:* Where true OCD exists after improvement in the eating disorder behaviors and thinking, most SSRIs (at higher-than-antidepressive doses) are equally effective, although some clinicians believe fluvoxamine is more specific for OCD. There are some contraindications in using fluvoxamine with concomitant prescription of certain antibiotics or antifungals, or in the presence of prolonged QT intervals.

4. *Substance abuse:* The first goal is to assess the role of substance abuse in the eating disorder. In perhaps one-third to one-half of cases of teenage girls with comorbid substance abuse, the substance abuse is closely related to the onset or self-treatment of the eating disorder. For example, some individuals with anorexia can allow themselves to eat more than minimal amounts of daytime food only when they have had several drinks just before bedtime. A substantial percentage of teenage women with bulimia who use methamphetamines or cocaine or abuse prescription stimulants depend on these drugs for suppression of hunger, for interruption of binge urges, and for mood improvement. Alcohol abuse or marijuana smoking may convert formerly binge-abstinent dieting behavior into overeating followed by compensatory purging. If there is no clear amelioration of the drug craving despite treatment of the eating disorder, then referral to in-

patient or outpatient drug rehabilitation, after treatment of the eating disorder, is the optimal approach. The initial treatment of this dual diagnosis is usually best accomplished in an eating disorder program because of the general capability of such programs to treat all psychiatric disorders. Substance abuse treatment programs generally do not treat the eating disorder effectively. Nicotine withdrawal can be accomplished skillfully without any feared increase in weight.

5. *Personality disorders:* The guideline here is long-term management according to the type of personality disorder. Patients with sensitive, persevering, anxious features generally respond to support, education, and CBT as part of their eating disorder treatment. Repeated confrontation with feared situations is often effective in social anxiety disorders. A common and sometimes challenging combination is the association of an eating disorder with a borderline personality disorder. These individuals respond best to care by skilled, experienced group and individual therapists with evidence-based programs in emotional management, such as DBT or the STEPPS program. True schizophrenia is almost always non-overlapping with a diagnosis of an eating disorder. Too often, soft diagnoses of schizophrenia have incorrectly been suggested as comorbid disorders.

There is some evidence, not universally agreed upon, that antidepressants may play a supplemental role in relapse prevention after a patient's weight has improved, independent of whether comorbid depressive symptoms are present. Tertiary antidepressants, such as venlafaxine and duloxetine, acting on noradrenergic as well as serotoninergic (and probably some dopaminergic) sites, may be used as a second choice for patients with treatment-resistant bulimia nervosa or for binge-eating disorders.

Studies have demonstrated that anorexia nervosa is associated with variable but usually significant changes in the brain itself In severe cases, the brain may appear on magnetic resonance imaging (MRI) to be indistinguishable from the brain of a person with Alzheimer's disease. Ventricles are enlarged and cortical substance is decreased. While patients with anorexia nervosa often have a surprising degree of accomplishment in school, as weight erodes they become increasingly unable to attend and to concentrate on written materials or sustain reasoning. Of concern is the demonstration that weight improvement is not immediately associated with complete restoration of normality in an MRI brain scan, especially in the gray matter. Work is under way in positron emission tomography, tension diffusion studies, and other brain imaging methods to localize the specific brain regions most affected by starvation so as to determine their response to treatment. Defining brain loci that may be vulnerable, predisposing sites in eating disorders is far in the future, if possible at all.

Treatment by Primary Care Physicians versus Specialized Programs

Persons with serious, chronic, or complex cases of eating disorders usually do best when referred to established programs. The benefits versus risks of referral, however, need to be weighed. Long-term continuity of treatment with an established primary care physician argues for keeping treatment as local as possible. But when weight is not restored steadily (at a rate of 1–2 lb/week) in a patient with anorexia nervosa who is receiving outpatient treatment by a primary care physician, or when bulimic symptoms are not improved despite the treatment methods described above, then referral to a specialized program, outpatient or inpatient, is required. The success of treatment is maximized by combining the skills of a primary care physician with concurrent psychotherapy by a psychologically trained colleague, whether a psychiatrist, social worker, psychologist, or nurse clinician. This partnership allows the primary care physician to monitor and treat the medical symptomatology and maintain a long-term relationship with the patient, while the psychologically trained person works with established methods of treating the core psychological dysfunction.

If motivated and educated in supportive psychotherapy methods, the primary care doctor may carry out both medical management and psychotherapeutic treatment. This may be especially important when OB-GYN specialists also act as primary care providers, which is often the case for women between the ages of 15 and 50 (Andersen and Ryan, 2009).

Genetics and Eating Disorders

Multiple studies document that genetics plays a substantial role in the onset and/or maintenance of eating disorders. This finding may be of comfort to families who have been accused of causing the eating disorder. For reimbursement advocacy, it may provide evidence that eating disorders are serious, genetically predisposed, psychiatric and medical disorders. The strongest support for genetics playing a role in eating disorders comes from twin studies and family studies. When one twin has an eating disorder,

Table 1.14. Genetics of eating disorders

- Twin studies: 3- to 5-fold increase in identical twins.
- Family studies: Substantially increased in families with affective spectrum disorder.
- Molecular studies: Minimal/modest progress despite intensive effort. Most likely multiple genes with variable penetrance are involved.
- Epigenetics: Evidence for an interactive effect of genetic vulnerability with life events during critical windows of development.
- Eating disorders "breed true": They are not *forme fruste* of OCD, depressive illness.

it is about four times as common for the other twin to suffer an eating disorder when the twins are identical than when they are disconcordant, fraternal twins (table 1.14).

Family studies show that an individual with a family history of the mood disorders spectrum, including depressive disorders, bipolar disorders, anxiety disorders, OCD, and substance abuse disorders, has a substantially increased probability of developing an eating disorder. Working from the family history method, there is no doubt that a predisposing genetic vulnerability to developing an eating disorder exists (Brandys et al., 2015; Scott-VanZeeland et al., 2014; Strober, Peris, and Steiger, 2014).

Working from the other end of the methods in genetics research involves uncovering a molecular genetic contribution to eating disorders. This method has proved unyielding in producing significant or persuasive results. Energetic studies with as many as 40 coauthors have foundered in their attempts to define specific molecular genetic contributions to these disorders. Eating disorders are undoubtedly polygenetic with variable penetrance.

An epigenetic approach, investigating the interaction of genetic vulnerability with sensitizing life events, holds the most hope for understanding these disorders. Epigenetics attempts to comprehend how environmental factors, often during critical developmental windows, interact with genetically vulnerable substrates to make an individual more likely to develop an eating disorder. Gone are the days of genes alone determining illness, with rare exceptions such as Huntington's disease. Genes have not changed significantly over recent centuries, but certain disorders such as eating disorders and autism spectrum disorders appear to be on the increase, meaning that environmental factors may play a large role. This is an encouraging finding because, generally, environmental changes respond more easily and quickly to intervention than do genetic vulnerabilities. Improved diagnosis may play a role in the increased prevalence of eating disorders, but environmental factors should not be dismissed.

Caring for the Caregivers

Studies show that those who care for family members with eating disorders suffer much like caregivers who struggle to help patients with Alzheimer's disease—as much or more so. Support, education, relief from blame, and respite care are at the core of helping caregivers of patients with eating disorders (table 1.15).

Families are relieved by understanding that while eating disorders are often serious and sometimes lethal, they also have a documented, proven chance to remit, resolve, or be substantially improved with comprehensive treatment—more so than early-onset schizophrenia, OCD, or autism spectrum disorders. Yet, the burden of caregiving is higher among caregivers of patients with eating disorders than among caregivers of patients with depression or schizophrenia (Martin et al., 2015). Family members receive additional relief when blame is taken off their shoulders (Salerno et al., 2016). Next, a substantial dose of psychoeducation on what is known about the origin, course, and treatment of eating disorders further helps families fear less and hope more. Hope, although not absolute certainty, is

---

Table 1.15. Preventing burnout by families and caring for caregivers

- Teach psychoeducational principles about the nature, course, diagnosis, treatment, and prognosis of eating disorders.
- Take the blame off the shoulders of families.
- Where appropriate, avoid hospitalization of teens by teaching and implementing family-based treatment when family is intact and willing.
- Plan respite care for caregivers, as with caregivers of patients with dementia or autism.
- Attempt to resolve alexithymia in parents, especially in fathers of males with eating disorders, to promote bonding and decrease emotional conflict. Develop a common language of accurate identification of emotional states and shared communication.
- Refer parents to supportive psychotherapy.
- Allow parents to set rules for leaving eating disorders at the door when adolescents/adults come home from the hospital.

---

reasonable and evidence-based. Understanding that their family member may be genetically vulnerable helps other family members realize that eating disorders are true illnesses, not willful self-choices or consequences of "refrigerator moms." Respite care may be very welcome once caregivers' guilt about self-care is diminished and self-nurturance is prescribed. In addition to improving parent-patient relationships, parents are encouraged to return to a more balanced relationship with the patient's siblings, who may have been neglected in the intense focus on helping the patient.

Finally, parents are empowered to ask patients who are still actively ill to leave their symptoms at the door when they come home. Supported and educated parents stop being enablers or codependent with patients suffering from eating disorders. When family members in family therapy (especially CBT-based) learn to accurately identify and express their feelings, specifically their mood states, so that all members of the family speak the same language, improved bonding and reduced conflict often occur.

Myths about Eating Disorders

Families with members who have eating disorders, as well as clinicians treating patients with these disorders, benefit by being aware that they may be holding on to myths about eating disorders. Such erroneous beliefs will interfere with the process of healing or convey undue pessimism. Table 1.16 provides a summary of these myths.

The Holy Grail: Primary Prevention

The optimum goal of medical practice is primary preventive intervention. Some historical examples are illustrative. Vaccination against common, previously almost universal childhood infectious diseases that resulted in severe morbidity and not insignificant mortality is now taken for granted. Methods to achieve safe water supplies, free from organisms causing epidemic infections such as cholera, are another highpoint in the history of medicine. Phenylketonuria and other aminoacidemias are routinely identified at birth and preventively treated. Pneumonia in the elderly has decreased with vaccination. New use of cigarettes in North America, Great Britain, Scandinavia, and some European countries (but not Asia) has declined following a combination of financial disincentives and psychoeducational efforts, with physicians leading the way in decreased smoking.

Table 1.16. Myths about eating disorders

Myth	Fact
Eating disorders are always chronic.	The large majority of cases are acute, and patients improve rapidly with skilled care, remitting in up to 75% of cases for younger patients.
Eating disorders are difficult to treat.	Eating disorders respond well at all levels of severity to an experienced multidisciplinary team approach; in mild cases, patients respond to 10–15 sessions.
Eating disorders always recur or reappear in a different form.	"Symptom substitution" has been disproved; recurrence is low with expert treatment.
"Normal" means no concerns about body weight, shape, or food, ever.	"Normative cultural distress" is a reasonable goal, with "lip service" about dieting.
Eating disorders are always severe.	Eating disorders occur on a spectrum of severity, with most cases being mild to moderate, often subclinical.
It always takes a village to treat an eating disorder.	Multidisciplinary team treatment is best for moderate to severe cases; a small, coordinated team usually suffices. For early, milder cases, an experienced single therapist is sufficient.
All families of patients with eating disorders are abnormal.	Families vary; most are worn out, worried, and have done their best. Distressed families are usually a consequence, not a cause.
Most males with eating disorders are gay.	Most males with eating disorders are heterosexual; younger males, asexual.
Eating disorders are a form of depression, OCD, or schizophrenia.	Eating disorders "breed true." They are not an indirect expression of other disorders.
Eating disorders are a result of past trauma.	Past trauma increases the probability of all psychiatric disorders, not specifically eating disorders.
Forcing patients with anorexia to eat works well.	Persuasion, by challenging cognitive distortions, supervised eating, healthy role models, is effective. Need for nasogastric tube is rare.

Table 1.16. (*continued*)

Myth	Fact
Finding the right medication is necessary.	Essential medication is normal food eaten normally. No medication has proved effective or necessary for anorexia nervosa; medication may be adjunctive for bulimia nervosa, binge eating.
You can scare patients into wellness.	Discovering the benefits of wellness works. Scare tactics are not effective; persuasion about seriousness is helpful.
Eating disorders are addictions.	While some similarities are logical, addiction to food is not possible; patients may be dependent on eating disorder behaviors for emotional regulation.
Eating disorders are purely psychiatric disorders.	Eating disorders begin with voluntary dieting, overvaluation of thinness; once established, they become medical disorders.
Eating disorders are entirely intentional, due only to our cultural and voluntary personal choices.	Eating disorders have a 50%–70% genetic contribution.
Eating disorders occur only in spoiled, white, suburban, upper-class teen girls.	Eating disorders are equal-opportunity illnesses, occurring at all ages (7–77), in both genders, in all ethnic and racial groups, in all locations.
Anybody can treat eating disorders.	Persons with eating disorders do better with clinicians trained specifically in eating disorder diagnosis and treatment; general competence is not enough.
Eating disorders involve delusions.	Delusions are uncommon. Most patients have strong, overvalued beliefs about the benefits of slimness or shape change.
Slow heart rate, low body temperature, and low blood pressure need immediate correction by specialists.	Many starvation symptoms self-improve with weight restoration and watchful waiting. Other symptoms, such as prolonged QT interval, need immediate attention.
The reproductive system is ruined.	With recovery, patients with anorexia nervosa rarely have permanent problems in gonadotropin functioning; "nothing is broken." The reproductive system is on pause, waiting for weight restoration.

Where primary prevention has not been widely effective, secondary preventive intervention through early diagnosis and treatment is an increasing reality. Many chronic, serious disorders that commonly afflict large numbers of people in westernized countries are yielding to a variety of secondary preventive and therapeutic interventions. Death from coronary artery disease has substantially decreased, as has death from the silent killer of hypertension, although both are still distressingly high.

The status of primary prevention for eating disorders is controversial, with substantial differences between countries and clinicians (table 1.17). Early intervention and increasingly effective treatments are not in dispute. Norway assigns an experienced nurse to encourage healthy athleticism and eating habits (primary prevention), as well as to identify early cases of eating disorders (secondary intervention). Other countries forego the opportunity for primary prevention. Two examples in the United States offer hope for primary prevention. Ballet schools that set a lower limit on weight for students to be eligible for continuing their studies appear to decrease the number of cases of anorexia nervosa. Some states and institutions have set lowest acceptable weights, lowest speeds of weight loss, and minimum final percentages of body fat acceptable for students engaging in wrestling. What is clear is that speaking to students about signs and symptoms of eating disorders encourages, rather than discourages, the beginning of eating disorders. Reducing risk factors may lead to benefits in reducing eating disorders (Greif, Becker, and Hildebrandt, 2015). School-age bullying is one specific risk factor that appears to be amenable to reduction (Copeland et al., 2015).

Table 1.17. Preventive intervention for eating disorders

- Currently, secondary intervention is the most proven approach: early diagnosis, prompt referral, experienced treatment to comprehensive goals.
- Primary prevention has some preliminary evidence:
  - Setting lowest acceptable weight in dance schools and wrestling programs limits severe weight loss because the result of falling below this weight is elimination from programs.
  - Families that eat the dinner meal together every day have fewer cases of eating disorder and fewer children with substance abuse.
  - Teaching signs and symptoms of eating disorders to schoolchildren probably increases the number of cases.

Information for Patients

It is essential for patients to know that organ functions will not be completely normal for 3–6 months after weight becomes normal. Attaining a healthy weight and resolving abnormal behaviors and cognitions is the *beginning* of comprehensive treatment, not the end. The goal is to plant flowers, not just to pick weeds—language for instilling, to the maximum degree possible, the sense of a life that is flourishing and resilient. Patients with bulimia nervosa may be reassured to know that urges to binge or purge are not, in themselves, indications of ineffective treatment. Continued reflux in formerly bulimic patients may indicate some incompetence of the gastro-esophageal junction.

The goal for dealing with persisting medical symptoms is prompt, effective, complete treatment so that we can help patients achieve changes in thinking and behavior without uncomfortable or serious medical symptomatology interfering with the process of psychological and behavioral change. Severe bloating, painful reflux, or severe hypothermia makes it difficult to concentrate in psychotherapy. Occasionally, a specialist may be needed for assessment and treatment of complex medical aspects.

There is increasing concern that low bone mineral density may be present in patients who have had as little as 6 months of amenorrhea. DEXA scans should be requested for patients with a history of 3 months of amenorrhea, 6 months of significant weight loss, or, for males (Mehler et al., 2008), low weight for 6 or more months. This information may be used psychotherapeutically. Other chapters in this book deal in more detail with medical evaluation and treatment of endocrine, gastrointestinal, cardiac, and bone symptomatology.

Summary of Diagnosis and Treatment

Primary care physicians can confidently diagnose eating disorders with a brief set of screening questions and a mental status examination, and can treat these disorders with clear, proven treatment goals and methods. Relatively recent cases of mild to moderate severity can be treated comprehensively by the primary care physician alone or in conjunction with psychologically trained colleagues. Medical assessment is important for establishing the severity of illness and treating significant medical complications, but not for diagnosis. The guideline is to "rule in" eating disorders, not to "rule out" all possible causes of weight loss or binge-purge.

Families respond well to a combination of education, support, and inclusion in the treatment process, according to the age of the patient and the needs of the family. Realistic optimism based on comprehensive treatment is entirely warranted. Every aspect of most eating disorders can be improved, especially with the up-to-date diagnostic and therapeutic skills of motivated medical and psychological clinicians.

Table 1.18 summarizes some take-away "pearls" regarding the diagnosis and treatment of eating disorders.

Hopes for the Near Future

Some hopes for the near future (the next decade) include:

1. Establishment of more eating disorder treatment centers that can comprehensively treat all such disorders no matter what the severity, employing a *continuum of care* including intensive medical care units, specialized inpatient units, a partial hospital (day) program, intensive and weekly outpatient diagnosis and treatment, and aftercare in residential settings that offer decreasing supervision as the transition to independent living is accomplished.

2. Endowment of more chairs devoted to eating disorders; the first and notable example is in Johns Hopkins Department of Psychiatry.

3. Closing the gap between molecular genetics and family genetics, through epigenetics, to improve our understanding of the mechanisms involved in predisposing and sustaining factors in the eating disorders.

4. Increasing the evidence for primary preventive intervention.

5. Wider teaching of simple methods for routine assessment of eating disorders diagnosis in primary care practice.

6. True legislative parity for health plan funding for the comprehensive treatment of patients with eating disorders until maximum improvement is attained.

7. Increased training of clinicians competent to use CBT, IPT, or DBT in the treatment of eating disorders.

8. Improved understanding of how males with eating disorders may benefit from different diagnostic methods and different treatment strategies.

Table 1.18. "Pearls" concerning diagnosis and treatment of eating disorders

- Large community studies indicate a female-to-male ratio for eating disorders of 1:2–4; the ratio of 1:10 in clinic reports is a false ratio. Implication: Many males are undiagnosed or avoidant of diagnosis and/or treatment. Anorexia nervosa in males is less ego-syntonic than in females. Screening criteria are often female-oriented.

- Dieting is normative for most females, without specific reasons; dieting in males usually begins for specific reasons; the desire for lean muscularity is normative.

- Diagnosis is made by history and mental state examination, not by ruling out all possible medical causes.

- Although most common in the teens and 20s, eating disorders can occur from 7 to 77 years of age. Remember to consider eating disorders in older women, males, minorities, and the mentally challenged.

- Females with anorexia are often proud of weight loss, but bulimic behavior is usually shameful or guilt-producing (ego-dystonic). The patient may test how judgmental you are before disclosing bulimia nervosa symptoms.

- The *DSM-5* and ICD-10 diagnoses are categorical diagnoses. In real life, amount of weight loss, drive for thinness, body image distortion, and fear of fatness are dimensional variables. There are many more subclinical cases of anorexia nervosa than cases meeting full categorical diagnosis. Compare asthma, high blood pressure, and hyperglycemia: all are treated short of severe symptomatology.

- Binge-eating disorder (binge eating without any compensation) occurs in about 25% of medically obese patients as a contributing factor to total weight burden. Assess symptoms of eating disordered thinking and behavior in all obese patients.

- Patients with binge-eating disorder most typically are older (30s–40s). Occurrence is about equal in males and females; may involve compulsive grazing as well as binges.

- Eating disorders in older patients are often complicated by concurrent medical or depressive symptoms as well as a failure to consider an eating disorder as diagnosis.

- Eating disorders are almost never "Lone Rangers." Once an eating disorder diagnosis is made, assess for the comorbid psychiatric disorders and medical consequences. Decide which are predisposing factors and which are secondary to the eating disorder.

- The most common contributing factor to eating disorders is dieting. *Diet* is a four-letter word.

- Approximately 8% of anorexia nervosa cases begin with involuntary weight loss; additional, voluntary weight loss is practiced only after initial weight loss from a medical or surgical cause inspires the idea and benefits of losing weight.

(continued)

Table 1.18. (*continued*)

- Younger patients with anorexia nervosa may try to fool the physician about prescribed weight restoration by carrying secret weights in their pockets or drinking noncaloric beverages before examination. An outside informant is essential.
- Primary care physicians can be fully competent to treat many cases of eating disorders, especially the earlier and milder cases that are most common.
- Males are usually preoccupied with attaining lean muscularity, and especially concerned with body shape from the waist up. Females are most commonly concerned with body shape from the waist down. In males, desire for shape change exceeds desire for weight change; in females, desire for weight change exceeds desire for shape change. Body image distortion is more complex in males than in females; males may desire (a) extreme thinness, (b) normal weight with extreme muscular definition, or (c) high weight with extreme muscular definition.
- An increased probability of gay orientation exists (18%–20%), but homosexuality is a factor in a minority of cases.
- Males usually perceive fatness and a need to start dieting at higher relative weights than females, who feel fat starting at 15%–17% below normal weight.
- Males may fear being told they have a girl's disease or a gay person's disease. They often delay coming in for diagnostic evaluation. Anorexia nervosa is generally ego-alien in males, often ego-syntonic in females; a high feeling of shame.
- Males are sometimes stigmatized by female patients with eating disorders as typical of problematic males in their past.
- Many health professionals are uneducated about eating disorders in males and often do not consider a diagnosis of eating disorders in male patients, or programs may not accept males—a form of gender discrimination.

9. Use of innovative electronic methods for diagnosis and treatment, such as the Internet for case finding, diagnosis, treatment, and follow-up.

10. Developing for all school-age children a "virtuous circle" of healthy nutritional patterns and the teaching of life-long programs in enjoyable exercise, using models found to work in other countries.

11. Identifying additional subpopulations highly vulnerable to eating disorders, such as children and adolescents with insulin-dependent diabetes mellitus, for whom primary prevention is possible.

12. Long-term studies to identify which methods of treatment have the most enduring and comprehensive results.

REFERENCES

American Psychiatric Association. 2013. *Diagnostic and Statistical Manual of Mental Disorders, 5th Edition: DSM-5.* Arlington, VA: American Psychiatric Association.

Andersen AE and Yager J. 2009. Eating disorders. In: Sadock BJ and Sadock VA, eds. *Kaplan & Sadock's Comprehensive Textbook of Psychiatry,* 9th ed. Philadelphia: Lippincott Williams & Wilkins, pp. 2128–49.

Andersen AE and Ryan GB. 2009. Eating disorders in the obstetric and gynecologic patient population. *Journal of Obstetrics and Gynecology* 114:1353–67.

Arcelus J, Mitchell AJ, Wales J, and Nielsen S. 2011. Mortality rates in patients with anorexia nervosa and other eating disorders. *Archives of General Psychiatry* 68:724–31.

Baran SA, Weltzin MD, and Kaye WH. 1995. Low discharge weight and outcome in anorexia nervosa. *American Journal of Psychiatry* 152:1070–72.

Beck D, Casper R, and Andersen AE. 1996. Truly late onset of eating disorders: A study of 11 cases averaging 60 years of age at presentation. *International Journal of Eating Disorders* 20:389–95.

Brandys MK, de Kovel CGF, Kas MJ, et al. 2015. Overview of genetic research in anorexia nervosa: The past, the present and the future. *International Journal of Eating Disorders* 48:814–25.

Bulik CM, Thornton L, Poyastro AP, et al. 2008. Suicide attempts in anorexia nervosa. *Psychosomatic Medicine* 70:378–83.

Citrome L. 2015. A primer on binge eating disorder diagnosis and management. *CNS Spectrums* 1:44–50.

Copeland WE, Bulik CM, Zucker N, et al. 2015. Does childhood bullying predict eating disorder symptoms? A prospective, longitudinal analysis. *International Journal of Eating Disorders* 48:1141–49.

Crisp AJ. 1995. *Anorexia Nervosa: Let Me Be.* New York: Routledge, Taylor and Francis Group.

Crow SJ and Nyman JA. 2004. The cost effectiveness of anorexia nervosa treatment. *International Journal of Eating Disorders* 35:155–60.

Dalle Grave R, El Ghoch M, Sartirana M, and Calugi S. 2016. Cognitive behavioral therapy for anorexia nervosa: An update. *Current Psychiatry Reports* 18:2.

Devlin MJ, Goldfein JA, and Dobrow I. 2003. What is this thing called BED? Current status of binge eating disorder nosology. *International Journal of Eating Disorders* 34(Suppl):S2–18.

Elzakkers IFFM, Danner UN, Hoek HW, et al. 2014. Compulsory treatment in anorexia nervosa: A review. *International Journal of Eating Disorders* 47:845–52.

Fairburn CG. 2008. Eating disorders: The transdiagnostic view and the cognitive behavioral theory. In: Fairburn CG, ed. *Cognitive Behavior Theory and Eating Disorders.* New York: Guilford Press, pp. 7–22.

Fairburn CG and Cooper Z. 2011. Eating disorders, DSM-5 and clinical reality. *British Journal of Psychiatry* 198:8–10.

Fairburn CG, Cooper Z, Doll HA, et al. 2013. Enhanced cognitive behavior therapy for adults with anorexia nervosa: A UK-Italy study. *Behaviour Therapy and Research* 51:R2–8.

Fichter MM and Quadflieg N. 2016. Mortality in eating disorders—results of a large prospective clinical longitudinal study. *International Journal of Eating Disorders* 49:391–401.

Gallucci G and Andersen AE. 2003. Eating and feeding difficulties in patients with intellectual and developmental disabilities: Four cases. *Mental Health Aspects of Developmental Disabilities* 6:3.

Gonçalves SF, Machado BC, and Martins A. 2014. Eating and weight/shape criticism as a specific life-event related to bulimia nervosa: A case control study. *Journal of Psychology* 148:61–72.

Greif R, Becker CB, and Hildebrandt T. 2015. Reducing eating disorder risk factors: A pilot effectiveness trial of a train-the-trainer approach to dissemination and implementation. *International Journal of Eating Disorders* 48:1122–31.

Haedt-Matt AA, Keel PK, Racine SE, et al. 2014. Do emotional eating urges regulate affect? Concurrent and prospective associations and implications for risk models of binge eating. *International Journal of Eating Disorders* 47:874–77.

Haynos AF, Snipes C, Guarda A, et al. 2016. Comparison of standardized versus individualized caloric prescriptions in the nutritional rehabilitation of inpatients with anorexia nervosa. *International Journal of Eating Disorders* 49:50–58.

Hilbert A, Pike KM, Goldschmidt AB, et al. 2014. Risk factors across the eating disorders. *Psychiatry Research* 220:500–506.

Keys A, Brožek J, Henschel A, Mickelsen O, and Taylor HL. 1950. *The Biology of Human Starvation*. Minneapolis: University of Minnesota Press.

Latner JD and Clyne C. 2008. The diagnostic validity of the criteria for binge eating disorder. *International Journal of Eating Disorders* 41:1–14.

Le Grange D, Lock J, Agras WS, et al. 2015. Randomized clinical trial of family-based treatment and cognitive behavioral therapy for adolescent bulimia nervosa. *Journal of the American Academy of Child and Adolescent Psychiatry* 54 886–94.

Machado BC, Gonçalves SF, Martins C, et al. 2014. Risk factors and antecedent life events in the development of anorexia nervosa: A Portuguese case-control study. *European Eating Disorders Review* 22:243–51.

Margolis R, Spencer W, DePaulo RJ, Simpson SG, and Andersen AE. 1994. Psychiatric comorbidity in eating disorder patients: A quantitative analysis by diagnostic subtype. *Eating Disorders* 2:231–36.

Martin J, Padierna A, Van Wijngaarden B, et al. 2015. Caregivers consequences of care among patients with eating disorders, depression or schizophrenia. *BMC Psychiatry* 15:124.

Marzola E, Knatz S, Murray SB, et al. 2015. Short-term intensive family therapy for adolescent eating disorders: 30-month outcome. *European Eating Disorders Review* 23:210–18.

Mehler PS, Sabel AL, Watson T, and Andersen AE. 2008. High risk of osteoporosis in male patients with eating disorders. *International Journal of Eating Disorders* 41:666–72.

Meier SM, Bulik CM, Thornton LM, et al. 2015. Diagnosed anxiety disorders and the risk of subsequent anorexia nervosa: A Danish Population Register study. *European Eating Disorders Review* 23:524–30.

Morgan JF, Reid F, and Lacey JH. 1999. The SCOFF questionnaire: Assessment of a new screening tool for eating disorders. *British Medical Journal* 319:1467–68.

Reas DL and Grilo CM. 2015. Pharmacological treatment of binge eating disorder: Update review and synthesis. *Expert Opinions in Pharmacotheraputics* 16:1463–78.

Redgrave GW, Coughlin JW, Schreyer CC, et al. 2015. Refeeding and weight restoration outcomes in anorexia nervosa: Challenging current guidelines. *International Journal of Eating Disorders* 48:866–73.

Rodin J, Silberstein L, and Striegel-Moore R. 1985. Women and weight: A normative discontent. In: TT Sonderegger, ed. *Psychiatry and Gender.* Lincoln: University of Nebraska Press, pp. 267–307.

Russell G. 1979. Bulimia nervosa: An ominous variant of anorexia nervosa. *Psychological Medicine* 9:429–48.

Salerno L, Rhind C, Hibbs R, et al. 2016. An examination of the impact of care-giving styles (accommodation and skillful communication and support) on the one year outcome of adolescent anorexia nervosa: Testing the assumptions of the cognitive interpersonal model in anorexia nervosa. *Journal of Affective Disorders* 191:230–36.

Scott-VanZeeland AA, Bloss CS, Tewhey R, et al. 2014. Evidence for the role of EPHX2 gene variants in anorexia nervosa. *Molecular Psychiatry* 19:724–32.

Steinhausen J-C, Jakobsen H, Helenius D, et al. 2015. A nation-wide study of the family aggregation and risk factors in anorexia nervosa over three generations. *International Journal of Eating Disorders* 48:1–8.

Strober M, Freeman R, and Morrell W. 1997. The long-term course of severe anorexia nervosa in adolescents: Survival analysis of recovery, relapse, and outcome predictors over 10–15 years in a prospective study. *International Journal of Eating Disorders* 22:339–60.

Strober M, Peris T, and Steiger H. 2014. The plasticity of development: How knowledge of epigenetics may advance understanding of eating disorders. *International Journal of Eating Disorders* 47:696–704.

Thornton LM, Mazzeo SE, and Bulik CM. 2011. The heritability of eating disorders: Methods and current findings. *Current Topics in Behavioral Neurosciences* 6:141–56.

Wilson GT. 2011. Treatment of binge eating disorder. *Psychiatry Clinics of North America* 34:773–83.

Woodside BD and Staab R. 2006. Management of psychiatric comorbidity in anorexia nervosa and bulimia nervosa. *CNS Drugs* 20:655–63.

2

The Role of the Multidisciplinary Team and Levels of Care in the Treatment of Eating Disorders

Craig Johnson, PhD, Kenneth Weiner, MD, Russell Marx, MD, Anne Marie O'Melia, MD, Philip S. Mehler, MD, and Cynthia Pikus, PhD

Common Questions

Which major disciplines are typically members of the treatment team for eating disorders?

What are the common psychologically based therapies that are evidence-based treatments for eating disorders?

Is there any way to know whether an eating disorder professional possesses the competencies necessary to be effective?

What is the core psychopathology of eating disorders?

Which medications are FDA-approved for the treatment of eating disorders?

Eating disorders (anorexia nervosa, bulimia nervosa, binge-eating disorder, avoidant/restrictive food intake disorder) are complex illnesses affecting both the body and the mind. Genetic, neurochemical, psychological, and sociocultural factors all contribute to the onset and maintenance of these disorders. The inherent nature of the illnesses together with the complex interactions of the biopsychosocial factors that underlie them speak to the need for multidisciplinary teams to provide treatment. In fact, guidelines developed by the American Psychiatric Association (APA) (2006), American Academy of Pediatrics (AAP) (2013), American Academy of Child and Adolescent Psychiatry (Lock and La Via, 2015), Society for Adolescent Health and Medicine (SAHM) (2015), Academy for Eating Disorders (AED) (2012), and American Dietetic Association (ADA) (2011) all emphatically recommend a multidisciplinary team approach to the treatment of eating disorders. The Joint Commission (JC) (2016) and the Commission on Accreditation of Rehabilitation Facilities (CARF) (2013) have recently established disease-specific standards for inpatient/residential treatment for eating disorders that mandate the use of a multidisciplinary treatment team (physicians, psychotherapists, dieticians, and nurses). In this chapter we review the composition, roles, and responsibilities of the multidisciplinary team, present the recommended criteria for different levels of care, and discuss how these affect standards of care for the various disciplines.

Case

Consider the number and types of disciplines involved in the care of the patient in this case.

R.G., a 27-year-old married female with a 15-year history of anorexia nervosa and multiple prior treatment stays in residential units, was admitted to treatment in an inpatient eating disorder program at a major medical center. She presented with marked restriction of food and fluids, self-induced vomiting when she ate normal meals, extreme fear of weight gain, and belief that she already looked too big, at 5 feet 6 inches and 75 pounds (58% of ideal body weight [IBW]; body mass index [BMI] of 12.1). R.G. also struggled with a comorbid anxiety disorder. She described conflict with her husband, stemming in part from her difficulty discussing her thoughts and feelings with him. Admission EKG indicated marked sinus bradycardia (heart rate in the high 30s), prompting a brief transfer to a medical floor for cardiac telemetry monitoring and initiation of nutrition rehabilitation with consultation from the eating disorder treatment team.

Once R.G.'s heart rate had increased into the 40s, she returned to the inpatient eating disorders unit. There, under the guidance of a registered dietician, she began following a prescribed meal plan with regular increases in caloric intake to support a weight restoration of 2–4 pounds per week. In the first few weeks of her stay, R.G. had repeated episodes of hypoglycemia; she initially refused to accept glucose tablets or IV dextrose, citing fear of additional calories, but ultimately, after an endocrine consult, was willing to comply with the IV until her blood sugars had stabilized. She was followed closely by the internist on the eating disorders unit, who also monitored the patient's labs biweekly to help avoid refeeding syndrome.

Throughout her stay in the inpatient eating disorder program, R.G. met with an individual therapist twice a week and participated in several therapy groups per day. Therapy focused on helping R.G. develop and practice skills for tolerating the distress she experienced as she restored her weight, as well as skills for managing her anxiety more generally. A family therapist met weekly with R.G. and her husband, focusing on improving the couple's communication skills.

After 10 weeks of inpatient treatment, R.G. stepped down to the partial hospitalization level of care in the same eating disorder program, at a weight of 104 pounds (80% of IBW; BMI 16.8). There she continued the weight restoration process with the support of the registered dietician and began practicing eating snacks, and then meals, at restaurants with staff supervision and participated in a weekly cooking group facilitated by an occupational therapist. Her psychotherapy shifted to include work on long-standing body image concerns, helping R.G. strengthen her sense of self and identity separate from her eating disorder, and relapse prevention work.

Diagnostic Categories for Eating Disorders

The most recent *Diagnostic and Statistical Manual of Mental Disorders*, *DSM-5* (APA, 2013), includes five diagnostic categories of eating disorders (table 2.1): Anorexia Nervosa, Bulimia Nervosa, Binge-Eating Disorder, Avoidant/Restrictive Food Intake Disorder, and Other Specified Feeding or Eating Disorder. Throughout this chapter, the generic term *eating disorders* refers to all of the diagnostic categories listed above.

Roles and Responsibilities of the Treatment Team

Medical physicians, psychiatrists, psychotherapists, dieticians, and nurses are the common core disciplines in the eating disorder treatment team. The level of care prescribed for the patient usually determines the level of involvement of each of these core disciplines. Additionally, the higher the level of care, the more involvement is needed from other disciplines such as occupational and activity therapists and educators, because these patients are generally more debilitated from the severity of their illnesses.

Medical Physicians

Internists, pediatricians, family practice physicians, and adolescent medicine physicians are the providers that assess and manage the medical conditions associated with eating disorders. Increased attention has been placed in recent years on the awareness of eating disorders among

Table 2.1. Eating disorder diagnostic categories (*DSM-5*)

Anorexia Nervosa

A. Restriction of energy intake relative to requirements, leading to a significantly low body weight in the context of age, sex, developmental trajectory, and physical health. *Significantly low weight* is defined as a weight that is less than minimally normal or, for children and adolescents, less than that minimally expected.

B. Intense fear of gaining weight or of becoming fat, or persistent behavior that interferes with weight gain, even though at a significantly low weight.

C. Disturbance in the way in which one's body weight or shape is experienced, undue influence of body weight or shape on self-evaluation, or persistent lack of recognition of the seriousness of the current low body weight.

Bulimia Nervosa

A. Recurrent episodes of binge eating. An episode of binge eating is characterized by both of the following:

    1. Eating, in a discrete period of time (e.g., within any 2-hour period), an amount of food that is definitely larger than what most individuals would eat in a similar period of time under similar circumstances.

    2. A sense of lack of control over eating during the episode (e.g., a feeling that one cannot stop eating or control what or how much one is eating).

B. Recurrent inappropriate compensatory behaviors in order to prevent weight gain, such as self-induced vomiting; misuse of laxatives, diuretics, or other medications; fasting; or excessive exercise.

C. The binge eating and inappropriate compensatory behaviors both occur, on average, at least once a week for 3 months.

D. Self-evaluation is unduly influenced by body shape and weight.

E. The disturbance does not occur exclusively during episodes of anorexia nervosa.

Binge-Eating Disorder

A. Recurrent episodes of binge eating. An episode of binge eating is characterized by both of the following:

    1. Eating, in a discrete period of time (e.g., within any 2-hour period), an amount of food that is definitely larger than what most people would eat in a similar period of time under similar circumstances.

    2. A sense of lack of control over eating during the episode (e.g., a feeling that one cannot stop eating or control what or how much one is eating).

B. The binge-eating episodes are associated with three (or more) of the following:

    1. Eating much more rapidly than normal.

    2. Eating until feeling uncomfortably full.

    3. Eating large amounts of food when not feeling physically hungry.

(continued)

Table 2.1. (*continued*)

---

    4.   Eating alone because of feeling embarrassed by how much one is eating.

    5.   Feeling disgusted with oneself, depressed, or very guilty afterward.

C. Marked distress regarding binge eating is present.

D. The binge eating occurs, on average, at least once a week for 3 months.

E. The binge eating is not associated with the recurrent use of inappropriate compensatory behavior as in bulimia nervosa and does not occur exclusively during the course of bulimia nervosa or anorexia nervosa.

Avoidant/Restrictive Food Intake Disorder

A. An eating or feeding disturbance (e.g., apparent lack of interest in eating or food; avoidance based on the sensory characteristics of food; concern about aversive consequences of eating) as manifested by persistent failure to meet appropriate nutritional and/or energy needs associated with one (or more) of the following:

    1.   Significant weight loss (or failure to achieve expected weight gain or faltering growth in children).

    2.   Significant nutritional deficiency.

    3.   Dependence on enteral feeding or oral nutritional supplements.

    4.   Marked interference with psychosocial functioning.

B. The disturbance is not better explained by lack of available food or by an associated culturally sanctioned practice.

C. The eating disturbance does not occur exclusively during the course of anorexia nervosa or bulimia nervosa, and there is no evidence of a disturbance in the way in which one's body weight or shape is experienced.

D. The eating disturbance is not attributable to a concurrent medical condition or not better explained by another mental disorder. When the eating disturbance occurs in the context of another condition or disorder, the severity of the eating disturbance exceeds that routinely associated with the condition or disorder and warrants additional clinical attention.

Other Specified Feeding or Eating Disorder

This category applies to presentations in which symptoms characteristic of a feeding and eating disorder that cause clinically significant distress or impairment in social, occupational, or other important areas of functioning predominate but do not meet the full criteria for any of the disorders in the feeding and eating disorders diagnostic class. The other specified feeding or eating disorder category is used in situations in which the clinician chooses to communicate the specific reason that the presentation does not meet the criteria for any specific feeding and eating disorder. This is done by recording "other specified feeding or eating disorder" followed by the specific reason (e.g., "bulimia nervosa of low frequency"). Examples of presentations that can be specified using the "other specified" designation include the following:

Table 2.1. (*continued*)

A. Atypical anorexia nervosa: All of the criteria for anorexia nervosa are met, except that despite significant weight loss, the individual's weight is within or above the normal range

B. Bulimia nervosa (of low frequency and/or limited duration): All of the criteria for bulimia nervosa are met, except that the binge eating and inappropriate compensatory behaviors occur, on average, less than once a week and/or for less than 3 months.

C. Binge-eating disorder (of low frequency and/or limited duration): All of the criteria for binge-eating disorder are met, except that the binge eating occurs, on average, less than once a week and/or for less than 3 months.

D. Purging disorder: Recurrent purging behavior to influence weight or shape (e.g., self-induced vomiting; misuse of laxatives, diuretics, or other medications) in the absence of binge eating.

E. Night eating syndrome: Recurrent episodes of night eating, as manifested by eating after awakening from sleep or by excessive food consumption after the evening meal. There is awareness and recall of the eating. The night eating is not better explained by external influences such as changes in the individual's sleep-wake cycle or by local social norms. The night eating causes significant distress and/or impairment in functioning. The disordered pattern of eating is not better explained by binge-eating disorder or another mental disorder, including substance use, and is not attributable to another medical disorder or to an effect of medication.

Unspecific Feeding or Eating Disorder

This category applies to presentations in which symptoms characteristic of a feeding and eating disorder that cause clinically significant distress or impairment in social, occupational, or other important areas of functioning predominate but do not meet the full criteria for any of the disorders in the feeding and eating disorders diagnostic class. The unspecified feeding and eating disorder category is used in situations in which the clinician chooses *not* to specify the reason that the criteria are not met for a specific feeding and eating disorder, and includes presentations in which there is insufficient information to make a more specific diagnosis (e.g., in emergency room settings).

Source: American Psychiatric Association, 2013.

physicians (AED, 2012). This is particularly important because early detection and intervention is associated with better outcomes (Forman et al., 2011), and physicians are often the first point of contact for patients. The extent of medical involvement by these providers is determined by the nature and extent of the patient's medical condition and the level of care. It is important that all members of the treatment team understand that psychosomatic complaints are common in this population. Medical tests and interventions must be judicious and be provided in conjunction with psychological interventions for management of physical discomfort and anxiety. Those with the most severe forms of the illness (e.g., those with BMI of <13 or marked electrolyte and acid-base aberrations resulting from excessive purging behaviors) may require daily medical visits early in the course of treatment.

Psychiatrists

Psychiatrists are usually responsible for medication management of the psychiatric conditions associated with eating disorders. Unfortunately, there is only a modest evidence base for the use of psychiatric medications for eating disorders (APA, 2006). There is, however, a good evidence base for the use of medications for treatment of other psychiatric illnesses that often co-occur with eating disorders, such as depression, anxiety, and obsessive compulsive disorder (National Institute for Clinical Excellence [NICE], 2004). Consequently, it is recommended that patients with eating disorders receive a psychiatric evaluation early in treatment. The extent of ongoing contact with the psychiatrist is then determined by the complexity of the medications recommended and the patient's level of care. Some psychiatrists also deliver psychotherapy, so the frequency of contact and length of sessions could be greater, as dictated by the nature of the psychotherapy being provided.

Many geographic areas do not have adequate access to psychiatrists. Family practice physicians, internists, and pediatricians will often fill this gap by taking responsibility for managing psychiatric medications. Conversely, some psychiatrists are highly informed about the medical management of patients with eating disorders and are comfortable with assuming that responsibility, except for patients with the most severe forms of the illness.

Psychotherapists

Currently, the primary evidence-based treatments for eating disorders are psychologically based. These include cognitive behavioral therapy (CBT), interpersonal therapy (IPT), and dialectical behavioral therapy (DBT) (NICE, 2004), and acceptance and commitment therapy (ACT) and family-based therapy (FBT) (APA, 2006; NICE, 2004). These psychotherapies may be delivered by psychiatrists (MD), clinical psychologists (PhD, PsyD), social workers (LCSW, LSW), and master's-level counselors/psychotherapists (LPC, LMFT). As with the other disciplines discussed here, the initial assessment is critical in determining how the psychotherapist proceeds in treating a patient with an eating disorder, including what psychotherapy approaches are to be used and in what modality (individual, family, and/or group therapy), and the length and frequency of sessions.

Dieticians

The irrefutable need for nutritional rehabilitation of patients with eating disorders has created an unprecedented opportunity for registered dieticians (RDs) to become core members of a behavioral health treatment team. Dieticians play a critical role in assessing the level of nutritional compromise and advising the rest of the treatment team and the patient on meal planning and meal supervision. Since food is often the "centerpiece" of these illnesses both psychologically and with respect to medical complications, all interactions with the patient that relate to food are important. Consequently, it is imperative that dieticians be fully integrated into the treatment team and fully trained in the medical and psychological complications of eating disorders and of nutritional rehabilitation (ADA, 2011).

Nurses

Nurses usually become involved in the treatment of patients with eating disorders at the inpatient, residential, and partial hospitalization program (PHP) levels of care. This is because as medical and psychiatric acuity increases, the need for more continuous supervision of the patient also increases. Registered nurses (RN) and other nursing staff (psychiatric technicians, nurses' aides, child care workers, and other milieu staff) are responsible for the overall supervision and safety of patients in 24-hour care (i.e., inpatient and residential care) and, to some extent, patients in PHP care. They are also largely responsible for implementation of the medical and psychiatric treatment plan. In many treatment settings, nursing staff also actively participate in delivering group therapies and in meal supervision.

Competency Certification

Currently there is only one organization that provides competency certification for different disciplines in the eating disorders field. The International Association of Eating Disorder Professionals (IAEDP) (2005) offers Certified Eating Disorder Specialist (CEDS) designation for physicians, psychotherapists, dieticians, nurses, and art/recreation/movement therapists. Membership in either the AED or IAEDP would indicate disease-specific interest, as would attending continuing education workshops and conferences specific to eating disorders. One can also simply ask the professional for detailed information about his or her experience in treating patients with eating disorders and overall philosophy of care.

Treatment Team Involvement and Levels of Care

Following an initial assessment, the patient usually receives a recommendation regarding level of care. As mentioned earlier, the roles and responsibilities of the various disciplines are largely determined by the level of care being provided. Figure 2.1 outlines usual standards of treatment for different disciplines at each level. The most common levels of care, and the roles of the various team members at each level, are summarized below.

Outpatient Care

Initial medical and psychiatric medication evaluations are recommended during the first outpatient visit, with follow-up visits with physician and psychiatrist as needed.

For adults with anorexia nervosa, psychotherapy sessions are typically provided once or twice a week. Family/couples therapy may be added if indicated. For children and adolescents with anorexia nervosa, a high level of family involvement as prescribed in FBT (Lock and Le Grange, 2013) is usually recommended; individual therapy for adolescents may be added as indicated.

For bulimia nervosa and binge-eating disorder, one or two psychotherapy sessions per week are provided, typically using CBT or IPT manualized treatment (Fairburn, 2008).

Outpatient treatment for adults with an eating disorder may also include weekly visits with a dietician for nutrition counseling. Monitoring of weight, if needed, is typically provided either by the RD or by the medical

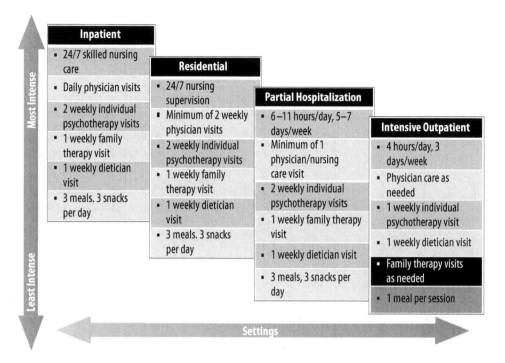

Figure 2.1. Standards of treatment for eating disorders by various disciplines at each level of care.

doctor. Manualized FBT with children and adolescents with anorexia nervosa does not require dietician involvement.

One challenge for most multidisciplinary outpatient teams is maintaining regular communication to ensure coordinated care. Because medical and psychiatric symptoms are often minimal at this level of care, team communication is often coordinated by the psychotherapist.

Intensive Outpatient Program

The patient in an intensive outpatient program lives at home and attends a treatment program for 2–4 hours per day, typically 3 days per week. Programming usually includes individual psychotherapy once a week, nutrition counseling with an RD once a week, various group therapies, and limited meal supervision provided by the therapist, dietician, or ancillary staff (two or three meals per week). Family/couples therapy may also be included. Initial medical and psychiatric medication evaluation are recommended, with follow-up visits with the physician and psychiatrist as needed.

Partial Hospitalization Program

The patient receiving care in a PHP lives at home and spends 6–12 hours per day, 5–7 days per week, at a hospital or clinic. Medical and psychiatric evaluations are required. Medical follow-up is provided as needed, including blood draws for phosphorus levels. Psychiatric follow-up is typically provided once or twice a week. Nursing care is provided as needed.

Programming usually includes individual, group, and family/couples therapy. Meal support (two or three meals and one or two snacks each day) is provided by milieu staff. Dieticians are responsible for evaluating the nutritional status of the patient, recommending a strategy for nutritional rehabilitation, and providing nutrition counseling and guidance, typically meeting with the patient once a week. This level of care can also include participation from other disciplines such as activity and occupational therapists and educators for child/adolescent programs.

The more intensive 7-days-a-week programs are often more effective—particularly in the early stages of treatment—at accomplishing weight gain and interruption of symptoms such as binge eating, purging, and excessive exercise. These more intensive programs will often reduce the days and hours expected of the patient once he or she demonstrates progress with symptom interruption.

Residential Treatment

In residential care, the patient resides in either a hospital facility or a homelike setting, receiving care and supervision 24 hours per day, 7 days per week. The involvement of medical providers, psychiatrists, and nurses is variable across residential facilities, but a certain segment of patients at this level of care may need frequent medical and psychiatric oversight. Programming usually includes individual, group, and family/couples therapy. Support and supervision at meals and snacks is provided by milieu staff. Physician visits are once a week and can be either medical or psychiatric. Psychotherapy is usually twice a week and may include family therapy. Dieticians are responsible for evaluating the nutritional status of the patient, recommending a strategy for nutritional rehabilitation, and providing nutrition counseling and guidance, typically meeting with the patient once or twice a week to accomplish 2–4 pounds of weight gain per week. Residential treatment may also include participation from other disciplines such as activity and occupational therapists and educators for child/ adolescent programs.

Inpatient Care

NONSPECIALIZED MEDICAL HOSPITALS / EMERGENCY CENTERS

These are general medical settings with providers who are often inexperienced in the medical and psychiatric management of eating disorders. The treatment team typically consists of nonspecialized hospitalist physicians and medical nurses. The goal is usually medical stabilization then return of the patient to an outpatient team or referral to either a general psychiatric hospital or a specialized eating disorders residential or inpatient program.

NONSPECIALIZED INPATIENT PSYCHIATRIC HOSPITAL

These general psychiatric settings are focused on crisis stabilization for all diagnostic groups, with an average length of stay of 3–7 days. The providers are typically inexperienced in addressing the medical and psychiatric challenges of weight restoration and symptom interruption for patients with eating disorders. The treatment team typically consists of a psychiatrist, psychotherapist, and nursing staff, and sometimes activity and occupational therapists. The goal is usually to quickly stabilize acute psychiatric symptoms and then return the patient to the outpatient team or refer him or her to a specialty eating disorders inpatient/residential program.

Clearly, medical or psychiatric acuity requires accessing the closest care available. However, nonspecialized, poorly informed treatment can result in medical ineffectiveness or even calamity as well as psychological trauma for patients with eating disorders, due to the inexperience factor. Rapid refeeding can be life threatening, and poorly conceived invasive medical procedures (e.g., nasogastric tubes without clear indication, total parenteral nutrition) and behavioral/psychological interventions (such as use of physical restraints and shame-based psychological interactions) can have long-lasting adverse iatrogenic effects. We highly recommend that specialized care be engaged as quickly as possible.

SPECIALIZED EATING DISORDERS MEDICAL
INPATIENT HOSPITAL

Housed within medical hospitals, these units are rare and specialize in treating the most medically complex eating disorders. The patient is hospitalized and the treatment is focused on medical stabilization with little emphasis on psychiatric or psychological symptoms. The treatment team on these units typically includes internists, subspecialist physicians, nursing staff, and RDs who oversee the patient's nutritional rehabilitation. Physicians, nurses, and dieticians have intensive daily contact and have been extensively trained in the intricacies of safely caring for this severely ill patient. A psychotherapist may be part of the team, but typically provides supportive sessions rather than in-depth psychotherapy, because the patient is often too weak or cognitively impaired by malnutrition to engage in this type of therapy. The goal is to medically stabilize, begin nutrition rehabilitation, effectuate weight gain to 65%–70% of IBW, and then refer the patient to typical eating disorder programs for more in-depth psychiatric and psychological treatment along with continued nutritional and weight restoration.

SPECIALIZED EATING DISORDERS INPATIENT
PSYCHIATRIC HOSPITAL

The patient resides in the facility and is under the continuous and intensive supervision of staff, 24 hours per day, 7 days per week. Staff members are experienced in the medical and behavioral challenges of treating this patient population. This level of care is usually indicated when the patient is below 75% of IBW or is acutely medically or psychiatrically ill, or when outpatient care or PHP attempts have failed to interrupt eating disorder symptoms. At this level of care, physicians are responsible for the overall care of the patient and typically lead the treatment team. At the inpatient level of care, a psychiatrist meets with the patient 7 days per week, and a medical provider sees the patient for an initial assessment and then as often as needed. Full-time supervision by nursing staff is also required. The nursing staff is responsible for ensuring the overall safety of the patient, communicates concerns to the medical and psychiatric physicians, and helps ensure that the treatment plan is being implemented. Nursing staff may also participate in providing group therapy and meal supervision. Milieu staff assist with implementing the individual treatment plan for each patient and with supervising patients at meals and in general. Psychother-apists are responsible for the patient's psychological treatment, which usu-ally includes twice-a-week individual therapy, once-a-week family/couples therapy, and group therapy several times a day. Psychotherapists may also participate in meal supervision. Dieticians are responsible for evaluating the patient's nutritional status, recommending a strategy for nutritional rehabilitation, and providing nutrition counseling and guidance, typically meeting with the patient once or twice a week to help achieve the goal of 2–4 pounds of weight gain per week. The dieticians also participate in meal supervision. The inpatient level of care can also include participation from other disciplines such as activity, art, or movement therapists and occupa-tional therapists. Educators for child/adolescent programs are usually nec-essary for younger patients so that they do not lose valuable school time.

Inpatient versus Residential Facilities

Licensed inpatient facilities have to meet the more stringent safety and treatment standards required for medical and psychiatric hospitals across the United States. These include standards for construction, infection control, food and medication management, and medical records. Inpatient facilities also require full-time nursing (RN/LPN) supervision and daily physician involvement. Some inpatient units are locked, and some can provide involuntary treatment when that is needed.

The licensure and regulatory requirements for the residential level of care are highly variable across states. Building and other safety requirements can be minimal. Nurse and physician involvement can also vary greatly and may be minimal.

The Joint Commission (JC, 2016) and the Commission on Accreditation of Rehabilitation Facilities (CARF, 2013) are the predominant regulatory organizations that accredit inpatient and residential psychiatric programs. Each has recently developed criteria specific to eating disorders that allow programs to achieve disease-specific accreditation. We would highly rec-ommend referring patients to programs that have met these standards, given their inherent increased focus on the care being provided.

Psychiatric Medications and Psychotherapy

Comprehensive treatment for patients with eating disorders si-multaneously addresses the medical/nutritional components of the illness (e.g., weight restoration, normalization of eating, treatment of medical complications) and the behavioral/emotional aspects of the disorder. In this section we focus on how treatment addresses the behavioral/emotional parts of the illness and expand on the role of the psychotherapist and psychiatrist within the treatment team.

At the core of the psychopathology of eating disorders are dysfunctional beliefs, emotions, and behaviors centering around food and weight, often including an overvaluation of the benefits of thinness, misinterpretation of normal digestive sensations, and efforts to lose weight or change body shape. Additionally, there is often marked fear and distress related to the prospect of changing these attitudes and behaviors. Surrounding these core symptoms are a variety of maladaptive factors that maintain the illness for the individual (e.g., lack of sense of self, low self-esteem, fears related to taking on adult responsibilities).

The psychiatrist and psychotherapist join efforts to help the patient to identify, challenge, and diminish the aforementioned eating disorder symptoms and maintaining factors and to move toward recovery, with a combination of psychotherapy, experiential relearning, and individualized medications. They also focus on comorbid conditions, with both psychotherapy and the judicious use of medications.

Psychiatric Medications

No medications are approved by the US Food and Drug Administration for the treatment of anorexia nervosa. As Mitchell et al. (2013) have said, "The treatment literature in anorexia nervosa consists of relatively few controlled pharmacotherapy studies in comparison to bulimia nervosa and binge-eating disorder. Controlled studies have generally shown a lack of efficacy for pharmacological interventions." The largest maintenance trial of fluoxetine for treatment of anorexia nervosa, reported by Walsh et al. (2006), randomized 93 patients to either 60 mg of fluoxetine or a placebo and found the medication not effective for preventing either relapse or depression.

The most promising class of medications for anorexia nervosa are second-generation antipsychotics ("atypicals"). Results of trials with first-generation antipsychotics pimozide and sulpiride showed that they did not significantly improve outcome. Second-generation antipsychotics in several large studies also showed a lack of significant weight gain for patients with anorexia nervosa. Trials of risperidone, olanzapine, and quetiapine have not shown great success. However, it is still thought that reduction in distorted thinking through the use of second-generation antipsychotics might eventually prove helpful, if larger studies can be done to identify subgroups of patients who might respond to these medications or to identify predictors of treatment response.

The only FDA-approved medication for bulimia nervosa is fluoxetine, which is indicated for acute and maintenance treatment of binge eating and vomiting behaviors in adult patients with moderate to severe bulimia nervosa. In three initial short-term studies, fluoxetine at 60 mg, but not 20 mg, was effective in reducing the number of binge eating and vomiting episodes. The largest maintenance trial, reported by Romano et al. (2002), lasted 52 weeks and showed greater efficacy for fluoxetine over placebo. The dropout rates were high for both arms of the study: 83% for the fluoxetine group and 92% for the placebo group. These very high dropout rates were mostly the result of illness relapse and patients' decisions, not adverse events. Also of note, as with most bulimia nervosa studies, the goal in this study was reduction of binge eating and purging behaviors, not abstinence.

Selective serotonin reuptake inhibitors (SSRIs) have been the most commonly studied medications for bulimia nervosa, and results show efficacy for fluoxetine (12 trials), fluvoxamine (3 trials), and sertraline (1 trial). Trials of tricyclic antidepressants such as desipramine and imipramine have also shown some efficacy; however, given their favorable side effect profile, SSRIs have been the more common first-line treatments. Other antidepressants examined include reversible monoamine oxidase inhibitors such as brofaromine and moclobemide, which did not show advantage over placebo. Another medication that has shown efficacy is the anticonvulsant topiramate (Hoopes et al., 2003). There are significant side effects, however, which can be somewhat attenuated by starting at a low dose and increasing slowly.

Binge-eating disorder is the most common of the eating disorders, and numerous medications have been examined for efficacy for this patient population. The only medication with FDA approval to treat binge-eating disorder is lisdexamfetamine dimesylate (Vyvanse), approved in 2015. The efficacy of Vyvanse in treating binge-eating disorder was demonstrated in two clinical trials that included 724 adults with moderate to severe binge eating (US Food and Drug Administration, 2015). Compared with the placebo group, participants taking the active drug showed a decrease in the number of binge eating days per week and had fewer obsessive/compulsive binge eating behaviors. The most common side effects in clinical trials were anxiety, dry mouth, insomnia, constipation, and increased heart rate. Vyvanse was approved in 2007 to treat attention deficit hyperactivity disorder (ADHD) in patients 6 years and older. Serious risks of stimulants like Vyvanse include psychiatric problems such as psychotic or manic symptoms as well as heart problems, including sudden death, stroke, and heart attack. Also of note, in the United States, Vyvanse is a Schedule II controlled substance showing a high potential for abuse and potential dependence. Although some patients lose weight when taking Vyvanse, it is not approved or recommended for weight loss. Vyvanse is a "pro drug," not active until absorption by the intestine and removal of L-lysine, converting the drug to dextroamphetamine. The exact mechanism of action is unknown, but in ADHD, enhancement of dopamine and norepinephrine has been shown in numerous brain areas.

Other classes of medication show some efficacy for treatment of binge-eating disorder. Mitchell et al. (2013) found that SSRIs "are reasonably effective agents in suppressing [or], albeit rarely, eliminating binge-eating disorder." These have included fluvoxamine, citalopram, escitalopram, and sertraline. Marcus et al. (1990) found fluoxetine to have additional benefit when added to behavioral modification for binge-eating disorder. In other studies, Ricca et al. (2001) found that fluoxetine did not confer added benefit over CBT alone, and Devlin et al. (2007) found fluoxetine showed a positive effect on depression but not on binge eating frequency in binge-eating disorder.

Another medication class that has shown some efficacy for treating binge-eating disorder is the selective norepinephrine reuptake inhibitors (SNRIs). McElroy et al. (2004) found positive effects for atomoxetine in reducing binge eating frequency, and Silveira et al. (2005) found a positive effect for reboxetine in lowering scores on the binge eating scale. Some older studies, done before publication of current criteria for binge-eating disorder, found a positive effect on binge eating by the tricyclics imipramine and desipramine (McCann and Agras, 1990; Laederach-Hoffman et al., 1999).

Two medications widely used in binge-eating disorder are the anticonvulsants topiramate and zonisamide. Both have shown decreases in binge eating episodes (Mitchell et al., 2013), and both can result in significant weight loss through poorly understood mechanisms. However, both can have significant side effects including sedation, cognitive difficulties, and kidney stones.

Finally, orlistat, a lipase inhibitor that partially blocks the absorption of ingested fat, has shown efficacy in some binge-eating disorder trials for weight loss, but it may be associated with uncomfortable diarrhea.

Psychotherapy

The goals for psychotherapy with persons who have eating disorders typically include helping the patient begin to make shifts in behaviors and attitudes, develop a stronger sense of identify apart from the illness, and engage fully in a meaningful life. Some therapy approaches focus on changing dysfunctional thoughts and beliefs, while others help patients accept difficult thoughts and change how they relate to those thoughts, thereby lessening their impact. The process of psychotherapy for patients with eating disorders involves taking a dual approach to the individual. On the one hand, the psychotherapist must have a clear, objective, evidence-based understanding of eating disorders, their comorbidities, and the treatments suited for this combination of challenges. On the other hand, the clinician must also establish a sensitive engagement with the patient to form a therapeutic alliance that allows the individual to understand the functions that the eating disorder is serving and, ultimately, to let go of the eating disorder and develop new, more adaptive coping mechanisms and skills for navigating difficult emotions and experiences.

The modest evidence base for psychotherapy for patients with eating disorders has been focused on outpatient treatment. FBT is recommended by the APA, the AAP, and England's NICE for the treatment of mild to moderate anorexia nervosa in children and adolescents. FBT is a 20-session manualized treatment delivered by a psychotherapist with specific family therapy training. The treatment is delivered to the entire family, with sessions once or twice a week. Seven randomized controlled trials support the efficacy of this treatment for children and teens with anorexia nervosa (Couturier, Kimber, and Szatmari, 2013; Lock, 2015; Lock and Le Grange, 2013).

CBT and IPT have been approved by the APA (2006) and NICE (2004) as recommended treatments for adults with bulimia nervosa and binge-eating disorder. These are 20-session, manualized treatments delivered by a psychotherapist in individual appointments that are typically held weekly and last for 45–60 minutes. Randomized trials have demonstrated the efficacy of these approaches compared with other treatments (Champion and Power, 2012; Watson and Bulik, 2012). Two randomized controlled trials using FBT have shown it to be effective in the treatment of adolescents with bulimia nervosa.

There is also growing evidence for the efficacy of some of the newer "third wave behavioral therapies" such as DBT and ACT in the treatment of adults with eating disorders (Bankoff et al., 2012; Juarascio, Forman, and Herbert, 2010; Lenz et al., 2014). These therapies focus on increasing awareness of one's experiences, shifting the way one relates to difficult experiences, and developing a life with purpose.

Several other adjunct interventions are commonly used in eating disorder programs, although they have not yet been empirically validated. One such approach is sensory modulation, initially developed by occupational therapists and often used with more severe forms of illness to help patients broaden their repertoire of skills for self-regulating in the face of difficult emotions or experiences. Patients with functional gastrointestinal symptoms resulting in food avoidance, rumination, or vomiting can be provided with behavioral interventions and instructed in the use of diaphragmatic breathing for symptom control. Another adjunctive approach is individual or group-based art therapy, in which making art provides an avenue for exploring and managing thoughts, feelings, and difficult experiences.

Group psychotherapy is an important component of most eating disorder treatment programs. Groups offer the experience of peer support and peer challenge, the opportunity to see parallels in the experience of others, and the opportunity to use peers who are further along in the treatment process as role models. Psychotherapy groups in an eating disorder program may include process groups (in which patients explore and share their thoughts, feelings, and relationships), skills-based groups (typically centered around a specific treatment model such as CBT, DBT, or ACT), body image groups (in which distorted perceptions of the body are explored and challenged), and psychoeducational groups (e.g., focusing on medication, medical issues, or nutrition). Many programs also include experiential groups such as supervised grocery shopping and cooking groups or restaurant outing groups. One category of experiential group that warrants special mention is the expressive arts groups, including art therapy, psychodrama, music group, and movement therapy. These allow patients opportunities to access emotions they might otherwise struggle to name and talk about.

Summary

Given the complexity of these illnesses, the biopsychosocial model and the multidisciplinary treatment team the foundation of state-of-the-art care for patients with eating disorders. Providers from numerous disciplines blend their skills to create the optimal recovery environment. The treatment delivered by this group of clinicians involves a combination of standard components (e.g., medical monitoring, nutritional rehabilitation, therapy groups) and individualized components (e.g., addressing the individual's life journey, family environment, and specific medical needs). Patients looking back on their care often cite "the team" as one of the most beneficial aspects of their treatment and one of the key catalysts in the recovery process. In sum, the assembly, integration, and ongoing collaboration of the multidisciplinary team form an invaluable aspect of the treatment for individuals with eating disorders.

REFERENCES

Academy for Eating Disorders (AED). 2012. *Critical Points for Early Recognition and Medical Risk Management in the Care of Individuals with Eating Disorders.* Reston, VA: Academy for Eating Disorders.

American Academy of Pediatrics (AAP). 2013. Policy statement: Identifying and treating eating disorders. *Pediatrics* 111:204–11.

American Dietetic Association (ADA). 2011. Position of the American Dietetic Association: Nutrition intervention in the treatment of eating disorders. *Journal of the American Dietetic Association* 111:1236–41.

American Psychiatric Association (APA). 2006. *Practice Guideline for the Treatment of Patients with Eating Disorders.* Arlington, VA: American Psychiatric Association.

———. 2013. *Diagnostic and Statistical Manual of Mental Disorders, 5th Edition: DSM-5.* Arlington, VA: American Psychiatric Association.

Bankoff SM, Karpel MG, Forbes HE, and Pantalone DW. 2012. A systematic review of dialectical behavior therapy for the treatment of eating disorders. *Eating Disorders* 20:196–215.

Champion L and Power MJ. 2012. Interpersonal psychotherapy for eating disorders. *Clinical Psychology and Psychotherapy* 19:150–58.

Commission on Accreditation of Rehabilitation Facilities (CARF). 2013. *Standards for Eating Disorder Programs.* CARF.org.

Couturier J, Kimber M, and Szatmari P. 2013. Efficacy of family-based treatment for adolescents with eating disorders: A systematic review and meta-analysis. *International Journal of Eating Disorders* 46:3–11.

Devlin MJ, Golsfein JA, Petkova E, Liu L, and Walsh BT. 2007. Cognitive behavioral therapy and fluoxetine for binge eating disorder: Two-year follow-up. *Obesity* 15:1702–9.

Fairburn CG. 2008. *Cognitive Behavioral Therapy and Eating Disorders.* New York: Guilford Press.

Forman SF, Grodin LF, Graham DA, et al. 2011. An eleven site national quality improvement evaluation of adolescent medicine-based eating disorder programs: Predictors of weight outcomes at one year and risk adjustment analyses. *Journal of Adolescent Health* 49:594e600.

Hoopes SP, Reimherr FW, Hedges DW, et al. 2003. Treatment of bulimia nervosa with topiramate in a randomized, double-blind, placebo-controlled trial. *Journal of Clinical Psychiatry* 64:1335–41.

International Association of Eating Disorders (IAED). 2005. *Certification Program for Eating Disorders.* IAEDP.com.

Joint Commission. 2016. New requirements for residential and outpatient eating disorders programs. *Joint Commission Perspectives* 36:4–9.

Juarascio AS, Forman EM, and Herbert JD. 2010. Acceptance and commitment therapy versus cognitive therapy for the treatment of comorbid eating pathology. *Behavior Modification* 34:175–90.

Laederach-Hoffman K, Graf C, Horber F, Lippuner K, Lederer S, Michel R, and Schneider M. 1999. Imipramine and diet counseling with psychological support in the treatment of obese binge eaters: A randomized, placebo-controlled, double-blind study. *International Journal of Eating Disorders* 26:231–44.

Lenz AS, Taylor R, Fleming M, and Serman N. 2014. Effectiveness of dialectical behavior therapy for treating eating disorders. *Journal of Counseling and Development* 92:26–35.

Lock J. 2015. An update on evidence-based psychosocial treatments for eating disorders in children and adolescents. *Journal of Clinical Child and Adolescent Psychology* 44(5):707–21

Lock J and La Via M. 2015. Practice parameter for the assessment and treatment of children and adolescents with eating disorders. *Journal of the American Academy of Child and Adolescent Psychiatry* 54:412–25.

Lock J and Le Grange D. 2013. *Treatment Manual for Anorexia Nervosa: A Family-Based Approach,* 2nd ed. New York: Guilford Press.

Marcus MD, Wing RR, Ewing L, Kern E, McDermott M, and Gooding W. 1990. A double-blind, placebo-controlled trial of fluoxetine plus behavior modification in the treatment of obese binge-eaters and non-binge eaters. *American Journal of Psychiatry* 147:876–81.

McCann UD and Agras WS. 1990. Successful treatment of nonpurging bulimia nervosa with desipramine: a double-blind, placebo-controlled study. *American Journal of Psychiatry* 147:1509–13.

McElroy SL, Guerdjikova A, Kotwal R, et al. 2004. Atomoxetine in the treatment of binge-eating disorder: A randomized placebo-controlled trial. *Journal of Clinical Psychiatry* 68:390–98.

Mitchell J, Roerig J, and Steffen K. 2013. Biological therapies for eating disorders. *International Journal of Eating Disorders* 46:470–77.

National Institute for Clinical Excellence (NICE). 2004. *Eating Disorders: Core Interventions in the Treatment and Management of Anorexia Nervosa, Bulimia Nervosa, and Related Eating Disorders: Clinical Guideline 9.* London: National Institute for Clinical Excellence. www.nice.org.uk/pdf/g009niceguidance.pdf.

Ricca V, Mannucci E, Mezzani B, et al. 2001. Fluoxetine and fluvoxamine combined with individual cognitive-behavior therapy in binge eating disorder: A one-year follow-up study. *Psychotherapy and Psychosomatics* 70:298–306.

Romano SJ, Halmi KA, Sarkar NP, Koke SC, and Lee SJ. 2002. A placebo-controlled study of fluoxetine in continued treatment of bulimia nervosa after successful acute fluoxetine treatment. *American Journal of Psychiatry* 159:96–102.

Silveira RO, Zanatto V, Appolinario JC, and Kapczinski F. 2005. An open trial of reboxetine in obese patients with binge eating disorder. *Eating and Weight Disorders* 10:93–96.

Society for Adolescent Health and Medicine (SAHM). 2015. Position paper of the Society for Adolescent Health and Medicine: Medical management of restrictive eating disorders in adolescents and young adults. *Journal of Health* 56:121–25.

US Food and Drug Administration. 2015. FDA news release. January 30.

Walsh BT, Kaplan AS, Attia E, et al. 2006. Fluoxetine vs placebo to prevent relapse in anorexia nervosa: Primary outcome of drug on time to relapse in 93 weight restored subjects. *JAMA* 295:2605–12.

Watson HJ and Bulik CM. 2012. Update on the treatment of anorexia nervosa: Review of clinical trials, practice guidelines and emerging interventions. *Psychological Medicine* 43:2477–2500.

3

Medical Evaluation of Patients with Eating Disorders

Kristine Walsh, MD, MPH, Jennifer McBride, MD, and Philip S. Mehler, MD

Common Questions

Are anorexia nervosa and bulimia nervosa associated with significant medical issues?

Are there specific physical signs, symptoms, or laboratory results that point to a diagnosis of anorexia nervosa or bulimia nervosa?

What questions need to be asked during an initial history and physical examination?

Which examinations are strongly recommended?

Which laboratory tests are strongly recommended?

Which examinations are optional?

How often do the examinations have to be repeated?

Case

M.P. was a 22-year-old female admitted to the residential unit of an eating disorder program for weight restoration. She gave a 12-year history of anorexia nervosa, restricting subtype. Her highest adult weight was 125 lb and her current weight was her lowest. She denied all forms of purging and had been subsisting on less than 500 kcal per day. Her review of systems endorsed cold intolerance, fatigue, constipation, chest pain, and low back pain. On physical examination she was noted to be in no distress. At 5 feet 6 inches tall her weight was 97 lb, putting her at 75% of ideal body weight (IBW). Blood pressure was 94/70 mm Hg and pulse was 52. There was lanugo hair growth on the sides of her face, a normal result on cardiac exam, hypoactive bowel sounds, and no edema. Laboratory results revealed a normal comprehensive panel and leukopenia (white cell count 2.3). The EKG showed sinus bradycardia at 50 with nonspecific ST changes. On the bone density scan (DEXA), the worst T score was −3.1 in her lumbar spine.

Background

This chapter presents a broad general overview of the medical evaluation that is appropriate for the patient with an eating disorder. Many of the medical issues dealt with here are covered in much greater detail in other chapters, as noted throughout this review.

Most of the medical complications of anorexia nervosa and bulimia nervosa result either from starvation and weight loss or from the mode and frequency of specific purging behavior. *Purging* indicates all forms of self-induced compensation for unwanted calories or methods to lower weight by loss of body fluids. This can be accomplished by (1) self-induced vomiting (which may be induced manually with an object such as a toothbrush, or by simply tightening abdominal muscles, or by ingesting ipecac); (2) laxative abuse; (3) diuretic abuse; or (4) ingestion of thyroid hormone or stimulant-type medications. The first two methods account for 90% of purging behaviors, followed by the other methods in descending order of frequency.

These are dangerous illnesses. Anorexia nervosa is a potentially life-threatening disorder and one of the most lethal psychiatric disorders. In a meta-analysis, the aggregate 10-year mortality rate for patients with anorexia nervosa was more than five times greater than for age-matched controls (Arcelus et al., 2011). About 20% of deaths resulted from suicide; the majority resulted from a direct effect of the illness. Bulimia nervosa is medically more benign than anorexia nervosa. However, its mortality rate is still twice that of age-matched controls, with most deaths attributable to serious electrolyte abnormalities due to purging behaviors (Crow et al., 2009). Specifically, death is usually caused by cardiac abnormality resulting from dangerous hypokalemia (low potassium) due to a purging behavior, or by suicide, which is generally a consequence of the common comorbid personality disorder.

Diagnosis

Most individuals who have an eating disorder will not present with symptoms directly attributable to the eating disorder and may attempt to hide evidence of disordered eating from the physician. This is especially true for individuals of normal weight who have bulimia nervosa. However, symptoms, signs, and laboratory results may provide appropriate clues for the alert clinician.

Symptoms

Most patients with an eating disorder are females in their teens or twenties, and they present for medical care with nonspecific complaints of feeling cold, tired, or "bloated" and experiencing constipation, gynecologic problems, swelling of the hands and feet, numbness and tingling, or nonspecific cardiopulmonary symptoms such as exertional fatigue, heart palpitations, or syncope (fainting) (table 3.1). If the physician misses these subtle clues, he or she can easily overlook the diagnosis.

Signs

The most common physical signs associated with anorexia nervosa and bulimia nervosa are listed in table 3.2 (Westmoreland, Krantz, and

Table 3.1. Symptoms in individuals with eating disorders

Anorexia nervosa	Bulimia nervosa
Amenorrhea	Irregular menses
Infertility	Heart palpitations
Irritability	Esophageal burning
Depression	Abdominal pain
Exertional fatigue	Abdominal bloating
Weakness	Fatigue
Headache	Headache
Dizziness	Constipation/diarrhea
Chest pain—palpitations	Rectal bleeding
Faintness	Swelling of feet
Dysphagia (difficulty swallowing)	Frequent sore throat
Constipation	Teeth sensitivity
Abdominal pain	Depression
Heartburn	Swollen cheeks
Feeling of "fullness" with eating	Numbness and tingling
Polyuria	Nosebleeds
Dry skin	
Intolerance of cold	
Low back pain	
Fragility fractures	

Table 3.2. Physical signs in individuals with eating disorders

Anorexia nervosa	Bulimia nervosa
Emaciation	Calluses on the back of the hand
Hypothermia	Salivary gland hypertrophy (swollen
Hyperactivity	cheeks)
Bradycardia (heart rate <60 beats/minute)	Erosion of dental enamel
Hypotension (blood pressure <90 mm Hg	(perimylolysis)
systolic)	Periodontal disease
Hypoactive bowel sounds	Dental caries
Dry skin	Facial petechiae (red dots on the face)
Pressure sores	Perioral irritation
Brittle hair	Mouth ulcer
Brittle nails	Hematemesis (vomiting blood)
Hair loss on scalp	Edema (ankle, periorbital)
"Yellow" skin, especially palms	Abdominal bloating
Lanugo hair growth on face	Cardiac arrhythmia
Cyanotic (blue) and cold hands and feet	Rectal prolapse
Leg edema	Hemorrhoids
Heart murmur (mitral valve prolapse)	

Mehler, 2016). In severe anorexia nervosa, the emaciation of the patient usually alerts the clinician to the diagnosis. However, individuals with anorexia usually try to conceal their low weight. Common strategies include wearing large pants and sweaters to mask their thinness and carrying hidden objects or ingesting water to artificially inflate their weight. Not infrequently, probably because of society's emphasis on thinness, health care professionals overlook the marked degree of emaciation and thus may fail to recognize the seriousness of the patient's condition.

People with anorexia nervosa have thinning scalp hair; lanugo hair growth (downy, fine hair), particularly on the face, neck, arms, back, and legs; and a yellowish tinge to the skin. There is often bradycardia, hypotension, and hypothermia, which may present as cold intolerance and an inability to compensate for changes in temperature. The hands and feet are frequently purplish-blue due to cyanosis and abnormalities of temperature regulation (acrocyanosis) (Strumia, 2009).

In contrast to people with anorexia, whose emaciation draws medical attention, people with bulimia nervosa often appear physically healthy. Because binge eating is often done secretively, most patients will not provide this information unless specifically asked. In addition, the associated behaviors of vomiting and of abuse of laxatives, diet pills, diuretics, or ipecac are often concealed from others due to guilt or shame and must be specifically inquired about during the history.

Certain signs are present on physical examination, however, and are of some utility in detecting occult bulimia nervosa (Sachs and Mehler, 2016). A common sign is the erosion of dental enamel in individuals who engage in self-induced vomiting. The erosion is particularly marked on the lingual surface of the upper teeth. This is referred to as perimylolysis (see chapter 11). Fillings or amalgams, which are relatively resistant to the gastric acid, appear to be raised above the level of the tooth surface. Other types of dental change include increased sensitivity to cold or hot temperatures and a possible increased rate of developing caries (Kisely et al., 2015). A second clinical sign is swelling of the salivary glands, particularly the parotid glands on the sides of the face, a few days after cessation of purging. This swelling is usually bilateral and painless, but can be pronounced (Park and Mandel, 2006). Patients sometimes refer to this as "puffy cheeks." It is seen in people with bulimia who engage in excessive amounts of self-induced vomiting and abruptly cease. A third sign of diagnostic utility is calluses on the dorsum of the hand as a result of irritation of the fingers by the teeth during repeated induction of self-induced vomiting (Russell's sign). This sign, specific to bulimia, may be more common early in the course of the illness; during later stages, patients often no longer require mechanical stimulation to induce vomiting and can simply turn their head, bend forward, and initiate vomiting.

In some patients, periorbital petechiae (small red dots around the eyes) may be seen shortly after a forceful vomiting episode, and there may be redness of the skin around the corners of the mouth as a result of irritation by acidic stomach contents. This is referred to as angular cheilosis. Fluid retention can be dramatic, particularly in the hands and feet, after withdrawal of laxatives or diuretics or cessation of excessive vomiting.

In both disorders, physical signs of past self-mutilation are not uncommon as part of the psychopathology of eating disorders, especially in bulimia nervosa associated with borderline personality disorder. Inquiry about this and an examination of the skin are important.

Laboratory Results

Unfortunately, objective, accurate, and specific measures of the severity of disordered eating behavior do not exist. Clinicians must therefore rely on the self-reports of their patients, who may not accurately describe the frequency of their eating disordered behaviors. There are not many consistently reliable screening laboratory tools for occult eating disorders. A good patient-doctor relationship, which sets the tone for candid responses to validated screening questions, is key. There are, however, some helpful clues on blood testing that may speak to the presence of an eating disorder (table 3.3).

Abnormally low serum potassium levels are highly specific for covert purging behaviors but are not highly sensitive (see chapter 5) (Mehler and Walsh, 2016). In general, the body has an impressive ability to maintain normal serum levels of potassium in the absence of severe gastrointestinal (GI) or renal losses of potassium. Pure dietary-induced hypokalemia is relatively rare in the absence of purging behaviors, which deplete the body's potassium stores. The serum bicarbonate level also is often abnormal in bulimia. High levels (>30 mEq/L) are most consistent with either self-induced vomiting or diuretic abuse; low levels are most consistent with acute diarrhea due to laxative abuse. Patients with purely restrictive anorexia nervosa are rarely at risk for hypokalemia, even if their weight is very

Table 3.3. Laboratory results that might point to a diagnosis of eating disorder

Anorexia nervosa (food-restricting subtype)	Bulimia nervosa
Hypercholesterolemia	Hyperamylasemia
Hypoglycemia	Hyponatremia
Elevated enzymes in liver function tests	Hypokalemia
Bradycardia (heart rate <60 beats/min)	Hypomagnesemia
Low white blood cell count (leukopenia)	Metabolic alkalosis
Low red blood cell count (anemia)	Non-gap metabolic acidosis
Low LH, FSH, estradiol, or testosterone levels	
Low thyroxine levels (T4)	
Hypophosphatemia (low phosphorus)	
Hyponatremia (low sodium)	
Osteopenia/osteoporosis	
Low leptin levels	

low, until they begin to refeed. In fact, generally, their blood chemistry values are remarkably normal, and they may die from anorexia nervosa–induced starvation with normal blood chemistry values, including a preserved serum albumin level. Therefore, the presence of a substantially low albumin level in anorexia nervosa should prompt the clinician to look for independent medical comorbidities. Severe hyponatremia (low sodium level) can result from diuretic abuse in a patient with bulimia who is further volume-depleted from vomiting or a patient with anorexia nervosa who is drinking even as little as 5–10 liters of water per day to obtain a "full" feeling without eating. If therapeutic correction of the serum sodium is too rapid, these patients risk developing the serious neurologic disorder known as central pontine myelinolysis.

Serum amylase levels are frequently raised above the normal range in people who vomit regularly. The hyperamylasemia is mostly salivary-based rather than pancreatic in origin and results from enlargement of salivary glands due to overeating and vomiting. As with potassium levels, the role of serum amylase measurements as a diagnostic test is limited. Nevertheless, amylase levels may correlate positively with frequency of binge eating and purging. Because an elevated amylase level can also be seen with acute pancreatitis, it is worthwhile to follow up with a lipase test. If the lipase level is normal, then one can conclude that the elevated amylase level is of salivary rather than pancreatic origin.

In summary, the presence of an abnormally low potassium value and an abnormally high serum amylase level, together with an elevated bicarbonate level, in an otherwise healthy young woman seems to be specific for frequent purging behavior. However, its sensitivity as a screening tool is poor. As with all patients, a careful history directed toward uncovering problem eating behaviors that might cause serious medical complications is the most important source of information, for which no laboratory tests can substitute—especially for patients in the right clinical setting who are between the ages of 13 and 30, when eating disorders are most prevalent.

Hypercholesterolemia has been noted in up to 50% of patients with anorexia nervosa but is probably clinically insignificant. It is most likely a reflection of an elevated "good" cholesterol subtype (HDL) rather than an elevated "bad" cholesterol subtype (LDL).

Elevations of liver transaminase levels can be seen both before refeeding in patients with severe anorexia nervosa and as a result of aggressive refeeding in dietary plans containing high-dextrose caloric sources (Nagata et al., 2015). Also in anorexia nervosa there may be abnormalities in the complete blood count (CBC). Leukopenia (low white count), anemia (low red count), and thrombocytopenia (low platelet count) may be present, especially as weight loss becomes more severe. In addition, results of endocrine-hormonal tests, such as estrogen, testosterone, cortisol, and thyroid levels, are often abnormal in anorexia nervosa.

Differential Diagnosis

In the food-restricting subtype of anorexia nervosa, the symptoms and signs are usually those that occur secondary to caloric restriction and weight loss. Many of the manifestations are similar to the complications observed in patients with starvation due to other causes, including fatigue, dizziness, and cold intolerance. However, there are a few important differences. For example, most starving patients will note lethargy and inability to exercise, whereas patients with anorexia may nevertheless continue to exercise excessively in attempts to lose weight. Patients with weight loss from other organic causes will express grave concern about their weight loss, while patients with anorexia will be unconcerned about their marked weight loss. Moreover, common causes of weight loss due to malabsorption will present with diarrheal symptoms, which are generally absent in anorexia nervosa, or with symptoms of adrenergic excess such as sweating and rapid heart rates, also absent in anorexia nervosa. The clinician should also bear in mind that the most common cause of substantial weight loss in young adolescent females in western societies is anorexia nervosa. Patients with anorexia nervosa are often spared the starvation-related complications of the inhabitants of developing countries (kwashiorkor and marasmus) because of their usual ingestion of vitamins, even though their total caloric intake is very low.

Especially for patients presenting with atypical features, clinicians should make a careful assessment to exclude other organic pathologies such as occult malignancies, chronic infections, diabetes, or malabsorption syndromes. Selected laboratory tests can facilitate the diagnosis of other illnesses, such as hyperthyroidism (TSH level), which may cause weight loss and simulate anorexia nervosa. Inflammatory bowel disease (IBD) affecting the intestine can cause abdominal pain associated with eating that may lead to food restriction, incorrectly suggesting a diagnosis of anorexia nervosa; however, the central psychopathology of anorexia (see chapter 1) and normal albumin levels are lacking in IBD. Other common psychiatric disorders are also associated with weight loss, such as depression, schizophrenia, substance abuse, somatoform disorders, and dissociative disorder. When starvation begins with self-induced vomiting and the patient endorses a drive for thinness with a morbid fear of weight gain, a purely medical cause is rarely found.

Similarly, a variety of other medical conditions may present with symptoms that are difficult to distinguish from those of bulimia nervosa. For example, illnesses such as IBD and connective tissue syndromes (scleroderma) may cause abnormal upper GI motility and result in many of the same symptoms as in people who have bulimia and abuse laxatives or engage in self-induced vomiting.

Generally speaking, these diagnoses can be made by a thorough medical history and physical examination together with laboratory screening tests. Complex and expensive work-ups are rarely indicated. The guiding principle is that a diagnosis of an eating disorder is made not by a "rule out" of all possible medical disorders but by confident determination of the presence of an eating disorder through a combination of focused physical examination, a thoughtful use of laboratory testing, and screening questions (Academy for Eating Disorders, 2016) (table 3.4).

Patients with eating disorders frequently complain about constipation. However, a detailed history of the patient's perception of constipation is required because constipation is differently defined by patients and physicians. Experts define constipation as having fewer than three bowel movements per week. Patients with bulimia often have unrealistic beliefs about the need to have frequent bowel movements. In bulimia nervosa, constipation is usually caused by dependence on stimulant laxatives, which can in the long run, albeit rarely, result in the death of the colonic wall myenteric nerve plexus and severe constipation. In anorexia nervosa, colonic motility is delayed due to lack of oral intake, even if there has never been abuse of stimulant laxatives (Mitchell and Crow, 2006) (see chapter 6).

Given the frequency of comorbid psychiatric conditions, a complete psychiatric evaluation should be performed to diagnose comorbid depression, substance abuse, and personality disorders. The patient should also be evaluated for impulsivity and suicidality.

Table 3.4. Differential diagnosis for anorexia nervosa and bulimia nervosa

Anorexia nervosa	Bulimia nervosa
Hyperthyroidism	Scleroderma or other connective tissue
HIV	disorders with GI involvement
Malabsorption	Infections
Addison's disease	Inflammatory bowel disease
Diabetes mellitus	Malabsorptive states
Malignancy, especially lymphoma,	Gastroesophageal disorder (GERD)
stomach cancer	Bowel obstruction
Irritable bowel syndrome	Esophageal stricture
Chronic infection, especially tuberculosis,	Peptic ulcer disease
AIDS, fungal disease	Gastric outlet syndrome
Hypothalamic lesion or tumor	Parasitic intestinal infection
Cystic fibrosis	Chronic pancreatitis
Superior mesenteric artery syndrome	Diabetes
Inflammatory bowel disease (Crohn's	Hypothalamic lesion or tumor
disease, ulcerative colitis)	Zenker's diverticulum
Parasitic intestinal infection	Brain tumor
Chronic pancreatitis	
Psychiatric disorders associated with	
weight loss	

Physical Examination

There are two distinct reasons for conducting a physical examination of patients with eating disorders. The first is to elicit the signs related to the medical complications of anorexia nervosa or bulimia nervosa and, in the process, to begin to define a treatment plan to stabilize patients medically (American Psychiatric Association, 2006). The second is to use the examination in a motivational context and to confront patients with objective medical evidence that the disordered eating behavior has adversely affected their physical health (see chapter 14). The information is particularly relevant for physicians in the light of the long-term increased mortality rate, especially for patients with severe anorexia nervosa. The facets of such a physical examination are summarized in table 3.5.

Obtaining accurate measures of a patient's height and weight to determine body mass index (BMI) and percent ideal body weight (IBW) and assessing the degree of emaciation are important. The IBW is easily calculated, starting with 100 pounds for a female 5 feet tall and then adding

Table 3.5. Physical examination for patients with eating disorders

Weight, height, BMI, % ideal body weight	Cardiac examination
Pulse and blood pressure	Abdominal examination
State of hydration	Extremity examination (edema and
Skin examination	cyanosis)
Neurologic examination (strength)	Musculoskeletal examination
Dental examination	(weakness)

5 pounds for each additional inch. Thus, if the patient is 5 feet 5 inches tall and weighs 100 pounds, she is 80% of IBW. For males, starting at 106 pounds and adding 6 pounds for each inch is the common approach. Severe anorexia nervosa is generally diagnosed for weights that are more than 25%–30% below IBW (see chapter 4). The patient's current weight should not be self-reported, because patients with eating disorders are often unreliable in self-estimations of body weight. The clinician should also attempt to establish the patient's premorbid weight.

Examination of the mucous membranes and skin turgor and, if indicated, measurement of orthostatic blood pressure help to assess the patient's state of hydration. An examination of the abdomen is necessary for patients with anorexia nervosa or bulimia. Inspection, auscultation, and light palpation are recommended. For most patients, further evaluation will not be necessary unless significant abnormalities are detected or serious complaints have been articulated.

For individuals with bulimia, a careful dental examination for evidence of dental caries and enamel erosion should be performed. The erosion has a characteristic pattern, tending to occur on surfaces that have maximum exposure to the vomitus, particularly the palatal surfaces of the maxillary teeth and the occlusal surfaces of posterior teeth, especially on the lingual sides (see chapter 11).

Pulse and blood pressure should be checked for all patients. Sinus bradycardia of fewer than 60 beats per minute is present in many patients with anorexia nervosa because of an energy-conserving slowing of the metabolic rate and vagal hyperactivity. Hypotension, with a blood pressure of less than 90/60 mm Hg, is often present in these patients, related to chronic volume depletion and cardiac changes, and may result in episodes of dizziness and frank syncope. Orthostatic blood pressure measurements should include supine and standing postures for those with excessive purging or for patients with anorexia nervosa (Sachs et al., 2016).

Laboratory Tests

Mandatory Tests

Several screening laboratory tests are indicated for all people who present with an eating disorder, and several specific procedures and ancillary tests are indicated in certain situations (table 3.6). The choice of laboratory tests at the initial evaluation will be guided by the results of the history and the physical examination. Most people with eating disorders should have a screening laboratory panel of blood tests. A complete blood count with differential, electrolytes, blood urea nitrogen (BUN), creatinine, blood glucose, calcium, phosphate, liver function tests, thyroid-stimulating hormone (TSH), and 25-hydroxy vitamin D, as well as testosterone in males, and a pregnancy test in females, are indicated for most people with eating disorders, especially those being admitted to a hospital inpatient, residential, or partial hospitalization program.

Low white and red blood cell counts can occur with anorexia nervosa, reflecting bone marrow suppression due to malnutrition. An increase in leukocyte counts signaling infections might be overlooked due to low baseline values. Therefore, increased vigilance is necessary with patients who have anorexia and are being evaluated for possible infections. Also, these patients may not manifest a fever in infectious states, because of the baseline hypothermia associated with anorexia nervosa.

Serum electrolytes should be checked routinely for all patients to detect possible electrolyte imbalances. Specifically, elevated serum bicarbonate

Table 3.6. Laboratory tests for patients with eating disorders

CBC with differential	T4, TSH levels
Serum electrolytes	Testosterone level (males)
Calcium, magnesium, phosphorus levels	Urinalysis
Liver function tests and albumin	Stool examination for occult blood if
Serum salivary amylase level	abdominal complaints or if anemia
Vitamin D (25-hydroxy)	is present
Prealbumin	EKG
Serum BUN, creatinine levels	Bone densitometry (DEXA)
Blood glucose level	

levels indicating metabolic alkalosis are frequently seen in patients who vomit regularly. Hypokalemia is often present in patients with bulimia. Because hypokalemia is a potentially life-threatening abnormality, electrolyte function should be evaluated for patients with bulimia who are actively purging. Furthermore, many patients with electrolyte abnormalities are clinically asymptomatic. Hypophosphatemia can lead to very serious complications and often develops during the early stages of refeeding of patients who have anorexia nervosa (see chapters 4 and 5).

Liver enzyme abnormalities are relatively uncommon among patients with eating disorders at near-normal weights. However, low body weight can cause hepatic damage, and hepatic dysfunction may occur in patients with anorexia nervosa more often than in the general population (Saito et al., 2008). Elevated liver enzymes, aspartate aminotransferase (AST) and alanine aminotransferase (ALT), occur in patients with more severe forms of anorexia nervosa. In particular, AST and ALT, as well as indirect bilirubin, may be increased during refeeding, especially if nutritional intake emphasizes foods with high glucose content (see chapter 4).

A disproportionate rise in BUN compared with creatinine may be caused by dehydration from diuretics, laxative abuse, or decreased fluid intake in patients with anorexia nervosa. Generally, this ratio is less than 20:1. Blood glucose often decreases with more severe weight loss in anorexia nervosa but is generally asymptomatic in the 40–60 mg/dL range. However, hypoglycemia is a bad prognostic sign in anorexia nervosa because it indicates depleted hepatic glycogen and glucose stores, necessitating urgent follow-up.

Because the symptoms and signs of both hyperthyroidism and hypothyroidism can mimic eating disorders, thyroid function tests are appropriate. Patients with anorexia nervosa might be misdiagnosed as having hypothyroidism. The pattern of thyroid indices in patients with anorexia is a normal or low T4, decreased T3, increased reverse T3, and normal TSH. This represents a physiologic adaptation to starvation that need not be treated with thyroid supplementation. It is referred to as the euthyroid sick syndrome. Patients may even abuse thyroid hormone therapy to further lose weight. Occasionally, TSH is mildly elevated, but it generally returns to normal a few weeks after refeeding is under way and thus should be rechecked before committing a patient to thyroid hormone replacement therapy.

Young people with insulin-dependent diabetes mellitus sometimes overdose their insulin to compensate for binges or underdose to create hyperglycemic-induced urinary frequency and weight loss. This is now being referred to as diabulimia (see chapter 10)

Given that conception can occur during recovery from anorexia nervosa even before the return of menstruation, a serum pregnancy test is recommended.

Optional Tests

The specific items of the history, the complaints of the patient, and the findings on physical examination should direct the physician to the need for further evaluation. This includes selective use of chest or abdominal X-rays, electromyography (EMG), examination of muscle enzymes (creatinine phosphokinase, CPK), computed tomography (CT) or magnetic resonance imaging (MRI) scans of the head, or GI endoscopy if there is evidence of GI blood loss or significant esophageal, gastric, or abdominal pain.

If abuse of diuretics or laxatives is suspected but is denied by the patient, urine samples to detect the surreptitious use of these agents may be considered in rare cases, as well as stool samples for phenolphthalein testing as evidence of laxative use. The presence of possible neurologic dysfunction may necessitate an electroencephalogram (EEG) or a head CT or MRI to rule out seizure disorder or structural brain illness, especially in atypical eating disorders.

Screening for osteoporosis should be an important standard part of the management of individuals with anorexia nervosa of more than one year's duration, and the results can often be used as a motivational tool. Ordering a dual-energy X-ray absorptiometry (DEXA) scan for measurement of bone density of hip and spine, for all men and women with a history of 9–12 months or more of anorexia nervosa, is good practice. These findings may be used to guide the physician in giving advice about the level of physical activity suitable for the patient and support recommendations for adequate calcium intake and full restoration of body weight to restore normal menstrual activity.

On the basis of the initial evaluation, judicious use of medical subspecialists to evaluate any identified major medical complications may be indicated. Certainly, at a minimum, a primary care physician who is well versed in the medical issues of these patients should be closely involved in their care.

An initial electrocardiogram (EKG) with a rhythm strip is desirable for any patient who has bulimia or has anorexia nervosa and is severely emaciated. It is good practice to obtain a baseline EKG for any patient with an eating disorder admitted to an inpatient or residential unit. The EKG commonly shows sinus bradycardia; low-amplitude P waves and QRS voltages, reflecting reduced cardiac size; nonspecific ST segment and T wave abnormalities; and occasionally, U waves associated with hypokalemia and hypomagnesemia. Dangerous QTc abnormalities may also be present (see chapter 5).

Ongoing Medical Management

The majority of the above-mentioned abnormalities and complications are fully reversible with weight restoration and cessation of purging behavior. Osteoporosis and cognitive functions may be the glaring exceptions. Careful, ongoing medical management is an essential component of the overall treatment plan for patients with eating disorders. The frequency and content of medical follow-up visits must be individualized for each patient, depending on the severity and chronicity of the eating disorder and the associated medical complications. Occasionally, patients who have severe anorexia nervosa or bulimia nervosa should be seen a few times per week during the early phases of their treatment plan or weight restoration program or when a nonmedical therapist expresses concern for the patient's appearance or new complaints.

Daily monitoring of weight, pulse, and blood pressure is strongly advised for all markedly underweight patients who have anorexia or are purging. For many patients with eating disorders, especially those who have bulimia, electrolyte abnormalities are the most prominent medical complication. The clinician should closely follow up on these patients to ensure adequate correction of electrolyte values, as well as patients with anorexia nervosa during the early phase of refeeding.

Follow-up evaluations should be performed more frequently if medical complications have been identified, if the patient with anorexia nervosa is being aggressively refed or is more than 25%–30% below IBW, if the patient's condition has deteriorated, or if medical interventions are planned that might affect these parameters. All health care workers caring for these patients must be aware that eating disorders pose serious medical risks and predispose the patient to development of serious medical complications. Thus, it is important to have close medical oversight as part of the multi-disciplinary treatment team.

Summary

Eating disorders can have a deleterious effect on many different body systems. It is imperative that patients with eating disorders have a health care provider who is well versed in the medical complications of eating disorders, especially as the prevalence of these disorders increases, and most especially as the severity of the disorder increases.

REFERENCES

Academy for Eating Disorders. 2016. *Critical Points for Early Recognition and Medical Risk Management in the Care of Individuals with Eating Disorders*, 3rd ed. Reston, VA: Academy for Eating Disorders.

American Psychiatric Association. 2006. *Practice Guideline for the Treatment of Patients with Eating Disorders*, 3rd ed. Arlington, VA: American Psychiatric Association, pp. 35–41.

Arcelus J, Mitchell AJ, Wales J, and Nielsen S. 2011. Mortality rates in patients with anorexia nervosa and other eating disorders: A meta-analysis of 36 studies. *Archives of General Psychiatry* 68:724–731.

Crow SJ, Peterson CB, Swanson SA, et al. 2009. Increased mortality in bulimia nervosa and other eating disorders. *American Journal of Psychiatry* 166:1342–1346.

Kisely S, Baghale H, Lalloo R, and Johnson NW. 2015. Association between poor oral health and eating disorders: Systematic review and meta-analysis. *British Journal of Psychiatry* 207:299–305.

Mehler PS and Walsh K. 2016. Electrolyte and acid-base abnormalities associated with purging behaviors. *International Journal of Eating Disorders* 49:311–18.

Mitchell JE and Crow S. 2006. Medical complications of anorexia nervosa and bulimia nervosa. *Current Opinion in Psychiatry* 19:438–43.

Nagata JM, Park KT, Colditz K, and Golden NH. 2015. Association of elevated liver enzymes among hospitalized adolescents with anorexia nervosa. *Journal of Pediatrics* 166:439–43.

Park MJY and Mandel L. 2006. Diagnosing bulimia nervosa with parotid swelling: Case report. *New York State Dental Journal* 72:36–39.

Saito T, Tojo K, Miyashita Y, et al. 2008. Acute liver damage and subsequent hypophosphatemia in malnourished patients: Case reports and review of literature. *International Journal of Eating Disorders* 41:188–92.

Sachs KV, Harnke B, Mehler PS, and Krantz MJ. 2016. Cardiovascular complication of anorexia nervosa: A systematic review. *International Journal of Eating Disorders* 49:238–48.

Sachs K V and Mehler PS. 2016. Medical complications of bulimia nervosa and their treat-
    ments. *Eating and Weight Disorders* 21:13–18.

Strumia R. 2009. Skin signs in anorexia nervosa. *Dermato-Endocrinology* 1:268–70.

Westmoreland P, Krantz MH, and Mehler PS. 2016. Medical complications of anorexia
    nervosa and bulimia. *American Journal of Medicine* 129:30–37.

4

Nutritional Rehabilitation: Practical Guidelines for Refeeding Patients with Anorexia Nervosa

Philip S. Mehler, MD

Common Questions

How is ideal body weight calculated for adults?

What classification is used to define the severity of anorexia nervosa and the need for inpatient versus outpatient treatment?

What is the "refeeding syndrome"? Which patients are at risk?

Are there general guidelines to follow in formulating a dietary plan when refeeding a patient who has anorexia nervosa?

How has the approach to refeeding evolved in the past decade?

What laboratory tests should be done and how often should they be checked when refeeding a patient who has anorexia nervosa?

How are caloric needs ascertained and calculated?

What physical findings should the clinician follow during the refeeding process?

What alternative nutritional approaches may help reverse the course of refractory, severe anorexia nervosa?

What are "enteral nutrition" and "total parenteral nutrition"? What is their role in anorexia nervosa?

What determines whether adequate calories are being provided for the nutritional rehabilitation of the patient with anorexia nervosa?

How does one approach a patient's lack of expected weight gain on a specified dietary regimen?

Refeeding the patient who has anorexia nervosa is essential to successful treatment. Judging by outcome studies from around the world, most experts agree that one cannot effectively treat anorexia nervosa without first restoring body weight. It is also clear that without a concerted refeeding effort no meaningful psychotherapy can take place, because these patients have starvation-induced cognitive deficits. Weight restoration, however, may be one of the most challenging and frustrating parts of the recovery process for many patients with anorexia nervosa, given the inherent nature of their illness.

Traditionally, centers that treat patients with moderate and severe degrees of anorexia nervosa have used a combination of behavioral techniques, cognitive restructuring, and a progressive program of oral caloric intake to achieve the goal of weight restoration. Different types of enteral feeding and total parenteral nutrition (TPN) may be indicated for rare, more refractory cases. Clinicians caring for these patients must be facile in the art of the refeeding process, given the multitude of potential clinical and biochemical caveats. Two cases illustrate some of these points.

Case 1

J.W., a 40-year-old female, had a 15-year history of anorexia nervosa. She was transferred to an inpatient eating disorder program after an apparent suicide attempt through self-inflicted stab wounds. On admission, she was found to be almost 40% below her ideal body weight (IBW) (height 5 feet 6 inches, weight 83 pounds). Significant laboratory data included a low hematocrit of 21% (normal range 38%–45%) secondary to recent blood loss, sodium of 127 mg/dL (138–143), and serum albumin of 3.4 g/dL (3.5–5.0). Her dietary history indicated an average intake of 400–600 kcal per day. She reported weekly use of laxatives and daily exercise of 1–2 hours' duration. Her predicted resting energy expenditure (REE) was 1,050 kcal per day, based on the Harris-Benedict formula.

J.W. was started on 1,000 kcal per day divided into three meals and progressed to 1,600 kcal per day during the ensuing 7 days. After the first week, she developed slight edema in her legs, which was thought to be secondary to her lacerations rather than a manifestation of the refeeding syndrome. Her liver function tests became slightly elevated (AST and ALT), and she had intermittent problems with asymptomatic hypoglycemia, with a nadir fasting venous blood sugar of 38 mg/dL (normal range 60–100). An evening snack was added.

By the end of the second week, her liver function tests began to improve and her edema resolved. Blood sugar levels remained low. Calories were progressively increased to 2,000 kcal per day, but her weight remained unchanged. An indirect calorimetry study was obtained. It calculated an REE of 911 kcal per day, which indicated that she should have been gaining weight on her current diet plan. J.W. subsequently admitted to covert excessive exercise during evening hours. Once this was addressed in her treatment plan, her hypoglycemia resolved, and she gained a total of 14 pounds over the next 4 weeks. She subsequently gained an additional 18 pounds after discharge on a dietary plan that provided 3,100 kcal per day, and she has maintained a weight of 105 pounds over the past 3 years. She did not, however, have resumption of her menses.

Case 2

S.C., a 41-year-old female, had a 20-year history of anorexia nervosa. She had had multiple unsuccessful inpatient admissions for treatment of this condition. Over the preceding 18 months, she had lost 29 pounds and was infected with a fungal pneumonia. In addition, she complained of cold intolerance, fatigue, and an inability to concentrate. She was therefore readmitted to an inpatient eating disorder unit for the treatment of her anorexia nervosa.

Despite intensive psychotherapy and a defined nutritional plan in the hospital's regimented eating disorder program, S.C., who was 5 feet 10 inches tall, remained at her initial admission weight of 89 pounds. She also developed purulent bronchitis caused by the virulent bacteria *Enterobacter* and *Klebsiella*. Because of her persistent refractory anorexia nervosa, with a body weight more than 40% below ideal, and her adamant refusal of a gastric tube, the decision was made to judiciously initiate therapy with an alternative mode of nutritional rehabilitation using TPN.

S.C. received a total of 9 weeks of TPN. When TPN was discontinued, she had gained 28 pounds, which she has maintained for the 2 years since the TPN was completed. The TPN, consisting of a solution containing 50% dextrose and an 8.5% amino acids solution, was started at a rate of 25 mL/ hour, and the infusion rate was cautiously advanced over the course of 5 weeks to achieve a maximum intake of 3,600 kcal per day. Calories were also partly derived from a 10% intralipid solution for the first week of TPN, which was then advanced to an every-other-day 20% infusion of 500 mL.

Laboratory values were checked every other day for the first 2 weeks, bi-weekly for the next 3 weeks, and weekly for the last 2 weeks of therapy. Aside from some minor elevations in serum liver transaminase levels, there were no other significant biochemical changes. During the course of the TPN, S.C. also worked intensely with a dietician to choose oral foods at each meal. By the time the TPN was discontinued, the number of calories she derived from oral feeding had increased from 300 to 2,700 kcal per day. During the last 2 weeks of TPN therapy, the rate of infusion was progressively reduced, and her weight gain was successfully maintained after 6 months of follow-up.

Background

In general, the nutritional needs and goals of individuals with anorexia nervosa are based on attaining their healthy IBW. For a female, IBW may be calculated as 100 pounds for 5 feet of height plus 5 pounds for each additional inch. For a male, the only difference in the calculation is to start at 106 pounds and use 6 pounds per additional inch. Thus, patients' condition can be classified as mild, moderate, severe, or critical based on whether they are 10%, 20%, 30%, or more below IBW. An alternative way of classifying patients is based on body mass index (BMI), which is calculated on the basis of height and weight and is readily available in tables for an array of heights and weights. Specifically, the BMI value is obtained by dividing an individual's weight in kilograms by height in meters squared. The utility of BMI is limited, however, in that it does not provide any measure of body composition or nutritional status (Yates, Edman, and Aruguete, 2004). In addition, standardized tables of "ideal body weight" may not be appropriate for use with adolescents. Normative data from the National Center for Health Statistics' height and weight tables may be better suited for adolescents 12–18 years of age.

When a patient is set to begin the refeeding process, there must be, from the onset, an earnest attempt to achieve agreement among caregiver, dietician, and patient as to what the range for target weight is going to be. Also, spending time educating a patient with anorexia nervosa about metabolism and how it may change during the process of weight restoration may prevent future difficulties and reduce stress for the patient. Generally, weight gain to or very near IBW is an acceptable goal, regardless of the mode of refeeding. Some view a healthy weight as being the weight at which normal menstruation occurred in the past. However, if amenorrhea persists, it may be necessary for the patient to achieve full IBW or even a little above it. Discharging patients before they reach a minimum normal weight is associated with an increased rate of readmission (Castro et al., 2004; Redgrave et al., 2005). Current practice is generally to admit a patient to the hospital for inpatient treatment, medical stabilization, and nutritional restoration when the patient's weight is more than 30% below IBW (American Psychiatric Association, 2006). This is both to minimize morbidity during the early stages of refeeding and because the rate of severe medical complications increases at these low weights (Gaudiani et al., 2012).

Refeeding Syndrome

Before describing the specifics of refeeding, it is important to consider a potentially catastrophic complication that can occur during this process. It is referred to as the refeeding syndrome (Solomon and Kirby, 1990). This syndrome occurs in significantly malnourished patients, those who have had marked caloric restriction, during the early phase of nutritional replenishment—whether by the oral, enteral, or parenteral route. The risk of the refeeding syndrome is directly correlated with the degree of weight loss resulting from the anorexia nervosa. Thus, patients who are more than 30% below IBW should initially be refed during an inpatient hospitalization (Bermudez and Beightol, 2004).

In the early twentieth century, the heart was believed to be immune to the effects of chronic malnutrition. However, during World War II, experiments were performed using conscientious objectors who voluntarily agreed to lose a certain percentage of their body weight. As a result of this weight loss, they developed low blood pressure and reduced cardiac size, as seen on a chest radiograph. This finding led to a progressive realization that the heart can be adversely affected by weight loss as well as by subsequent refeeding. There is an even earlier reference to the refeeding syndrome in the famed novel *The Count of Monte Cristo*, by Alexandre Dumas, first published almost 175 years ago: "He turned his eyes toward the still steamy soup that the jailor had put on the table, raised the bowl and drank. Then he had the courage to stop, for he had heard of shipwrecked survivors found depleted by hunger, dying from eating gluttonously, overly substantial food."

The mechanism of the potential cardiovascular collapse in the refeeding syndrome is multifactorial. First, the reduced heart mass that accompanies weight loss makes it difficult for the heart to handle the increase in total circulatory blood volume that accompanies refeeding. The end result of this can be heart failure. Even though the heart mass does revert toward normal with weight gain, the first few weeks of refeeding require more attention to a patient's cardiovascular status (Lamzabi et al., 2015). Studies in anorexia nervosa have shown diminished cardiac output as a result of heart muscle atrophy that accompanies unhealthy weight loss (Goldberg, Comerci, and Feldman, 1988).

Second, changes in serum levels of phosphorus as well as potassium and magnesium are key variables in the refeeding syndrome. The mechanism by which hypophosphatemia (low phosphorus levels) develops during refeeding is mainly due to the glucose content of the food. The glucose load increases insulin release, which in turn drives phosphorus and potassium into the intracellular space. There is also an incorporation of phosphorus into newly synthesized tissues and high-energy compounds during refeeding. The resultant low serum phosphorus levels are accompanied by depletion of the high-energy compound adenosine triphosphate (ATP), which impairs the contractile properties of the heart and can evolve into congestive heart failure (fig. 4.1). Refeeding-induced hypophosphatemia can also result in diaphragmatic muscle fatigue and respiratory failure. Other sequelae of refeeding-induced hypophosphatemia include red blood cell membrane disruption (hemolysis), skeletal muscle injury (rhabdomyolysis), and seizures. Rhabdomyolysis is diagnosed by the finding of an abnormally high serum level of the muscle enzyme creatinine phosphokinase (CPK). Low levels of serum potassium and magnesium can also cause cardiac irritability and arrhythmias, along with skeletal muscle weakness.

The best predictor of risk for developing refeeding hypophosphatemia is BMI; the lower the BMI, the greater the risk (Brown, Sabel, and Mehler, 2015). Clinicians must regularly check phosphorus levels, perhaps daily, for the first 1–2 weeks of refeeding and replenish phosphorus levels with either powdered phosphorus or the pill form. There is no need for prophylactic phosphorus. Rather, the need is to assiduously monitor blood levels closely and replace phosphorus when low, while increasing calories.

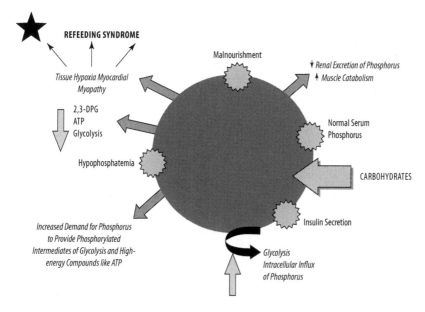

Figure 4.1. Refeeding hypophosphatemia.

Practical Tips for Refeeding

The medically worrisome refeeding syndrome is preventable (table 4.1). The older dictum on dietary calorie repletion to "start low, advance slow" has changed, with most studies supporting a more aggressive refeeding plan (Golden et al., 2013; Redgrave et al., 2015). But caution should still be exercised, especially for patients with severely low BMIs. The caloric requirements for the female patient with anorexia nervosa can be accurately calculated with the Harris-Benedict equation for basal energy expenditure (BEE):

$$BEE = 6.55 + (9.6 \times \text{body weight in kg}) + (1.8 \times \text{height in cm}) - (4.7 \times \text{age in years})$$

Dieticians are familiar with this calculation. Alternatively, BEE can be measured by indirect calorimetry, a relatively simple procedure involving a breathing test. It is available in many hospitals through the nutrition department. Calorimetry is based on measurement of carbon dioxide production and oxygen consumption. The BEE value basically reflects the energy used when the body is at rest; in clinical practice the terms BEE and REE

Table 4.1. Strategies to avoid refeeding syndrome

- Identify patients at risk (e.g., any patient who is chronically malnourished, is severely underweight, or has not eaten for 7–10 days).
- Measure serum electrolyte levels and correct abnormalities *before refeeding*.
- Obtain serum phosphorus and electrolyte values every day for the first 5–7 days, or until not falling, and thereafter at a reduced regular interval.
- Attempt to slowly increase daily caloric intake by 300–400 kcal every 3–4 days until the level of caloric intake is sufficient to produce adequate weight restoration.
- Clinically monitor the patient carefully for the development of complications.

are used interchangeably (Cuerda et al., 2007). The BEE must be multiplied by an activity factor (1.2–2.0) to determine total energy expenditure (TEE). In general, TEE exceeds BEE or REE by 10%–60%, depending on how active the patient is. The TEE should generally not be the starting point of caloric repletion. Rather, it is a target to achieve days to weeks after the initiation of refeeding. The REE measured by indirect calorimetry gives a slightly lower value for caloric needs than the values estimated by the Harris-Benedict formula. But, in reality, a beginning caloric intake of 1,400–1,800 kcal per day is a reasonable starting point and obviates the need for calorimetry or other calculations.

Although it is very important for patients to experience a significant degree of weight gain to maximize recovery, the optimal dietary intervention for effectuating this is unknown. There has been a distinct and surprising paucity of research on nutritional interventions in critical illness and in anorexia nervosa, and thus the rigorous evidence base is lacking (Haynos et al., 2016; Taylor, 2016). The usual goal is a weight gain of 3–4 pounds per week as an inpatient and 1–2 pounds for outpatients. Several approaches have been promoted (Mittnacht and Bulik, 2015). The main tenet is to check blood chemistry values frequently in the early stages of the refeeding process. Caloric levels usually begin at approximately 1,400–1,800 kcal per day and are increased by 300–400 kcal every 3–4 days. The treatment corollary of this is to individualize intake based on the achieved rate of weight gain. Augmenting the diet with a liquid supplement in the early stages of refeeding to achieve the prescribed daily calorie goal is an effective strategy for weight gain. Most patients require a caloric range that peaks at 3,000–3,600 kcal per day, but some may require upward of

4,000 kcal per day. It may be difficult to define precisely the factors that consistently correlate with the number of calories needed to gain one pound. In general, starved patients who have anorexia nervosa are metabolically inefficient and may require a little more than the expected 3,500 kcal, beyond the expected caloric needs to restore a pound of body weight.

Some simple general rules to follow (summarized in table 4.2) are:

1. Caloric intake should rarely exceed 70–80 kcal/kg of body weight.
2. For the patient who has more severe anorexia, begin a diet at 30–40 kcal/kg.
3. Protein intake should generally not exceed 2 g/kg of body weight, but at very low body weights this is often exceeded.
4. Meal planning should be individualized.
5. Macronutrient distribution should be approximately 50% carbohydrate and 25% protein and fat.
6. Weight gain should be in the range of 3–4 pounds per week for inpatient and residential patients.

Males generally peak at 4,000 kcal per day and females at 3,500 kcal per day. All approaches require vigilant clinical and laboratory monitoring and individualization of the dietary plan depending on the rate of weight gain and the laboratory and clinical course of the patient (table 4.3).

Currently, on most eating disorder units, caloric intake is being increased faster than in years past. These increases should always be guided by the patient's actual pattern of weight gain rather than the standard goal of 3–4 pounds per week. It is not uncommon, however, to see no weight gain or only 1–2 pounds of weight gain during the first weeks of nutritional repletion. Drastic increases in dietary calories should not be instituted in response to this. Rather, judicious consideration of covert purging behaviors

---

Table 4.2. Guidelines for refeeding patients with anorexia nervosa

- Nutritional rehabilitation should be individualized.
- Start refeeding at 30–45 kcal/kg/day.
- Intake should rarely exceed 70–80 kcal/kg/day.
- Limit protein intake when possible to less than 2.0 g/kg/day.
- Aim for 3–4 pounds/week of weight restoration for inpatients and 1–2 pounds/ week for outpatients.

Table 4.3. Practical guidelines for refeeding

- Start at 1,400–1,800 kcal/day.
- Advance by 300–400 kcal every 3–4 days.
- Maximum is usually around 3,500 kcal/day for females and 4,000 kcal/day for males.
- Monitor clinical examination and phosphorus/electrolyte levels closely.
- Begin with low-lactose, low-fiber diet.

or other complications should be undertaken. Similarly, caloric intake must be modified occasionally because of changes in REE during the course of refeeding, and such modifications will affect the rate of weight gain. Change in REE of the patient with anorexia nervosa seems to be a real phenomenon: REE is often lower in these patients early in the refeeding process than at later stages (Forman-Hoffman, Ruffin, and Schultz, 2006). This may be attributable to reversion to a euthyroid state from euthyroid sick syndrome. It is possible that these changes contribute to the difficulty of ongoing, sustained weight gain during the latter stages of refeeding (Salisbury et al., 1995). Caloric requirements for weight restoration are best determined by monitoring an individual's rate of weight gain. Given this dynamic process, caloric requirements may have to be recalculated if weight gain is not achieved as expected during the refeeding process, or consideration must be given to potential confounding sources of weight loss such as covert exercise or other modes of purging.

Potential Complications

From a clinical standpoint, rates of weight gain greater than 3–4 pounds per week are usually not nutritionally sound or sustainable and may represent edematous fluid retention or retained bowel contents due to constipation. Aside from the aforementioned numeric guide to weight gain, some clinical parameters should be closely followed. Specifically, vital signs contribute useful daily information. Individuals with anorexia nervosa generally have bradycardia ([[60 beats per minute). Although there are other potential reasons for tachycardia (]]100), the presence of an elevated supine heart rate, especially during the early stages of refeeding—even if just in the 80–90 range—can be a harbinger of the refeeding syndrome and cardiac compromise. Thus, even if patients technically do not have tachycardia, a sudden sustained increase in the pulse to greater than 80–90 deserves evaluation, given the typical baseline heart rates of 50–60 beats per minute in these patients. Daily monitoring of vital signs is clearly valuable during the first weeks of the refeeding process.

Checking for the presence of edema in the shin areas is another worthwhile practice during early refeeding; its presence can be an ominous sign. However, edema may also occur as a minor complication: during the early stages of refeeding, insulin secretion normally increases, which, in turn, induces sodium retention by increasing kidney tubular sodium reabsorption (Yucel et al., 2005). Low-sodium diets should not be used as part of the nutritional plan, however, as there is emerging evidence that this may have deleterious effects on levels of aldosterone secretion (Doukky et al., 2016). These clinical findings deserve a thorough medical evaluation, with consideration given to decreasing the rate of refeeding. In addition, because of the delayed stomach emptying and prolonged colonic transit time found in the severe stages of anorexia nervosa, these patients often complain of abdominal bloating and constipation (Trees et al., 2016). A bowel regimen, with a very minimal amount of fiber and adequate hydration, may help alleviate these symptoms during the early refeeding process (see chapter 6).

A multitude of potential fluid and electrolyte aberrations can occur during the refeeding process, especially early on and in cases of more severe anorexia nervosa. As the body shifts from a catabolic to an anabolic state, potassium, phosphorus, and magnesium are incorporated into the newly synthesized tissues and used for intermediary metabolism; this phenomenon can cause low serum levels of potassium, phosphorus, and magnesium. Phosphorus is the key electrolyte in the refeeding syndrome (O'Connor and Nicholls, 2013). Frequent initial monitoring of the patient's blood chemistry values can avert these problems. Early in the refeeding process, checking serum chemistry values every day or every other day is a reasonable plan. These checks can be reduced to weekly once the patient has consistently gained weight and has a relatively stable blood profile. Ultimately, with continued weight gain and stable laboratory results, monitoring can be even less frequent. However, the major emphasis should be on serum phosphorus levels because, again, refeeding hypophosphatemia is the main chemical cause of the refeeding syndrome.

Alternative Modes of Refeeding

Although progressive oral refeeding is the basic mode of refeeding for patients with anorexia nervosa, there are alternatives to this traditional mode. The oral refeeding plan, with a strict behavioral protocol, is nearly always the first choice because it provides a less invasive and more therapeutic method of treatment. The dietary goal must be to move from the reduced-calorie approach of anorexia nervosa to a truly balanced nutritional program with adequate calories to balance energy expenditures and the patient's developmental stage, while avoiding "underfeeding."

There are definite indications for enteral feedings and even parenteral feedings in anorexia nervosa (Mehler, 2008). These alternative modes of refeeding, however, are not a panacea for the treatment of this disorder, and they cannot be recommended as routine therapy for these patients. Some potential criteria for their use are (1) persistent failure to restore weight with other standard dietary therapies, (2) life-threatening weight loss, (3) worsening psychological state despite standard treatments, and (4) medical comorbidities. A patient's odds of recovery decline as the time spent continuously ill with anorexia nervosa lengthens, and thus, on rare occasions, these alternative modes of weight restoration might be reasonable.

Controlled studies of nutritional treatments for anorexia nervosa are essentially nonexistent. Enteral nasogastric (NG) feedings or percutaneous endoscopic gastrostomy-based (PEG) feeding have both been used for refractory cases of anorexia. Both of these enteral modes of nutritional delivery use liquid supplements that contain 1–1.5 kcal/mL. The only difference is whether the tube that delivers the enteral feed is inserted at the bedside through the nose and down the esophagus into the stomach or inserted surgically through the skin above the stomach and advanced into the stomach and secured. These two modes of enteral feeding can be used as a 24-hour continuous flow of supplement, or just nocturnally, or as a bolus feed, which takes only 5–10 minutes to push in, with the daily caloric amount divided into two or three rapid feeds. Dieticians are invaluable in calculating the rates and amounts of enteral feeds necessary to achieve weight gain. The advantage of bolus and nocturnal enteral feeds is that the patient is not tied to the pump all day long. The disadvantage is that the bolus mode may cause gastric discomfort and diarrhea and thus be less well tolerated. Anecdotally, although some physicians favor these modes of refeeding, patients often find them unpleasant, and some clinicians view them as psychologically harmful. Also, with enteral feeds, patients may complain of gastric fullness that diminishes appetite for foods. These problems are less associated with parenteral nutrition, which is nutritionally comparable. However, parenteral nutrition is more expensive and is also fraught with catheter-related complications. There are no randomized trials to guide the use of parenteral versus enteral nutrition in anorexia nervosa. These different modes of nutritional support have been compared in other medical patients. Recent evidence indicates that the parenteral route may not be more dangerous than the enteral route (Harvey et al., 2014).

Although standard protocols exist, parenteral nutrition must be viewed as a treatment modality prescribed only for severe and refractory cases, with utmost discretion and on an individual basis. It is beyond the scope of this chapter to discuss all of its specifics. Although TPN is a powerful tool and has been used successfully for patients with anorexia nervosa who have comorbid gastrointestinal issues that preclude oral caloric intake (Mehler and Weiner, 2007), its administration may be associated with mechanical, infectious, and metabolic difficulties. It is therefore best reserved for use in medical centers with expertise in dealing with such potential difficulties and for patients whose condition is truly refractory to more traditional refeeding programs. Also, either enteral or parenteral nutrition should rarely supplant the expectation that the patient will resume normal and adequate oral eating.

Summary

Although nutritional support of the malnourished patient is a most important component of the care plan for individuals with anorexia nervosa, nutrition regimens can cause adverse effects if used injudiciously. Because rapid refeeding can result in a catastrophic sequence of events, caution and restraint must be used when initiating therapy, together with careful monitoring of blood chemistry values and the patient's pattern and rate of weight gain. A well-balanced, nutritional, oral diet plan is generally the optimal approach for refeeding malnourished patients with anorexia nervosa. Clearly, the approach to refeeding has become more aggressive. This is mostly appropriate if tempered with assiduous monitoring and clinical evaluations, especially early in the refeeding program. Yet, many unresolved questions remain about this critical treatment paradigm for patients with anorexia nervosa. At this time we must be ever vigilant and circumspect as the tapestry of evidence is woven in this critically important field.

REFERENCES

American Psychiatric Association. 2006. Practice guideline for the treatment of patients with eating disorders, third edition. *American Journal of Psychiatry* 163:4–54.

Bermudez O and Beightol S. 2004. What is refeeding syndrome? *Eating Disorders* 12:251–56.

Brown C, Sabel A, and Mehler PS. 2015. Predictors of refeeding hypophosphatemia. *International Journal of Eating Disorders* 48:898–904.

Castro J, Gila A, Puig J, Rodriguez S, and Toro J. 2004. Predictors of rehospitalization after total weight recovery in adolescents with anorexia nervosa. *International Journal of Eating Disorders* 36:22–30.

Cuerda C, Ruiz A, Velasco C, Breton I, Camblor M, and Garcia-Peris P. 2007. How accurate are predictive formulas calculating energy expenditure in adolescent patients with anorexia nervosa? *Clinical Nutrition* 26:100–106.

Doukky R, Avery E, Mangla A, et al. 2016. Impact of dietary sodium restriction on heart failure outcomes. *Journal of the American College of Cardiology* 4:24–35.

Dumas A. 1844 (1996). *Count of Monte Cristo*. New York, NY: Modern Library.

Forman-Hoffman VL, Ruffin T, and Schultz SK. 2006. Basal metabolic rate in anorexia nervosa patients: Using appropriate predictive equations during the refeeding process. *Annals of Clinical Psychiatry* 18:123–27.

Gaudiani J, Sabel A, Mehler PS, and Mascolo M. 2012. Severe anorexia nervosa outcomes from a medical stabilization unit. *International Journal of Eating Disorders* 45:85–92.

Goldberg SJ, Comerci GD, and Feldman L. 1988. Cardiac output and regional myocardial contraction in anorexia nervosa. *Journal of Adolescent Health Care* 9:15–21.

Golden NH, Keane-Miller C, Sainani KL, et al. 2013. Higher calories in hospitalized adolescents with anorexia nervosa is associated with reduced length of stay and no increased rate of refeeding syndrome. *Journal of Nutritional Health* 53:573–75.

Harvey SE, Parrott F, Harrison DA, et al. 2014. Trial of the route of early nutritional support in critically ill adults. *New England Journal of Medicine* 371:1673–84.

Haynos AF, Snipes C, Guarda A, et al. 2016. Comparison of standardized versus individualized caloric prescriptions in the nutritional rehabilitation of inpatients with anorexia nervosa. *International Journal of Eating Disorders* 49:50–58.

Lamzabi I, Syed S, Reddy VB, et al. 2015. Myocardial changes in a patient with anorexia nervosa: A case report and review of literature. *American Journal of Clinical Pathology* 143:734–37.

Mehler PS. 2008. Use of total parenteral nutrition in severe anorexia nervosa complicated by gastrointestinal illness. *Current Nutrition and Food Science* 4:41–43.

Mehler PS and Weiner KL. 2007. Use of total parenteral nutrition in the refeeding of selected patients with severe anorexia nervosa. *International Journal of Eating Disorders* 40:285–87.

Mittnacht AM and Bulik CM. 2015. Best nutrition counseling practices for the treatment of anorexia nervosa: A Delphi study. *International Journal of Eating Disorders* 48:111–22.

O'Connor G and Nicholls D. 2013. Refeeding hypophosphatemia in adolescents with anorexia nervosa: A systematic review. *Nutrition Clinical Practice* 28:358–64.

Redgrave GW, Coughlin JW, Schreyer CC, et al. 2015. Refeeding and weight restoration outcomes in anorexia nervosa: Challenging current guidelines. *International Journal of Eating Disorders* 48:866–73.

Salisbury JJ, Levine AS, Crow SJ, et al. 1995. Refeeding, metabolic rate, and weight gain in anorexia nervosa: A review. *International Journal of Eating Disorders* 17:337–45.

Solomon SM and Kirby DF. 1990. The refeeding syndrome: A review. *Journal of Parenteral and Enteral Nutrition* 14:90–97.

Taylor BE. 2016. Guidelines for the provision of nutrition support in critically ill patients. *Critical Care Medicine* 44:390–98,

Trees N, Beaty L, Gusimano C, et al. 2016. Gastrointestinal complications of refeeding in anorexia nervosa. *Journal of Nutritional Biology* 1:49–60.

Yates A, Edman J, and Aruguete M. 2004. Ethnic differences in BMI and body/self-dissatisfaction among whites, Asian subgroups, Pacific Islanders and African-Americans. *Journal of Adolescent Health* 34:300–307.

Yucel B, Ozbey N, Polat A, and Yager J. 2005. Weight fluctuations during early refeeding period in anorexia nervosa: Case reports. *International Journal of Eating Disorders* 37:175–77.

5

Evaluation and Treatment
of Electrolyte Abnormalities

Margherita Mascolo, MD, and Philip S. Mehler, MD

Common Questions

Which patients with eating disorders develop electrolyte abnormalities? How common are these abnormalities?

Who is at risk of developing electrolyte abnormalities?

Which electrolyte abnormalities are most common in patients with eating disorders?

Is a particular pattern of electrolyte abnormalities associated with a specific mode of purging behavior?

What are the available classes of abused diuretics? How do they differ?

What is pseudo-Bartter's syndrome? How is this condition managed?

How is edema avoided and/or treated during the correction of electrolyte abnormalities in patients with bulimia nervosa?

How should the clinician treat the fluid and electrolyte abnormalities encountered in these patients?

What is the optimal treatment for severe hypokalemia?

What are the critical levels of potassium, sodium, and bicarbonate that necessitate a patient's emergency hospitalization?

Case

L.V., a 29-year-old female with a long history of AN-BP (anorexia nervosa, binge and/or purge subtype), presented to an inpatient eating disorder unit for medical stabilization and the beginning of weight restoration. She had a long history of anorexia nervosa that began when she was in high school, at the age of 14. She was on the cross country team in high school, and in an effort to train more aggressively and build her endurance, she began a strict exercise regimen. She concomitantly and gradually restricted her caloric intake to the point of consuming only about 800 kcal per day. Following a traumatic event, her disordered eating behaviors changed and she began to binge and subsequently purge through self-induced vomiting of all ingested calories. She had been to multiple eating disorder treatment facilities but had relapsed following each treatment course.

L.V.'s illness was further complicated by frequent visits to the emergency department, when not in treatment, because of weakness, dizziness, near syncope, and palpitations. Her work-up consistently revealed hypokalemia, metabolic alkalosis, and hypochloremia. Treatments in emergency departments consisted of aggressive resuscitation with intravenous fluids, electrolyte replacement, and discharge to home. Her outcome after emergency room visits was always the same: she gained 10–20 pounds of edema weight within a few days. This aggravated her body dysmorphia, further traumatized her, and made her very resistant to entering any kind of treatment facility for fear of edema formation and rapid weight gain.

At the time of admission to the inpatient unit, L.V. had been purging 10–15 times daily and had been treated in the emergency department 2 days prior, for palpitations and dizziness. On the day of admission she was found to be tachycardic to 115 beats per minute and hypotensive to 85/50 mm Hg. She was 5 feet 5 inches tall and weighed 93 pounds. Examination revealed an emaciated woman with enlarged parotids and dry mucous membranes. Results from her cardiac, pulmonary, and abdominal examination were normal, but she had striking lower extremity edema up to the mid-thighs bilaterally.

Laboratory tests revealed a normal complete blood count and normal liver function. However, her potassium level was low, at 2.6 mmol/L (normal 3.5–5.0); her bicarbonate level was high, at 38 mmol/L (normal 22–28); and her chloride was low, at 94 mmol/L (normal 101–112). She was given gentle intravenous hydration with normal saline at a rate of 50 mL per hour, potassium repletion, and spironolactone 50 mg per day, and began a progressive oral nutrition plan of 1,400 kcal.

Within one day of hospitalization, L.V.'s vital signs improved, her electrolytes had normalized, and her IV fluids were stopped. Over the next 2

weeks, she was compliant with treatment and her kilocalories were gradually increased up to 2,600 daily. The edema almost completely resolved and
the spironolactone was discontinued. This was the first time in her life
that she had entered treatment and had experienced gradual resolution of
her edema instead of its worsening.

Frequency

Patients with anorexia nervosa of the restricting subtype (AN-R)
may have abnormalities in their liver transaminase levels (aspartate aminotransferase, AST; alanine aminotransferase, ALT) and bone marrow
dysfunction evident from their blood counts. However, laboratory analysis should show normal electrolytes, even for patients with extremely low
body weight (Mehler, 2001). Conversely, patients who engage in purging
behaviors as part of their eating disorder, whether in the form of vomiting, diuretic misuse, or laxative abuse, commonly have electrolyte abnormalities. This is true for patients with the binge and/or purge subtype of
anorexia nervosa and for those with bulimia nervosa. A study by Crow
and others (1997) documented the frequency of fluid, electrolyte, and acid-
base disturbances encountered in patients with bulimia. Almost 50% had
electrolyte abnormalities. The most common abnormality was an elevated serum bicarbonate (metabolic alkalosis), present in 27.4% of the
patients. Other abnormalities observed were hypochloremia (low chloride;
23.8%), hypokalemia (low potassium; 13.7%), decreased serum bicarbonate
(8.3%), and hyponatremia (decreased sodium; 5.4%). There are complex
interrelationships among electrolytes, and an abnormality in one should
prompt further investigation and measurement of other electrolytes (Connan, Lightman, and Treasure, 2000). In Miller et al.'s study (2005) of the
prevalence of common medical findings in an outpatient eating disorders
population, 24% of the cohort exhibited purging behaviors; overall, the
most common electrolyte abnormalities were hypokalemia and hyponatremia. Hypokalemia was present in 20% of the study participants, and
48% of them reported a history of regular purging; hyponatremia was
present in 7% of the participants. Thus, despite discordant data on the
most frequent metabolic abnormality seen in eating disorders of the purging variety, the top three most common disturbances remain hypokalemia, metabolic alkalosis, and hyponatremia. Table 5.1 shows the normal
laboratory ranges for the electrolytes that are most frequently altered by

Table 5.1. Normal serum electrolyte ranges in laboratory tests

Electrolyte	Concentration range (mmol/L)
Bicarbonate (HCO_3^-)	22–28
Chloride (Cl^-)	101–112
Potassium (K^+)	3.6–5.2
Sodium (Na^+)	138–147

purging behaviors. Another observed abnormality is hypomagnesemia (low magnesium), which is most commonly seen in individuals who have bulimia and abuse diuretics. It is generally accompanied by hypokalemia because the two cations are handled in a similar fashion by the kidney.

Electrolyte abnormalities are very infrequent in patients who have anorexia nervosa without associated purging behavior. Gentile et al. (2011) evaluated 38 common laboratory tests for patients with anorexia nervosa, all of whom had a BMI below 17.5. The study found that 60% of the patients indeed had no abnormalities on laboratory chemistry evaluation of their blood. Unlike patients with bulimia, patients with restricting anorexia nervosa do not have a metabolic alkalosis along with the elevated BUN levels. In fact, if hypokalemia, hypochloremia, or a metabolic alkalosis is present in a patient who supposedly has anorexia nervosa, it is most likely due to a coexistent covert purging behavior disorder that the patient is attempting to conceal (Wolfe et al., 2001). This is an important clinical fact. The presence of a low albumin level in a patient thought to have pure anorexia nervosa, or the finding of electrolyte abnormalities, should prompt a thorough search for additional causes aside from the diagnosis of anorexia nervosa (Krantz et al., 2005).

Clinical Manifestations

The most common electrolyte abnormalities encountered in patients with purging behaviors are, as noted above, hypokalemia, hyponatremia, metabolic alkalosis, and hypochloremia; rarely, patients may present with hypomagnesemia and hypocalcemia (low calcium) (Stheneur, Bergeron, and Lapeyraque, 2014). There is no specific constellation of presenting symptoms that allows the clinician to diagnose such abnormalities based on history and physical examinations alone, given that the clinical manifestations of electrolyte abnormalities are nonspecific and vague. The most common patient complaints accompanying marked aberrations in electrolytes include weakness, fatigue, dizziness, constipation, myalgias, paresthesias, and depression.

Hypokalemia (<3.6 mmol/L) causes generalized muscle weakness, cramping, paresthesias, and fatigue, as well as constipation and, occasionally, heart palpitations. If severe (<2.5 mmol/L), it can also cause rhabdomyolysis (muscle breakdown), significant cardiac arrhythmias, and sudden death. Indeed, hypokalemia is extremely dangerous, especially when potassium is very low, and in females is associated with an elevated risk of death (Janson et al., 2015). In a study of patients who presented to an emergency department and were diagnosed with hypokalemia, only 49% of those with severe hypokalemia were symptomatic; their most common symptoms were weakness and muscle pain. Typical electrocardiographic (EKG) changes resulting from hypokalemia may include flat or inverted T waves, ST-segment depression, and prominent U waves, which can exceed the amplitude of the T waves. Cardiac complications and EKG abnormalities due to hypokalemia are rare if the potassium level exceeds 3 mmol/L and the decrease has occurred slowly—unless there is concomitant heart disease, in which case complications increase when serum potassium is less than 3.9 mmol/L. The finding of hypokalemia in an otherwise healthy young female is highly specific for the presence of a covert eating disorder. Thus, besides replenishing potassium, there should be inquiry about the potential cause of the hypokalemia.

Hyponatremia in the eating disorders population can be a consequence of dehydration, such as in purging disorders (due to fluid loss in emesis, stool, and diuretic effect), as well as a result of water loading or excessive water intake (free water intake exceeding water excretions). Dehydration is most common, seen with purging behaviors; water loading is mostly found in cases of restricting anorexia nervosa, as a result of low solute load in the kidney and an inability to clear free water. Symptoms in mild to moderate hyponatremia (120–135 mmol/L) can be vague, such as nausea, vomiting, headache, and confusion. In severe hyponatremia, when the sodium level is below 120 mmol/L, the symptoms can range from delirium to impaired consciousness, seizures, and cardiopulmonary collapse (Henry, 2015).

Metabolic alkalosis is generally asymptomatic; however, when moderate to severe (serum bicarbonate >35 mmol/L) it may cause compensatory respiratory adaptations in which patients take fewer and shallower breaths

(Feldman et al., 2012). This leads to symptoms of tachypnea and, when prolonged, respiratory insufficiency.

Hypomagnesemia may also complicate these symptoms and contribute to arrhythmias and sudden death. Although hypomagnesemia and hypocalcemia are less common in bulimia, they can, when severe, also result in tetany.

Pathophysiology

Metabolic alkalosis is one of the most common metabolic abnormalities in patients with bulimia nervosa. In those who have a metabolic alkalosis due to active purging through diuretic abuse or self-induced vomiting, the serum bicarbonate level, which is normally 22–28 mmol/L, ranges between 30 and 40 mmol/L. The more severe the metabolic alkalosis, the more likely it is that the purging behavior is self-induced vomiting.

The pathogenesis of this metabolic alkalosis varies according to the particular mode of purging behavior. With self-induced vomiting, the metabolic alkalosis develops in part because of the acid lost directly in the vomitus. More importantly, however, vomiting also leads to loss of sodium chloride (NaCl) and water. This results in a state of decreased intravascular volume (hypovolemia) resulting from dehydration. The body's adaptive response to a state of dehydration (to prevent fainting) is to stimulate the kidney's renin-angiotensin-aldosterone axis. This aids in sodium and water retention through the function of aldosterone, in an effort to prevent hypotension and syncope. Aldosterone, a hormone produced in the adrenal glands, acts on the kidneys to increase salt absorption and bicarbonate reabsorption at the expense of potassium and hydrogen. It thus leads to worsening metabolic alkalosis and hypokalemia as the body preferentially reabsorbs salt and water and, in exchange, wastes potassium and acid in the urine. This type of metabolic alkalosis is occasionally referred to as a "contraction alkalosis," or a sodium chloride–responsive metabolic alkalosis, as it is primarily due to a state of dehydration or volume "contraction" and is corrected with an infusion of saline. This entire cascade is the body's normal protective response to prevent dehydration and its symptoms, such as hypotension, dizziness, and syncope, in the presence of ongoing and frequent purging.

The metabolic alkalosis seen with surreptitious use of diuretics is also the result of intravascular volume depletion. Three main classes of diuretics are available on the market: thiazides, loop, and potassium-sparing diuretics. Thiazide diuretics (such as hydrochlorothiazide and metolazone) inhibit sodium and chloride reabsorption in the distal renal tubule, resulting in natriuresis and kaliuresis (sodium loss and potassium loss in the urine) and thus hypovolemia. Therefore, the typical electrolyte abnormalities are hyponatremia, hypokalemia, and the metabolic alkalosis. Loop diuretics (such as furosemide) act in the kidney's loop of Henle to block sodium reabsorption, which also leads to natriuresis, kaliuresis, and hypovolemia Lastly, potassium-sparing diuretics (such as spironolactone) act on sodium channels in the kidney. Thus, although natriuresis and a decrease in vascular volume are achieved, there is no potassium loss in the urine (Mascolo, Chu, and Mehler, 2011). These are all prescription diuretics and most often are abused by health professionals who have access to such medications. Over-the-counter (OTC) diuretics are much less potent and less likely to cause major electrolyte aberration. The active ingredients in OTC diuretics are caffeine, ammonium chloride, and/or pamabrom. The side effect common to all classes of diuretics abused by patients with eating disorders is hypovolemia. In general, the metabolic alkalosis seen with diuretics is milder than that resulting from vomiting, which, again, is associated with the most severe cases of metabolic alkalosis. A good rule to remember is that serum bicarbonate concentrations greater than 38 mmol/L are almost always due to self-induced vomiting. Elevated serum bicarbonate levels can also be a useful covert laboratory finding when a patient is denying purging behaviors, and this finding is almost always indicative of excessive vomiting or abuse of diuretics.

The constellation of laboratory abnormalities found in patients who purge by self-induced vomiting or diuretic abuse—namely, metabolic alkalosis, hypokalemia, and hypochloremia resulting from a state of dehydration—is known as pseudo-Bartter's syndrome (Bahia et al., 2012). In 1962, Frederic Bartter and colleagues described a syndrome of hypokalemia, hyponatremia, hypochloremia, and metabolic alkalosis with an associated hyperaldosterone state in two adolescents. This syndrome was later discovered to be due to defects in electrolyte transporters that lead to hypovolemia and thus upregulation of the renin-angiotensin-aldosterone axis. Although the biochemical changes that result from purging are the same as those described by Bartter, the electrolyte transporter in patients with eating disorders is intact—thus the name pseudo-Bartter's syndrome.

Although laxatives are an ineffective means of weight control, their abuse is fairly common, with studies reporting a prevalence of 10%–40% in people with eating disorders (Roerig et al., 2010). Self-induced vomiting and abuse of stimulant laxatives probably account for upward of 80% of all purging behaviors. Whereas purging by means of vomiting or diuretic abuse always leads to metabolic alkalosis, laxative abuse can give the initial picture of either a metabolic alkalosis or a mild metabolic acidosis. Significant acute diarrhea typically causes a hyperchloremic metabolic acidosis (also called a nongap acidosis) as a result of the large amount of bicarbonate lost in the stool. However, the acid-base abnormality seen with chronic laxative abuse is more commonly a metabolic alkalosis, with low serum chloride and potassium levels; this is consistent with pseudo-Bartter's syndrome resulting from volume depletion and dehydration due to loss of diarrheal fluids. The alkalosis tends to be mild, with bicarbonate levels in the range of 30–34 mmol/L, whereas the hypokalemia is usually more marked. The primary reason for hypokalemia is the loss of potassium in the diarrheal stools.

The typical serum and urinary electrolyte findings in the three types of purging behaviors discussed above are summarized in tables 5.2 and 5.3. Engaging in purging once or twice a week may not cause any significant electrolyte disorder, and thus the finding of normal electrolytes does not completely rule out the presence of symptoms of bulimia. The corollary of this is that the finding of an abnormally low potassium level or an elevated bicarbonate level is not consistent with a patient's report that he or she rarely purges or that the purging behaviors have receded (Mehler, 2001). Therefore, appropriate medical assessment of a patient with bulimia should always include obtaining a serum electrolyte panel.

Table 5.2. Serum electrolyte levels in purging disorders

| Purge type | Serum level | | | | |
	Sodium	Potassium	Chloride	Bicarbonate	pH
Vomiting	High, low, or normal	Low	Low	High	High
Laxatives	High, low, or normal	Low	High or low	High or low	Low or high
Diuretics	Low or normal	Low	Low	High	High

Table 5.3. Urinary electrolyte levels in purging disorders

	Urine level		
Purge type	Sodium	Potassium	Chloride
Vomiting	Low	High or low	Low
Laxatives	Low	Low	Normal or low
Diuretics	High	High	High

Fortunately, the diagnosis of electrolyte abnormalities is usually straightforward. A set of electrolytes with serum magnesium and amylase can be tested in blood drawn as part of the clinical evaluation, and this analysis is readily available in all laboratories. It is always wise to conduct an EKG to look for changes secondary to significant hypokalemia, hypomagnesemia, and hypocalcemia. As mentioned above, the common EKG changes seen with a decreased serum potassium are T-wave flattening, U waves, and ST-segment depression. Hypomagnesemia, hypokalemia, and hypocalcemia can cause a prolonged QT interval and nonspecific T-wave changes. The prolonged QT interval can precipitate serious ventricular arrhythmias, especially as the QTc increases above 480 milliseconds. If there is a need to differentiate between the several types of purging behaviors, measurement of serum and urine electrolytes can be helpful. In general, once again, metabolic alkalosis (elevated bicarbonate level) indicates vomiting or diuretic abuse, and a metabolic acidosis (low bicarbonate level) indicates laxative abuse, although chronic laxative abuse leads to metabolic alkalosis. It may be necessary in some cases, when there is a suspicion of laxative abuse despite the patient's denial, to check the feces or urine for phenolphthalein, an ingredient in some laxatives. Similarly, when there is suspicion of diuretic abuse, a laboratory can test the urine for the presence of common diuretics.

Treatment

Treatment of the metabolic abnormalities observed in eating disorders requires an understanding of the pathophysiology of these problems, as outlined above. There are two important concepts to keep in mind. First, because potassium is primarily an intracellular cation, the serum measurement can be misleading in estimating the true degree of *total* body potassium depletion. As a general rule, for each drop in serum potassium

Table 5.4. Total body potassium deficits

Serum potassium concentration (mmol/L)	Potassium deficit (mmol/L)
3–3.5	100–150
2–3	200–300
<1.5	400–600

of 0.3 mmol/L, there is a deficit in total body stores of more than 100 mEq (Asmar, Mohandas, and Wingo, 2012). Rough estimates of total body potassium deficits are shown in table 5.4. A common mistake is to underestimate the amount of potassium necessary to correct hypokalemia, and thus replacement is prolonged and delayed.

The main treatment to correct hypokalemia is replacement of potassium in either of two ways: the intravenous (IV) route or the oral route. There are no clearly defined potassium levels for which IV replacement is indicated, but if the patient is hemodynamically unstable due to hypokalemia or if the serum level is below 2.5 mmol/L, it is generally recommended to replace potassium intravenously. Intravenous replacement requires cardiac monitoring, and the infusion should run no faster than 20 mmol per hour. Cardiac monitoring is required because IV potassium may lead to overcorrection of the deficit and deadly arrhythmias, and it thus warrants hospital-level care. The most common side effects of IV replacement are overcorrection of hypokalemia and burning at the site of infusion. When potassium is replaced intravenously, repeat serum potassium level checks should follow each 30 mEq infusion.

Three salts are available for oral repletion of potassium: potassium chloride, potassium phosphate, and potassium bicarbonate. Potassium phosphate has minimal amounts of potassium and is mainly used to replenish low phosphorus levels. Potassium bicarbonate is very rarely used and usually only in settings of concomitant hypokalemia and metabolic acidosis. Of the three salts, potassium chloride is the most common formulation used to treat hypokalemia; it is available as a tablet and a liquid. The liquid form is less expensive but has an unpleasant taste and may lead to further nausea and emesis. Two slow-release tablets are available of which one has a wax matrix and the other is a microencapsulated tablet. Each is fairly well tolerated, although the risk of ulceration and bleeding of the gastrointestinal tract is slightly higher with the wax matrix formulation

Table 5.5. Oral potassium preparations

Preparation	mEq per tablet (or other preparation)
K-Dur (KCl)	10 or 20
K-Tab (KCl)	10
Micro-K Extencaps (KCl)	8 or 10
Slow-K (KCl)	8
K-Lor Powder Packets (KCl)	20
Polycitra-K Oral Solution (K citrate)	10/tsp (5 mL)
Rum-K syrup (KCl)	20/2 tsp (10 mL)

(Gennari, 1998). In general, the rule of thumb is that for each 10 mEq of oral potassium replacement, the serum potassium level should increase by 0.1 mmol/L. Note that the total body store deficit mentioned above (for each drop in serum potassium of 0.3 mmol/L the deficit in total body store is >100 mEq) should not be used as a guide by which to replace potassium. It does not take account of the complicated intracellular shifts of potassium and would lead to overcorrection of this delicate electrolyte. Rather, replacement should be based on the actual serum level, with the understanding that 10 mEq of any formulation will raise the serum potassium level by about 0.1 mmol/L. Table 5.5 lists common oral potassium formulations.

The second concept to keep in mind when treating hypokalemia due to purging behaviors is that efforts to replenish potassium are less effective if the coexisting metabolic alkalosis induced by dehydration is not also addressed and treated. This is because dehydration resulting from any purging behavior stimulates aldosterone production, which not only causes a metabolic alkalosis but also leads to ongoing renal potassium excretion. Cessation of purging behavior is the first step in treatment, followed by rehydration with IV or oral sodium-containing solutions in an effort to reduce aldosterone secretion and aid potassium repletion. The metabolic alkalosis in patients who abuse diuretics or engage in self-induced vomiting, with resultant volume contraction and elevated bicarbonate levels, is thus termed *chloride-responsive*. This means that normal saline, which contains water and sodium chloride, is the appropriate corrective treatment. Intravenous infusions of sodium chloride restore intravascular volume and lead to a reduction in excessive aldosterone secretion. The efficacy of potassium repletion will be abrogated if the dehydration state is not also corrected. Treatment of severe metabolic alkalosis (>33–35 mmol/L) with sodium-containing fluids usually needs to be done intravenously at a *slow* rate of 50–75 mL per hour for 1–2 L of fluid. Milder cases can be successfully treated with aggressive oral hydration using fluids other than plain water, such as bouillon.

A word of caution here: Excessive amounts of IV saline (>2 L per day), given at a rapid rate of infusion, can lead to marked edema formation and volume overload. It takes about 1–2 weeks following cessation of purging behaviors and restoration of normal plasma volume for the body to naturally downregulate the excessive secretion of aldosterone (the hormone driving the reabsorption of sodium and loss of potassium) (Schrier, Masoumi, and Elhassan, 2010). Therefore, with high ambient serum aldosterone levels, the IV saline is avidly reabsorbed by the kidney, a process that can also contribute to the body's rapid retention of salt and water with resultant edema. In fact, the edema can be severe during the early period after purging behaviors are discontinued, even without the use of IV fluids, because of persistently increased serum aldosterone levels. As mentioned above, this constellation of symptoms is termed pseudo-Bartter's syndrome. Table 5.6 highlights key points and treatment.

Some individuals with purging disorders who need to frequent emergency rooms for electrolyte replacement therapy may be reticent to seek additional help if their previous visits were punctuated by development of significant edema due to rapid infusions of IV saline. The formation of edema is very distressing, especially for a population of patients that suffer from body dysmorphia. Emergency department staff, who are used to rapid infusion of IV saline to treat adults with other states of dehydration such as gastroenteritis, must be warned about the dangers of this practice when applied to patients with purging behaviors (Trent et al., 2013). In fact, these misguided treatments often prevent patients with purging disorders from seeking timely treatment despite feeling ill from their

Table 5.6. Pseudo-Bartter's syndrome

- Syndrome is characterized by hypokalemia and metabolic alkalosis.
- Volume depletion plays a central role.
- Efficacy of potassium repletion is abrogated unless volume is restored.
- Restore volume with IV normal saline slowly (50–70 mL/hour).
- Edema may be alarming to the patient.
- Risk dissipates by 2–3 weeks after cessation of purging.

dehydration and electrolyte derangements. This delay may contribute to the increased standardized mortality rate for bulimia nervosa—nearly twice that of age-matched controls (Smink, Van Hoeken, and Hoek, 2012). Generally, the edema can be minimized, if not prevented, during this period with leg elevation for 10–15 minutes a few times a day and, when IV fluids are necessary, a slowed infusion of saline; a detailed explanation to the patient of the distressful but transient nature of the resultant edema is helpful (Mehler and Linas, 2002). To reiterate, given the sodium-avid state that results from purging behaviors, when IV fluids are necessary the rate should not exceed 50–75 mL per hour until the serum bicarbonate level is less than 30 mmol/L, at which point the IV infusion can be discontinued.

In addition to cessation of purging behaviors, restoration of volume status, and correction of electrolytes, there is one more important treatment modality that can minimize or prevent the formation of edema in this patient population. Paradoxically, it is through the use of a diuretic, a potassium-sparing one: spironolactone. Spironolactone is an aldosterone antagonist that competitively inhibits the action of aldosterone at the receptor level. It thus can block the action of aldosterone in the initial phases of treatment while the body naturally ceases its overproduction (Lainscak et al., 2015). The action of spironolactone is threefold: it not only blocks the action of aldosterone, as just noted, but also is potassium-sparing, thus aiding in treatment of hypokalemia, and is a mild diuretic, thus aiding with edema formation and treatment (Mascolo, McBride, and Mehler, 2015). A starting dose of 25 mg daily, for 1–2 weeks, can be initiated at the onset of cessation of purging behaviors. This can be increased as needed up to 200 mg as a single daily dose if edema worsens or there is rapid weight gain. Note that patients who have any degree of renal compromise should have their electrolytes closely monitored if spironolactone is used, given its potassium-sparing effect and potential for development of hyperkalemia.

A further word of caution when replenishing a dehydrated patient: If the patient also has significant hyponatremia (serum sodium <120 mmol/L), the saline infusion should be slow so that during the initial 24 hours, the serum sodium is corrected to only approximately 125–130 mmol/L. More aggressive correction of the serum sodium level may result in a devastating neurologic complication termed *central pontine myelinolysis*. A targeted rate of correction that does not exceed 4–6 mmol/L in 24 hours is recommended (Sterns, 2015). In addition, although a healthy person with normal kidney function would need to drink a large amount of plain water (25–30 L) to adversely dilute serum sodium and experience marked, symptomatic hyponatremia as a result, patients with anorexia nervosa are different. Their ability to tolerate water is severely limited by their extremely limited solute intake, as seen in older men and women who live on tea and toast and are thus unable to excrete a diluted urine. For patients with anorexia nervosa, amounts as little as 5–7 L per day can cause hyponatremia (Caregaro et al., 2005).

In addition to the central role of volume depletion in the treatment of hypokalemia associated with severe self-induced vomiting and diuretic abuse, undetected magnesium deficiency can also cause refractory potassium repletion. Magnesium deficiency should especially be considered in those individuals whose primary means of purging is the use of potent diuretics such as the loop, thiazide, and potassium-sparing diuretics mentioned above. The majority of diuretics cause some loss of magnesium in the urine (Tamargo, Segura, and Ruilope, 2014). Since magnesium and potassium hold the same charge, they, in effect, competitively inhibit each other for absorption. Thus, ongoing magnesium deficiency, if not treated, can impair efforts at potassium repletion. The most effective way to replenish magnesium is with magnesium sulfate through the IV route. Oral magnesium oxide is not well absorbed and can lead to diarrhea. which perpetuates the dehydrated state.

Summary

Metabolic abnormalities are common in patients with eating disorders, especially those who engage in purging behaviors, including self-induced vomiting, diuretic abuse, and laxative abuse. Metabolic alkalosis and hypokalemia are the most common abnormalities encountered clinically. The treatment of these metabolic derangements requires cessation of purging behaviors, repletion of electrolytes, and treatment of the volume contraction that causes hyperaldosteronism. A clinician who has the correct skills and a familiarity with treating these potentially dangerous electrolyte disorders in this patient population is essential for all but the mildest abnormalities.

REFERENCES

Asmar A, Mohandas R, and Wingo CS. 2012. A physiologic approach to the treatment of a patient with hypokalemia. *American Journal of Kidney Disease* 60:492–97.

Bahia A, Mascolo M, Gaudiani JL, and Mehler PS. 2012. PseudoBartter syndrome in eating disorders. *International Journal of Eating Disorders* 45:150–53.

Bartter FC, Pronove P, Gill R, and MacCardle RC. 1962. Hyperplasia of the juxtaglomerular complex with hyperaldosteronism and hypokalemic alkalosis: A new syndrome. *American Journal of Medicine* 33:811–28.

Caregaro L, Di Pascoli L, Favaro A, Nardi M, and Santonastaso P. 2005. Sodium depletion and hemoconcentration: Overlooked complications in patients with anorexia nervosa. *Nutrition* 21:438–45.

Connan F, Lightman S, and Treasure J. 2000. Biochemical and endocrine complications. *European Eating Disorders Review* 8:144–57.

Crow SJ, Salisbury JJ, Crosby RD, and Mitchell JE. 1997. Serum electrolytes as markers of vomiting in bulimia nervosa. *International Journal of Eating Disorders* 21:95–98.

Feldman M, Alvarez NM, Trevino M, and Weinstein GL. 2012. Respiratory compensation to a primary metabolic alkalosis in humans. *Clinical Nephrology* 78:365–69.

Gennari JF. 1998. Hypokalemia. *New England Journal of Medicine* 339:451–58.

Gentile MG, Manna GM, Pastorelli P, and Oltolini A. 2011. Laboratory evaluation in patients with anorexia nervosa: Usefulness and limits. *La Clinica Terapeutica* 162:401–7.

Henry DA. 2015. In the clinic: Hyponatremia. *Annals of Internal Medicine* 163(3):ITC 1–19.

Jansen HK, Brabrand M, Vinholt PJ, Hallas J, and Lassen AT. 2015. Hypokalemia in acute medical patients: Risk factors and prognosis. *American Journal of Medicine* 128:60–67.

Krantz MJ, Lee D, Donahoo WT, and Mehler PS. 2005. The paradox of normal serum albumin in anorexia nervosa: A case report. *International Journal of Eating Disorders* 37:278–80.

Lainscak M, Pelliccia F, Rosano G, et al. 2015. Safety profile of mineralocorticoid receptor antagonists: Spironolactone and eplerenone. *International Journal of Cardiology* 200:25–29.

Mascolo M, Chu ES, and Mehler PS. 2011. Abuse and clinical value of diuretics in eating disorders: Therapeutic applications. *International Journal of Eating Disorders* 44:200–202.

Mascolo M, McBride J, and Mehler PS. 2015. Effective medical treatment strategies to help cessation of purging behaviors. *International Journal of Eating Disorders* 49:321–27.

Mehler PS. 2001. Diagnosis and care of patients with anorexia nervosa in primary care setting. *Annals of Internal Medicine* 134:1048–59.

Mehler PS and Linas S. 2002. Use of a proton-pump inhibitor for metabolic disturbances associated with anorexia nervosa. *New England Journal of Medicine* 347:373–74.

Miller KK, Grinspoon SK, Ciampa J, Hier J, Herzog D, and Klibanski A. 2005. Medical findings in outpatients with anorexia nervosa. *Archives of Internal Medicine* 165:561–66.

Roerig JL, Steffen KJ, Mitchell JE, and Zunker C. 2010. Laxative abuse: Epidemiology, diagnosis, and management. *Drugs* 70:1487–503.

Schrier RW, Masoumi A, and Elhassan E. 2010. Aldosterone: Role in edematous disorders, hypertension, chronic renal failure, and metabolic syndrome. *Clinical Journal of the American Society of Nephrology* 5:1132–40.

Smink FRE, Van Hoeken D, and Hoek HW. 2012. Epidemiology of eating disorders: Incidence, prevalence, and mortality rates. *Current Psychiatry Reports* 14:406–14.

Sterns RH. 2015. Disorders of plasma sodium: Causes, consequences, and correction. *New England Journal of Medicine* 372:55–65.

Stheneur C, Bergeron S, and Lapeyraque AL. 2014. Renal complications in anorexia nervosa. *Eating and Weight Disorders* 19:455–60.

Tamargo J, Segura J, and Ruilope LM. 2014. Diuretics in the treatment of hypertension. Part 2: Loop diuretics and potassium-sparing agents. *Expert Opinion on Pharmacotherapy* 15:605–21.

Trent SA, Moreira ME, Colwell CB, and Mehler PS. 2013. ED management of patients with eating disorders. *American Journal of Emergency Medicine* 31:859–65.

Wolfe BE, Metzger ED, Levine JM, and Jimerson DC. 2001. Laboratory screening for electrolyte abnormalities and anemia in bulimia nervosa: A controlled study. *International Journal of Eating Disorders* 30:288–93.

6

Gastrointestinal Complications

Philip S. Mehler, MD

Common Questions

What clues from a gastrointestinal (GI) history and physical examination are helpful during both early (occult) and later stages of eating disorders?

What GI symptoms occur with early weight loss?

What common abnormalities found on laboratory testing may signal the presence of an eating disorder?

What symptoms and signs develop as weight loss becomes more severe and can frustrate weight restoration?

What treatment strategies can be used for common GI symptoms (bloating, early satiety, fullness) that may interfere with nutritional rehabilitation?

How do GI symptoms improve with time and weight gain? How can this be used to reassure patients?

What can you tell patients about the long-term effects of anorexia nervosa on the GI tract?

When are GI studies, such as upper or lower endoscopy, barium studies, or nuclear medicine testing, indicated?

What role is there for medications to help treat various GI complications of anorexia nervosa and bulimia nervosa?

Case 1

W.H., a 19-year-old female, presented with pure restricting anorexia nervosa, having had a 20-pound weight loss (height 5 feet 6 inches; original weight 115 pounds) and now 70% of ideal body weight. She had no prior history of intestinal disease. At the nadir of her weight loss, she complained of epigastric bloating and constipation. Physical examination revealed a normal abdomen, no evidence of distention, and hemoccult-negative stool.

Inpatient multidisciplinary treatment enabled W.H. to gain 25 pounds over a 10-week period. She was reassured that the bloating and constipation would improve with time and weight restoration. Fiber, which can often increase bloating, was avoided in her diet so as not to worsen her complaint of bloating. Her bloating and constipation spontaneously improved without the use of laxatives or need for any GI studies.

Case 2

A.D., a 25-year-old female with bulimia who was undergoing outpatient psychotherapy, continued intermittent self-induced emesis twice a day. She had no weight loss and did not engage in laxative use.

A.D. complained of sore throat, hoarseness, dyspepsia, and intermittent odynophagia. She was empirically treated with omeprazole 20 mg once a day. The hoarseness, dyspeptic symptoms, and sore throat resolved after 4 days, and the odynophagia after 2 weeks. One month later she denied any swallowing problems. With intensive psychotherapy, her purging ceased, as did all of the aforementioned symptoms. She was concerned about the previous difficulty with swallowing and wondered if additional testing was necessary. Her omeprazole was discontinued, and her symptoms did not recur.

Background

People who have eating disorders commonly complain of gastrointestinal symptoms (Salvioli et al., 2013). Such symptoms are often a consequence of the eating disorder rather than an etiologic factor in the disorder. However, early in the course of the illness, GI complaints may so preoccupy the patient and the physician that they interfere with and deflect attempts at psychological treatment. There may even be some question as to whether a primary GI disease exists in addition to the eating disorder. Moreover, an eating disorder may exacerbate a preexisting intestinal disease, especially irritable bowel syndrome, which is one of the most commonly encountered GI disorders in the general population and may overlap with eating disorders (Perkins et al., 2005).

The primary care physician and the primary therapist may be confronted with a wide spectrum of GI complaints in patients with eating disorders. To care for these patients, clinicians should be somewhat familiar with several germane GI topics:

1. The prevalence of GI symptoms in eating disorders
2. The time course of the evolution of these GI symptoms during illness and recovery
3. The effect of GI symptoms on treatment
4. Possible long-term GI sequelae for individuals who recover from eating disorders
5. Therapeutic modalities available to treat these GI issues

Both anorexia nervosa and bulimia nervosa are associated with specific GI symptoms that are uniquely attributable to the food restriction and weight loss or the purging behaviors, respectively, that characterize these two eating disorders. An initial complete medical history and physical examination are part of the evaluation for patients with eating disorders. It is important to elicit a thorough history of relevant GI disease and current symptoms. A history of gastroesophageal reflux (acid reflux), for example, may be exacerbated by weight gain or the self-induced vomiting of bulimia and may require aggressive treatment. Similarly, patients with preexisting irritable bowel syndrome may develop worsening symptoms of pain or altered bowel patterns at some time during the refeeding process. Patients with irritable bowel syndrome who are already inherently predisposed to focus on intestinal complaints may develop slowed GI motility due to ongoing weight loss, which often causes them to develop more severe bloating or constipation and frustrates weight restoration.

Anorexia Nervosa

Table 6.1 lists common GI symptoms associated with the weight loss in anorexia nervosa that generally improve with weight gain (Norris et al., 2016). Patients with anorexia nervosa who present to gastroenterologists are often heavy consumers of health information because they are hoping to diagnose organic causes for their litany of somatic complaints (Emmanuel et al., 2004). It is important to neither summarily dismiss nor repeatedly evaluate a patient's GI complaints, as both approaches, if inju-

Table 6.1. Common gastrointestinal symptoms with anorexia nervosa

▪ Bloating	▪ Nausea	▪ Abdominal pain
▪ Fullness	▪ Constipation	▪ Distention
▪ Early satiety		

diciously applied, can be laden with deleterious risks for the recovery of these patients. There is a complex interplay between the GI system and eating disorders, given the inextricable connection between food and the body system that digests the food.

Gastroparesis

With pure food restriction, once a weight loss of approximately 10%–20% occurs, there is often universal development of gastroparesis (Weterle-Snolinska et al., 2015). *Gastroparesis* refers to delayed emptying of the stomach due to impairment of antral stomach contractions that impedes grinding of the food. But the threshold for amount of weight loss needed to cause gastroparesis is not known. A shorter duration of anorexia nervosa seems to portend less likelihood of developing gastroparesis. Bloating and early satiety are the main symptoms and may be severe. Figure 6.1 illustrates gastric dilation. If the patient complains of severe left upper quadrant pain, significant vomiting, or early satiety in the setting of abdominal distention during the early phase of refeeding, gastric dilation should be screened for with an abdominal X-ray to avoid gastric rupture (Mascolo et al., 2015). The bloating can be worsened by a high-fiber diet, such as the vegetarian diet that these patients often adopt. Once gastroparesis develops, early satiety, nausea, bloating, and even acid reflux and vomiting that is no longer self-induced may occur in patients with anorexia nervosa (Perez, 2013). This may hamper attempts at weight restoration. Although the bloating and early satiety generally improve with weight restoration, improvement often takes many weeks to months, and its natural history is not well defined in anorexia nervosa. Therefore, it is crucial to offer reassurance to these patients that their symptoms are indeed inherent to their weight loss and the refeeding process, and to instruct them to avoid legume-type foods and excessive fiber, which promote gas and distention. This will enable them to understand that their symptoms will pass with time and that they are not "causing" the pain by eating. Likewise, patients should be informed that refusal to eat and regain

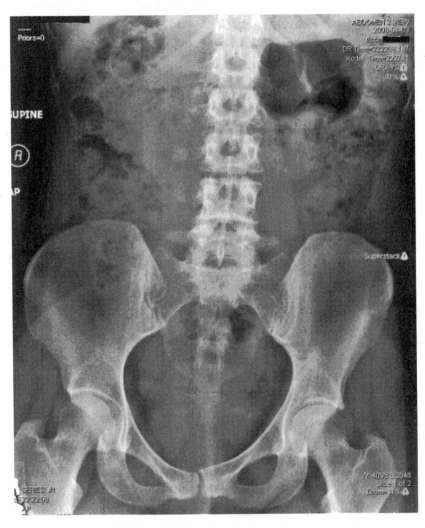

Figure 6.1. Gastric dilation.

weight will only delay the improvement and ultimate resolution of their symptoms.

Useful approaches to the problem of gastroparesis-induced bloating in patients with anorexia include the following:

1. Use of liquid food supplements as a portion of the daily calories (one can of supplement three times per day for a total of 750–1,000

calories) for the first week or two of refeeding, since gastric emptying of liquids is generally normal even in severe anorexia nervosa.

2. Ingestion of liquid components rather than solids earlier in the meal, which generally results in less bloating, so that the patient is able to continue eating.

3. Division of the daily caloric intake into two or three snacks and three smaller meals per day, so that meal-induced bloating will not result in termination of a meal and loss of a major portion of the daily caloric intake.

4. Use of small particle–sized foods (Olausson et al., 2014).

Working with a registered dietician experienced with patients who have anorexia nervosa is important to effectively deal with these refeeding GI issues (Trees et al., 2016).

Gastroparesis induced by weight loss generally improves with partial weight restoration. Thus, the severe bloating initially complained of, which often prevents patients from eating adequate calories with their meal, progressively improves with weight gain for most individuals. A significant improvement often occurs with moderate weight gain; in general, gastroparesis largely resolves with weight restored to 85% of ideal body weight. However, for patients with residual psychopathologic distress, symptoms of bloating may remain despite refeeding (Benini et al., 2004). Thus, in rare cases, it may be necessary to obtain a nuclear medicine gastric-emptying study to formally investigate prolonged gastroparesis-type symptomatology after refeeding and weight restoration.

Metoclopramide is a medication that stimulates stomach contraction and hastens emptying of the stomach. In a dose of 2.5–5 mg, 30 minutes before meals and perhaps also at bedtime, it is clinically useful in treating bloating and early satiety secondary to delayed gastric emptying in anorexia nervosa (Camilleri et al., 2013). It is also a well-established antiemetic medication. Caution must be exercised when using metoclopramide, however, because it can exacerbate neck cervical muscle spasm (torticollis) and, rarely, can cause tardive dyskinesia, especially at higher doses and in older patients. Macrolide antibiotics such as erythromycin or azithromycin are occasionally added to or used in place of metoclopramide. This dual use may be of added benefit for refractory symptoms (Moshiree et al., 2010).

Gastroesophageal Reflux

Gastroesophageal reflux (heartburn, acid reflux) often begins in patients with anorexia nervosa, perhaps secondary to gastroparesis. It also generally improves with time as weight is restored. In contrast to the gastric emptying abnormalities noted above, however, esophageal emptying has been found to be normal in anorexia nervosa. Therefore, esophageal complaints in patients with restricting anorexia nervosa are often of a functional nature. Gastroesophageal reflux usually requires histamine-2 antagonists (such as ranitidine 150 mg twice a day) or a proton-pump inhibitor (omeprazole 20–40 mg per day). The maintenance dosage usually used for peptic ulcer disease (only a nighttime dose) is often inadequate to control symptoms secondary to reflux. Any patient with persistent vomiting, reflux symptoms, or dysphagia that does not respond after 3 weeks of treatments should probably undergo an upper endoscopy procedure to evaluate for peptic ulcer disease or for ongoing severe esophageal inflammation. Inflammation can progress over years to esophageal carcinoma, especially if the patient has true esophageal reflux disease.

One additional concern, especially in patients with more severe forms of anorexia nervosa, is the possibility of *dysphagia* (difficulty swallowing), frustrating patients' ability to complete their meal plan. The pharyngeal muscles can atrophy with weight loss and result in the development of dysphagia. Consultation with a speech therapist may be of help (Holmes, Gudridge, and Mehler, 2012).

Gallstones, though rare, should also be considered in the differential diagnosis of patients with anorexia nervosa who have vomiting and/or right upper quadrant pain, given the known increased incidence of gallstones in patients with weight loss. However, if no right upper quadrant pain accompanies the vomiting, gallstones are less likely. A right upper quadrant abdominal ultrasound is a simple way to exclude the presence of gallstones.

Constipation

Constipation invariably accompanies the weight loss of anorexia nervosa, even in patients who have never abused stimulant laxatives. Persons with weight loss are expected to have fewer bowel movements due to an overall slowed GI transit time. They may incorrectly respond to their perceived problem with constipation by starting to use bulking, fiber-containing laxatives or dangerous stimulant laxatives. This may worsen the constipation by inducing bloating and distention, or through diarrheal losses of potassium, or by making the bowel dependent on stimulant laxatives. Because individuals often take laxatives in the mistaken belief that they will produce substantial weight loss, it is useful to educate patients that laxatives act in the colon, after caloric absorption has already occurred, and are thus ineffective as a means of weight loss. Others may take laxatives because they mistakenly believe that their abdominal pain is due to decreased bowel movements. Patients may need frequent reassurance that there is nothing fundamentally wrong with their bowels other than a need for weight restoration. They must be encouraged to focus on the expected return, over weeks, to their prior bowel pattern as weight is restored. Generally, with weight restoration and refeeding, normal bowel transit time resumes in less than one month (Chun et al., 1997). Anorectal dysfunction and anal muscle weakness documented by manometry are sometimes seen in patients with weight loss and can contribute to the bowel complaints. Rectal prolapse has also been described in anorexia nervosa. These conditions also resolve with time and nutritional rehabilitation (Mitchell and Norris, 2013).

Treatment options for constipation, in addition to education and progressive weight restoration, include (1) adequate water intake; (2) fiber in very low doses (10 g per day), avoiding the high doses that can cause bloating; (3) polyethylene glycol powder, at a dose of 1–2 capfuls one to three times per day; or (4) lactulose, a nonabsorbable synthetic disaccharide (similar to polyethylene glycol products in efficacy and mode of action), 30–60 mL once or twice per day. If lactulose is used, it is useful to tell patients that although this medication tastes sweet, it is devoid of calories because it is not absorbed. Lactulose reaches the colon in an unaltered form and, because it is highly osmotic, draws water into the bowel, resulting in a bowel movement. Polyethylene glycol products work in a similar manner and have a long record of efficacy for gut cleansing in preparation for colonoscopy and surgery (Rankumar and Rao, 2005). (See table 6.2 for a classification of laxative therapies.)

In general, it is best to avoid the use of any stimulant laxatives that contain senna, cascara, or bisocodyl, given the potential for long-term abuse and dependence after weight restoration. Long-term use of stimulant-type laxatives may cause direct damage to colonic nerve cells and result in refractory constipation. This syndrome is termed the *cathartic colon syndrome*.

Table 6.2. Classification of laxative therapies

Class	Mechanism of action	Site of action	Example
Osmotic	Attracts/retains water in intestinal lumen, increasing intraluminal pressure	Small intestine and colon	Magnesium hydroxide (saline osmotic) Lactulose Polyethylene glycol
Irritant or peristaltic (use with caution)	Direct action to stimulate myenteric plexus, and alters water and electrolyte secretion	Colon	Senna Bisacodyl Cascara Phenolphthalein
Bulk or hydrophilic	Holds water in stool and causes mechanical distention	Small and large intestines	Methylcellulose Psyllium Dietary bran
Stool softener	Softens stool by facilitating a mixture of fat and water (largely ineffective)	Colon and rectum	Docusate

Rarely, early in the refeeding process, a glycerin suppository or a stimulant-type laxative may be necessary to "jump-start" normal peristaltic motion in the bowel, but should always be used in a limited, judicious manner. New medications such as lubiprostone, which are approved for constipation-type irritable bowel syndrome, have not been specifically studied in anorexia nervosa but, anecdotally, may be of use for a brief period for early bouts of constipation.

Abdominal Pain

Abdominal pain is a frequent complaint in anorexia nervosa. It is generally diffuse, unaccompanied by tenderness, and more consistent with irritable bowel syndrome. "Functional" symptoms seem to be common in anorexia nervosa and generally improve slowly over time and with weight restoration. Persistent pain may need further evaluation. Abdominal pain accompanied by diarrhea should be evaluated to rule out fecal impaction, infectious causes, and other pathology, especially if accompanied by fever, extreme pain, or an elevated white blood cell count. However, the weight loss of anorexia nervosa itself can cause villous atrophy in the small intestine and reduce the intestinal surface area needed for proper digestion. This, in turn, can cause diarrhea soon after eating. It is diagnosed by the finding of a low serum diamine oxidase level (Takinoto et al., 2014).

Laboratory studies are occasionally worthwhile for patients with eating disorders who are experiencing abdominal pain. Iron-deficiency anemia may indicate significant GI disease or inability to absorb oral iron. Elevated amylase levels are almost always due to a salivary source resulting from excessive vomiting and are not indicative of pancreatitis. This can be confirmed by a lipase measurement, which is elevated in pancreatitis but normal when amylase elevation is due to a salivary source, as seen with purging. In some rare cases, however, the refeeding process, if too aggressive, can induce refeeding pancreatitis early in the course of the process. Malnutrition by itself can cause, on rare occasions, idiopathic pancreatitis that presents like typical pancreatitis with epigastric pain, nausea, and vomiting. In addition, gallstone pancreatitis can develop because gallstones develop with weight loss; these patients typically have extremely high amylase measurements (>1,000 mg/dL) along with elevated lipases. They require a cholecystectomy because of their risk of recurrent gallstone pancreatitis. Asymptomatic gallstones, probably due to weight loss, do not generally warrant urgent surgery.

A supine and upright simple abdominal X-ray may be useful to exclude bowel distention when symptoms of constipation persist after an adequate trial of medications aimed at alleviating constipation (fig. 6.2). The absence of excessive stool on these radiographic studies provides proof that bowel function is normal and no longer deserves ongoing concern. This is especially helpful because the interplay of functional GI disorders is significantly prevalent in patients with anorexia nervosa.

Elevated Liver Transaminase Levels

Routine blood tests for liver enzymes (AST and ALT) often show abnormalities in patients with anorexia nervosa (Rosen et al., 2016). Weight loss and malnutrition can produce mild elevation of these transaminases (AST/ALT) due to apoptosis, or programmed cell death, of hepatic cells. This is more common at lower BMIs and in patients with greater risk of refeeding hypophosphatemia (Brown et al., 2015). Mild transaminase elevations can also occur early in the course of refeeding if dextrose calories

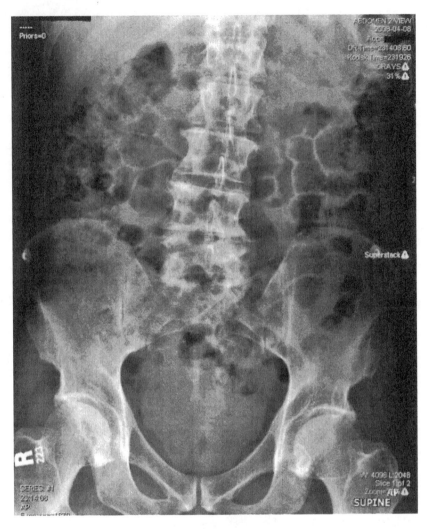

Figure 6.2. Excessive stool in colon.

are excessive and are causing steatosis, a fatty liver. These elevations usually resolve and normalize if the composition of the diet is changed to fewer glucose-based calories or the daily caloric intake is decreased by 300–500 kcal. A higher level of caloric intake can then be reintroduced at a later date once the liver tests have normalized. Rarely, the transaminases may be markedly elevated with severe anorexia nervosa even before refeeding has started, and this may be a sign of serious multiorgan failure

(De Caprio et al., 2006). Nutritional support should result in improvement. Rarely, a simple right upper quadrant ultrasound may be indicated if the transaminases are rapidly increasing or are approaching a level of 1,000 U/L. In general, as opposed to the finding in alcoholic liver disease, the ALT level is more abnormal than the AST level in the apoptosis of anorexia nervosa.

Superior Mesenteric Artery Syndrome

One other rare syndrome to be aware of in people with anorexia nervosa is the superior mesenteric artery (SMA) syndrome. It results from compression of the third portion of the duodenum between the aorta and the vertebral column posteriorly and the SMA anteriorly. Anything that narrows the normal angle between the aorta and the SMA can cause entrapment of the duodenum as it passes between these vessels. The SMA is normally kept in place by a fat pad; reduction in the fat pad due to weight loss narrows the angle. Patients with anorexia nervosa who have the SMA syndrome typically complain of intermittent vomiting and upper quadrant abdominal pain soon after starting to eat. With a weight gain of as little as 5–10 pounds and regrowth of the fat pad, tolerance of normal feeding can be restored. The diagnosis is made by upper GI series tests or by an abdominal CT scan, with the radiologist made aware of the diagnosis being considered. Once diagnosed, treatment involves either the use of a soft liquid oral diet or the placement of a nasogastric or nasojejunal tube until symptoms abate. Surgery probably has no role for SMA due to anorexia nervosa (Pottorf et al., 2014).

Bulimia Nervosa

Bulimia nervosa leads to a different set of GI symptoms (table 6.3). Severe GI reflux symptoms—heartburn, spontaneous vomiting, acid regurgitation, chest pain, dysphagia, and nocturnal choking when lying supine—and their complications often occur in bulimia. These symptoms are due to self-induced vomiting and weakening of the lower esophageal sphincter, which is normally a one-way valve that prevents stomach acid from moving up into the esophagus. These reflux symptoms may be among the few clues to the ongoing illness. Spontaneous vomiting is the effortless return of stomach contents into the mouth without retching. Food-restricting patients who do not have bulimia may also develop reflux due

Table 6.3. Common gastrointestinal symptoms associated with bulimia

Vomiting-related
  Heartburn
  Odynophagia
  Dysphagia
  Hoarseness
  Sore throat
  Hematemesis (vomiting bright red blood)
Laxative-related
  Diarrhea
  Abdominal cramping
  Constipation
  Hematochezia (passing bright red blood per rectum)

to weight loss–induced gastroparesis, but reflux in these cases generally involves only reflux into the distal esophagus and thus is milder. By contrast, in patients who induce vomiting, the acid contents travel up through the entire esophagus and mouth, and these patients are more likely to complain of more severe dyspeptic symptoms and the symptoms of reflux. Specifically, acid-induced inflammation of the vocal cords may produce hoarseness (which persists for several days after even a brief exposure of the vocal cords to acid), laryngitis, sore throat, or cough. These patients may also have symptoms of *odynophagia* (painful swallowing) or dysphagia also caused by the acid-induced esophageal inflammation or secondary to stricture formation.

A cessation of self-induced vomiting without concomitant acid-suppressing medication may not alleviate these symptoms. In addition, patients often do not respond to antacids. Rather, they need either higher-dose histamine-2 blockers (ranitidine 150–300 mg twice a day) or proton-pump inhibitors (omeprazole 20–40 mg once or twice a day). Prokinetic agents such as metoclopramide are also effective for controlling the reflux symptoms in patients with bulimia. In general, trials have established the superiority of the proton-pump inhibitors over the histamine-2 receptor antagonists for gastroesophageal reflux disease.

Because of the incessant exposure of their esophageal mucosa to acidic vomitus, patients with bulimia are at risk for Barrett's esophagus, a precancerous transformation of the lining mucosa of the esophagus. Therefore, the presence of refractory heartburn-type symptoms unresponsive to 4–6 weeks of a high-dose proton-pump inhibitor suggests the need for an upper endoscopy. Barrett's esophagus is discovered in some patients who undergo upper endoscopy for symptoms of gastroesophageal reflux disease, but many patients with Barrett's esophagus do not have typical symptoms of reflux. There is no current test other than an upper endoscopy to establish the diagnosis. Therefore, endoscopy may be reasonable for patients who have bulimia with a long-standing history of self-induced vomiting, but this is less strongly endorsed than previously (Spelcher and Souza, 2014).

Individuals with bulimia nervosa who purge through laxative abuse have a distinct set of GI problems. The diarrhea that commonly occurs during periods of excessive laxative use results in blood chemistry abnormalities along with dehydration and dizziness (see chapter 5). The bigger problem, however, involves trying to help the patient stop the abuse of laxatives. This is difficult because, if stimulant laxatives have been abused, the bowel may have become dependent on them, and cessation of their use can result in rebound constipation and fluid retention (cathartic colon syndrome). The result is a dilated, atonic colon, which is manifested by slowed or absent transit through some or all segments of the colon. Basically, the colon becomes an inert tube, incapable of propagating fecal material. This leads to hard, infrequently passed stools and, rarely, a state of refractory constipation. It is always difficult to convince patients to stop using laxatives, given their psychological dependence on laxatives and anxiety about losing the feeling of weight control (albeit inaccurate) that laxatives give them (Kovacs and Palmer, 2004).

Clinicians need to help patients understand that the range of normal bowel function, as defined by the Rome III criteria, includes as a minimum just three bowel movements per week. Also, as noted earlier in the chapter, it is important to point out that laxatives are an ineffective means of achieving weight loss because most caloric absorption occurs in the small intestine, well before the site in the colon where laxatives act.

Restoration of normal bowel function may take a few weeks. Patients should be encouraged to completely cease their use of stimulant laxatives. There is no scientific basis to support a gradual tapering off, because ongoing exposure to stimulant laxatives might harm the neurons that oversee bowel peristalsis. Patients must be made to understand that patience is a key virtue when attempting to become independent from stimulant laxatives. If constipation lasts more than 3–4 days, a short course of a mild

Table 6.4. Ancillary treatments for constipation

- Ample hydration and judicious exercise
- Distraction-free 10–15 minutes on the toilet rather than sitting and straining
- Elevating the legs onto a footstool during defecation
- Substitution of less-offending laxatives
- Measured small amount of fiber rather than undefined high-fiber diet
- *Tailoring medications to the complaint!*

nonstimulating laxative (see table 6.2), together with ample oral fluids, is important. Daily polyethylene glycol should also be started as soon as the decision is made to cease stimulant laxatives. An occasional glycerin suppository may be needed early in the "detox" process. Patients should be strongly discouraged from using diuretics for the temporary fluid retention that may occur with cessation of laxative abuse. Although diuretics will lessen edema formation, when they are stopped, the edema will recur to a greater degree than before due to pseudo-Bartter's syndrome (see chapter 5). In fact, moderate fluid intake is a useful adjunct for reestablishing normal bowel function, along with osmotic laxatives such as polyethylene glycol, which are safe and effective with regard to integrity of bowel function (DiPalma et al., 2007). As noted above for constipation in anorexia nervosa, lubiprostone may be efficacious for treating chronic constipation. A judicious amount of exercise is also beneficial for normal bowel function (table 6.4).

Table 6.5 presents some useful guidelines for the treatment of patients with anorexia nervosa or bulimia nervosa who have GI complications.

Summary

The gastrointestinal system is adversely affected by both anorexia nervosa and bulimia nervosa. With anorexia nervosa, the complications are mostly manifested during food restriction but become more prominent as the patient begins the process of refeeding. Similarly, the effects of bulimia on the GI system are present during purging behaviors and during the treatment phase when purging tendencies are being controlled. Thus, it is important for clinicians to become familiar with the GI complications of anorexia nervosa and bulimia because effective treatment and prophylaxis will increase the chances of successful treatment.

Table 6.5. Guidelines for care of patients with eating orders who have GI complaints

- It is important to reassure the patient that the intestinal symptoms generally improve with weight gain.
- Educating patients about the physiological basis for their constipation may help to decrease laxative abuse.
- Lack of improvement in GI symptoms should lead to consideration of an ongoing occult illness and/or underlying primary GI disease.
- Prokinetic agents may be useful for some patients who have bloating associated with weight loss. Metoclopramide (2.5–5 mg before meals and at bedtime) is often effective.
- Constipation is best treated with polyethylene glycol (1–3 tablespoons per day).
- Symptomatic reflux may be treated with histamine-2 blockers (such as oral cimetidine 400–800 mg or ranitidine 150–300 mg) twice a day. Proton pump inhibitors (such as omeprazole 20 mg once or twice a day) are probably more effective.
- Gallstones may develop due to weight loss but are often not the cause of the patient's pain. Surgery should not be undertaken routinely.
- Mild elevations in serum liver enzymes (ALT/AST) should resolve with weight gain and adjustments in caloric intake. If they do not, further evaluation is needed to exclude hepatitis B or C, autoimmune hepatitis, hemochromatosis, or Wilson's disease.
- Avoid barium and endoscopic GI studies for most patients unless their symptoms fail to improve with psychiatric recovery or if iron deficiency anemia is present.

REFERENCES

Benini L, Todesco T, Dalle Grave R, et al. 2004. Gastric emptying in patients with restricting and binge/purging subtypes of anorexia nervosa. *American Journal of Gastroenterology* 99:1448–54.

Brown CA, Sabel AL, Guadiani JL, and Mehler PS. 2015. Predictors of hypophosphatemia during refeeding of patients with severe anorexia nervosa. *International Journal of Eating Disorders* 48:898–904.

Camilleri M, Parkman HP, Shafi MA, et al. 2013. Clinical guideline: Management of gastroparesis. *American Journal of Gastroenterology* 108:18–37.

Chun AB, Sokol MS, Kaye WH, et al. 1997. Colonic and anorectal function in constipated patients with anorexia nervosa. *American Journal of Gastroenterology* 92:1879–83.

De Caprio C, Alfano A, Senatore I, et al. 2006. Severe acute liver damage in anorexia nervosa: Two case reports. *Nutrition* 22:572–75.

DiPalma JA, Cleveland MV, McGowan J, et al. 2007. A randomized, multi-center, placebo-controlled trial of polyethylene glycol laxative for chronic treatment of chronic constipation. *American Journal of Gastroenterology* 102:1436–41.

Emmanuel AV, Stern J, Treasure J, et al. 2004. Anorexia nervosa in gastrointestinal practice. *European Journal of Gastroenterology and Hepatology* 16:1135–42.

Holmes S, Gudridge TA, and Mehler PS. 2012. Dysphagia in severe anorexia nervosa and potential therapeutic interventions. *Annals of Otolaryngology, Rhinology, and Laryngology* 121:449–56.

Kovacs D and Palmer RL. 2004. The associations between laxative abuse and other symptoms among adults with anorexia nervosa. *International Journal of Eating Disorders* 36:224–28.

Mascolo M, Dee E, Townsend R, et al. 2015. Severe gastric dilation in anorexia nervosa. *International Journal of Eating Disorders* 48:532–34.

Mitchell N and Norris M. 2013. Rectal prolapse associated with anorexia nervosa. *Journal of Eating Disorders* 1:39.

Moshiree B, McDonald R, Hon WE, and Toskes PP. 2010. Comparison of effect of azithromycin versus erythromycin in patients with gastroparesis. *Digestive Disease Science* 55:675–83.

Norris M, Harrison ME, Isserlin L, et al. 2016. Gastrointestinal complications associated with anorexia nervosa: A systematic review. *International Journal of Eating Disorders* 49:216–37.

Olausson EA, Storsud S, Grundin H, et al. 2014. A small particle sized diet reduces gastrointestinal symptoms in patients with gastroparesis. *American Journal of Gastroenterology* 109:375–85.

Perez ME. 2013. Effect of nutritional rehabilitation on gastric motility in adolescents. *Journal of Pediatrics* 163:867–72.

Perkins SJ, Keville S, Schmidt U, et al. 2005. Eating disorders and irritable bowel syndrome: Is there a link? *Journal of Psychosomatic Research* 59:57–64.

Pottorf BJ, Husain FA, Hollis HW, and Lin E. 2014. Laparoscopic management of SMA syndrome. *JMA Surgery* 149:1319–22.

Ramkumar D and Rao SS. 2005. Efficacy and safety of traditional medical therapies for chronic constipation: Systematic review. *American Journal of Gastroenterology* 100:936–71.

Rosen E, Gaudiani J, Sabel A, and Mehler PS. 2016. Liver dysfunction in patients with severe anorexia nervosa. *International Journal of Eating Disorders* 49:153–60.

Salvioli B, Pellicciari A, Lero L, et al. 2013. Audit of digestive complaints in patients with eating disorders. *Digestive and Liver Disease* 45:639–44.

Spelcher SJ and Souza LF. 2014. Barrett's esophagus. *New England Journal of Medicine* 371:836–45.

Takinoto Y, Yoshiuchi R, Shimodaria S, et al. 2014. Diamine oxidase activity levels in anorexia nervosa. *International Journal of Eating Disorders* 47:203–5.

Trees N, Beaty L, Gusimano C, et al. 2016. Gastrointestinal complications of refeeding in anorexia nervosa. *Journal of Nutritional Biology* 1:49–60.

Weterle-Snolinska K, Banasiuk M, Oziekiewicz M, et al. 2015. Gastrointestinal motility disorders in patients with anorexia nervosa. *Psychiatria Polska* 49:721–29.

7

Cardiac Abnormalities and Their Management

Katherine Sachs, MD, Philip S. Mehler, MD, and Mori Krantz, MD

Common Questions

Why do patients with anorexia nervosa suffer sudden cardiac death?

What are "normal" vital signs for patients with anorexia nervosa?

Why do patients with anorexia nervosa have bradycardia?

What degree of bradycardia is cause for concern and needs additional monitoring?

When do vital sign abnormalities revert to normal in anorexia nervosa?

What EKG abnormalities are seen with anorexia nervosa?

What is the significance of heart palpitations in patients who have bulimia nervosa?

Case

K.L. was a 21-year-old female with a 6-year history of anorexia nervosa. She denied purging behaviors. Her chief complaint was dyspnea of 3 months' duration. She had had occasional chest pain with both rest and exertion. She denied fainting or use of ipecac. There was no family history of premature coronary artery disease. Her exercise tolerance had diminished over the preceding 2 years, but she remained active and jogged 2 miles per day. She had been in an eating disorder program for 2 weeks. A refeeding program was initiated, and K.L. had gained 3 pounds. Her physical examination was notable for a blood pressure of 80/50 mm Hg, a pulse of 48, and a respiratory rate of 10. She was 5 feet 4 inches tall and weighed 93 pounds (78% of ideal body weight). Physical examination revealed a cardiac midsystolic click, a soft holosystolic murmur, clear lungs, no edema, and normal abdomen.

Blood electrolytes revealed normal potassium, magnesium, and bicarbonate levels. An EKG showed sinus bradycardia with a heart rate of 50 beats per minute, normal QTc interval, and no ST-T wave changes; QRS voltage was reduced in the limb leads. Her chest X-ray on admission showed an enlarged cardiac silhouette. In view of the cardiac examination and chest X-ray, an echocardiogram was ordered. It revealed mitral valve prolapse with billowing of the mitral valve, a normal left ventricular ejection fraction, and no segmental wall motion abnormalities. A small to moderately sized circumferential pericardial effusion was noted without evidence of tamponade. K.L. was educated about mitral valve prolapse and continued to refeed successfully. She had no recurrence of chest pain or dyspnea as she gained a total of 16 pounds. On repeat echocardiographic evaluation 3 months later, the pericardial effusion was substantially reduced; the cardiac click and murmur were no longer audible on physical examination.

Background

Anorexia nervosa has the highest mortality rate of any psychiatric disorder (Arcelus et al., 2011). Of the litany of medical complications that contribute to the increased mortality rate for patients with anorexia nervosa, cardiovascular complications have historically been considered the most ominous. As research in this field has progressed, it has become well established that significant cardiac structural, conduction, repolarization, and hemodynamic changes do indeed occur. Despite this increased understanding, however, the relationship of these changes to sudden death remains speculative and is as yet unsubstantiated by rigorous data. Nevertheless, an awareness of structural and physiologic changes is important for clinicians caring for patients with anorexia nervosa.

Hemodynamics

Two of the most prominent and consistent findings in patients with anorexia nervosa are resting bradycardia (heart rate <60 beats per minute) and hypotension (systolic blood pressure <90 mm Hg). In addition to thinness, bradycardia may be the most common presenting sign of anorexia nervosa, and in the correct context it should alert the clinician to the possibility of an eating disorder (Grover, Robin, and Gharahbaghian, 2012). The bradycardia of anorexia nervosa generally resolves, with heart rates increasing into the normal range of 60–90 beats per minute, as weight is restored to a level greater than 85%–90% of ideal body weight; it may resolve even earlier with a stable pattern of nutritional replenishment and progressive weight gain (Shamim et al., 2003). Many patients believe that their low resting heart rates are attributable to their perceived physical fitness. It is important to educate patients on this important distinction. While truly conditioned athletes have low heart rates at rest with only small increases with exertion, malnourished patients who have anorexia nervosa have low resting heart rates but, due to diffuse weakness and debilitation, become tachycardic with even minimal exertion.

While sinus bradycardia is generally well tolerated and asymptomatic, when combined with the often seen orthostatic blood pressure changes, symptoms of presyncope or even frank syncope can occur. It is reasonable to strongly consider admission to an inpatient unit for telemetry monitoring for any patient with recent syncope, with a resting heart rate of less than 40 beats per minute, or with bradycardia other than sinus (Sachs et al., 2016). Resolution of orthostatic changes often lags behind normalization of the resting heart rate and may persist beyond the refeeding phase until significant weight restoration is achieved.

Although clinicians might find comfort in a "normal" heart rate, a "relative tachycardia" (pulse 70–100 at rest) in a patient with severe malnutrition due to anorexia nervosa may have more concerning implications, including occult infection (Derman and Szabo, 2006). Indeed, because resting bradycardia is such a constant finding in nutritionally depleted patients with severe anorexia, these "normal" heart rates, even if not strictly in the elevated range (pulse >100), are likely to be either a side effect of medication or an impending medical complication and should be viewed as a warning sign in need of expert medical evaluation (Krantz and Mehler, 2004). Finally, despite resting bradycardia, hospitalized patients with anorexia nervosa, during the early phases of weight restoration, often manifest rapid cardioacceleration with simple activities of daily living. This phenomenon remains under active investigation, but it generally normalizes as weight restoration proceeds, especially as weight approaches 90% of ideal body weight.

Though formal studies are lacking, there is anecdotal evidence of an increased prevalence of the positional orthostatic tachycardia syndrome

(POTS) among patients with anorexia nervosa. This condition is a form of dysautonomia that is typified by excessive tachycardia upon change in position from supine to standing that may be accompanied by a wide array of other symptoms. Distinguishing POTS from the expected orthostatic changes that occur with malnutrition can be difficult. However, an increase in heart rate with standing of more than 30 beats per minute may alert the clinician to a possible diagnosis of POTS. If these changes do not improve as expected with weight restoration, further investigation such as tilt table testing may be warranted.

Autonomic Dysfunction

The progressive bradycardia seen with increasing severity of anorexia nervosa has been an ongoing area of scientific inquiry on the influence of the parasympathetic and sympathetic nervous systems on cardiac function. Some researchers have hypothesized that increased vagal tone as part of an adaptive energy-conservation response leads to a decreased resting heart rate (Casiero and Frishman, 2006). However, the data show that this relationship is not as clear as would be theoretically expected. Some studies have found a marked reduction in both parasympathetic and sympathetic tone in patients with anorexia nervosa (Rechlin et al., 1998). Others have demonstrated an increase in parasympathetic activity with unchanged sympathetic tone (Galetta et al., 2003).

Autonomic changes in anorexia nervosa have generally been evaluated using the surrogate marker of heart rate variability. The moment-to-moment fluctuations in heart rate reflect the underlying stability of autonomic nervous system function through the integration of sympathetic and parasympathetic modulation. In limited studies of other patient populations, changes in heart rate variability were associated with increased mortality (Hon and Lee, 1963; Kleiger et al., 1987). Despite a number of studies on this topic in the literature on anorexia nervosa, however, the findings have not been consistent, often resulting in contradictory conclusions (Mazurak et al., 2011). The complex nature of this disease, along with the likely changes in autonomic function with disease progression, presumably accounts for these inconsistencies (Nakai et al., 2015). Further studies more precisely stratified to the duration of illness and subtype of anorexia nervosa are needed to further clarify this issue (Melanson et al., 2004).

Rhythm

Significant concern has centered on the potential propensity for patients with anorexia nervosa to develop QT interval prolongation, which can lead to torsade de pointes, a life-threatening ventricular arrhythmia that can degenerate into ventricular fibrillation. QT interval prolongation and torsade de pointes were long hypothesized to account for the risk of sudden death in anorexia nervosa (Cooke et al., 1994; Isager et al., 1985). As more data have been gathered, however, it seems much less certain that QT interval prolongation is inherent to anorexia nervosa; rather, it may be due to extrinsic factors such as electrolyte abnormalities, including hypokalemia, or the effects of medications such as psychotropics, anxiolytics, macrolide antibiotics, and antiemetics (Krantz et al., 2012). More recent studies suggest that after accounting for confounding variables, QT interval prolongation is indeed not an inherent abnormality in anorexia nervosa and therefore may not independently increase the risk of sudden cardiac death in these patients. Thus, current teachings suggest that the finding of QT prolongation in a patient with anorexia nervosa should prompt a search for potential independent causes.

The risk of torsade de pointes increases exponentially when the rate-corrected QT (QTc) interval exceeds 500 milliseconds (Bednar, Harrigan, and Ruskin, 2002), with antidepressants, antiemetics, gastrointestinal prokinetic agents, antipsychotics, and antibiotics being the most frequent offending agents. However, regardless of the underlying contributors, patients presenting with a prolonged QTc interval warrant careful monitoring. Individuals with a QTc exceeding 500 milliseconds should be admitted to an inpatient unit for telemetry monitoring, whereas those with a QTc below 470 milliseconds should have daily EKG monitoring (Sachs et al., 2016). Assiduous monitoring of electrolytes is critical also, especially for patients with a history of bulimia nervosa or the binge-purge subtype of anorexia nervosa. Given the known heightened risk for malignant arrhythmias caused by electrolyte abnormalities in these patients, a complaint of palpitations should prompt both investigation of electrolytes and cardiac monitoring.

Another marker of increased arrhythmic risk is a measure known as QT dispersion. This is defined by inter-lead variation in QT segment length on a routine 12-lead EKG. Normally, the length of the QT interval is similar in each of these leads. QT dispersion refers to the difference between the maximum QT interval and minimum QT interval occurring in any of the 12 leads. QT dispersion reflects heterogeneous ventricular depolarization and, when abnormally increased, may indicate a heightened propensity to develop serious ventricular arrhythmias, as has been shown to occur following myocardial infarction (Furukawa et al., 2006).

Over the past several years, increased QT dispersion has been found in young women with anorexia nervosa before refeeding (Mont et al., 2003). These patients may have a twofold or greater increase in QT dispersion, and this finding inversely correlates with resting metabolic rate; thus, there is a decrease in QT dispersion with refeeding and increased metabolic rate (Krantz et al., 2005). A newer marker derived from continuous Holter monitoring, the QT variability index, may also be abnormal in anorexia and resolve with weight restoration (Koschke et al., 2010). If prospectively validated, this index could eventually serve as a parameter for risk stratification of patients. Regardless, QT dispersion is a widely available and inexpensive measure that may reflect both metabolic status and the potential for arrhythmia.

Though ventricular arrhythmias are the most feared consequence of repolarization changes found in some patients with anorexia nervosa, conduction abnormalities including high-grade atrioventricular (AV) block may also, albeit rarely, occur. Sinus bradycardia is both common and expected, but in rare cases can progress to development of a second-degree AV block or junctional escape rhythm (Kanbur et al., 2009; Kossaify, 2010). A case of persistent junctional escape rhythm that was extinguished with exercise has been described (Krantz et al., 2011). The finding that bradycardia is easily overcome with exercise suggests that the elevated parasympathetic tone in anorexia is an adaptive physiologic response and is not pathologic in origin.

Structural Abnormalities

Substantial weight loss is accompanied by shrinkage of both skeletal and cardiac muscle. Chronic starvation results in ventricular wall muscle atrophy, reduced left ventricular mass index, and reduction in chamber dimensions (Docx et al., 2014). Reduction in chamber volumes can lead to annular laxity and subsequent mitral valve prolapse, despite no inherent pathology of the valves. Rarely, mitral valve prolapse can be associated with benign chest pain and could account for the symptomatology occasionally present in these patients, as described in the case study that opens this chapter.

The most prominent and consistently documented cardiac structural change in anorexia nervosa is reduction in left ventricular myocardial mass. This change has been suggested to relate to alterations in thyroid hormone levels, although such an association remains speculative (Carlomagno et al., 2011). The documented left ventricular structural changes have raised questions about the possibility of resulting functional changes. It seems that while overall left ventricular systolic function is preserved, changes in the geometry of the left ventricle may adversely affect both cardiac performance and remodeling (Almeida-Jones et al., 2014). Despite these recognized changes, a direct association between anorexia nervosa and heart failure has not been described, although the refeeding syndrome, if left untreated, can lead to a reversible form of acute decompensated heart failure. Additionally, abuse of syrup of ipecac for the purpose of inducing vomiting, as may be seen in bulimia nervosa or the binge-purge subtype of anorexia nervosa, can lead to a potentially irreversible cardiomyopathy due to the direct cardiotoxic properties of its ingredient alkaloid, emetine. However, with the markedly reduced availability of ipecac, ipecac-related cardiomyopathy has become an extremely rare finding.

In addition to the gross changes in myocardial mass, recently described microscopic changes of myocardial fibrosis may have more ominous consequences. Magnetic resonance imaging has shown evidence of fibrosis and scarring in the myocardium of patients with anorexia nervosa, not present in matched controls (Oflaz et al., 2013). These findings may correlate with those observed histologically in an autopsy report (Lamzabi et al., 2015). Myocardial scarring, even on a microscopic level, could provide a substrate for malignant arrhythmias, potentially accounting for the heightened risk of sudden death in this disease.

Finally, pericardial effusion is now known to occur in chronic anorexia nervosa. In a study of adolescents, 22% of patients had pericardial effusions, most of which resolved following refeeding (Docx et al., 2010). Despite the unexpected prevalence of this finding, nearly all patients with pericardial effusions were asymptomatic, and only one case of tamponade is described in the literature (Kircher et al., 2012). Given the benign nature of pericardial effusion, echocardiography should be considered primarily when there is clinical concern about a large pericardial effusion, such as an increased cardiac silhouette on chest X-ray or low-voltage QRS or electrical alternans on EKG, and for patients with hemodynamic instability, elevated jugular venous pressure, or complaint of prominent dyspnea on exertion.

In the past there was concern that the observed mortality in anorexia nervosa was a consequence of abnormal lipid metabolism leading to premature atherosclerosis and myocardial infarction. However, autopsy studies published more than 30 years ago found no evidence of obstructive coronary disease (Isner et al., 1985). Despite isolated case reports of acute coronary syndrome and myocardial infarctions in this patient population, atherosclerotic heart disease is not considered to be a specific cause of morbidity for patients with anorexia nervosa (Abuzeid and Glover, 2011). Some of the debate on this issue has stemmed from conflicting data on lipid abnormalities in this population, with some studies citing harmful slowed LDL-cholesterol transport, and others reporting elevated total cholesterol due to high levels of beneficial HDL-cholesterol (Mehler, Lezotte, and Eckel, 1998; Weinbrenner et al., 2004). It appears that anorexia nervosa and its associated weight loss may actually be protective against other risk factors for atherosclerosis and ischemic heart disease, as these patients have a significantly decreased risk for development of type 2 diabetes (Ji, Sundquist, and Sundquist, 2016) and generally are not hypertensive. Further studies are needed to better elucidate the subtleties of lipid metabolism, including particle size, particle number, and cholesterol efflux. This will allow enhanced prediction of global 10-year atherosclerotic risk for these patients. In the meantime, there seems to be no medical role for routine periodic lipid monitoring for patients who have anorexia nervosa (Sachs et al., 2016), beyond the more widely recommended initial screening for familial hyperlipidemia (Stone et al., 2014).

Despite this seemingly decreased risk for atherosclerotic vascular disease, it is important to remember that patients with anorexia nervosa are not immune to the development of conditions such as hypertension and hyperlipidemia, particularly with advancing age. These patients should be treated according to general clinical guidelines. However, while weight-based dosing of cardiovascular medications such as antihypertensives and statins is not recommended for adults, it is nevertheless important to keep in mind both the low body weight of these patients and their risk for decreased left ventricular mass. Medications such as beta-blockers, calcium channel blockers, and angiotensin converting enzyme inhibitors may be safely and effectively used, but lower starting doses should be selected, with slow and cautious titration.

Summary

Cardiac complications are likely to contribute to the morbidity and mortality seen in patients with anorexia nervosa and, to a lesser extent, those with bulimia nervosa. Most of the cardiac complications accompany the severe malnutrition associated with advanced stages of these eating disorders. A thorough cardiac history and meticulous physical examination should be performed, and basic chemistry panels, a baseline EKG, and orthostatic vital signs should be obtained for all patients after the first visit, to screen for abnormalities that need ongoing evaluation and treatment.

Anorexia nervosa is known to be associated with a number of serious cardiac complications. The vast majority of these issues resolve with timely weight restoration and do not lead to permanent sequelae. These cardiac abnormalities not only are present in the untreated state but can arise as a result of the refeeding process. With bulimia nervosa, most of the cardiac problems are due to electrolyte abnormalities related to purging behaviors. Despite these known and well-described changes, the true underlying cause of sudden death seen in this condition remains uncertain. Previous theories, such as ventricular arrhythmias due to inherent repolarization changes, seem more uncertain in the light of new data. Future studies are under way on long-term arrhythmia monitoring and assessment of chronotropic abnormalities associated with weight restoration.

REFERENCES

Abuzeid W and Glover C. 2011. Acute myocardial infarction and anorexia nervosa. *International Journal of Eating Disorders* 44:473–76.

Almeida-Jones ME, Suntharos P, Rosen L, et al. 2014. Myocardial strain and torsion quantification in patients with restrictive-type anorexia nervosa. *Journal of the American Society of Echocardiography* 27:B41–42.

Arcelus J, Mitchell AJ, Wales J, and Nielsen S. 2011. Mortality rates in patients with anorexia nervosa and other eating disorders: A meta-analysis of 36 studies. *Archives of General Psychiatry* 68(7):727–31.

Bednar M, Harrigan E, and Ruskin J. 2002. Torsades de pointes associated with nonanti-arrhythmic drugs and observations on gender and QTc. *American Journal of Cardiology* 89:1316–19.

Carlomagno G, Mercurio V, Ruvolo A, et al. 2011. Endocrine alterations are the main determinants of cardiac remodeling in restrictive anorexia nervosa. *ISRN Endocrinology* doi: 10.5402/2011/171460.

Casiero D and Frishman WH. 2006. Cardiovascular complications of eating disorders. *Cardiology Review* 14:227–31.

Cooke RA, Chambers JB, Singh R, et al. 1994. QT interval in anorexia nervosa. *British Heart Journal* 72:69–73.

Derman T and Szabo CP. 2006. Why do individuals with anorexia die? A case of sudden death. *International Journal of Eating Disorders* 39:260–62.

Docx MK, Gewillig M, Simons A, et al. 2010. Pericardial effusions in adolescent girls with anorexia nervosa: Clinical course and risk factors. *Eating Disorders* 18:218–25.

Docx M, Simons A, Ramet J, Weyler J, Thues C, and Mertens L. 2014. Predictors of diminished corrected left ventricular mass index in female anorexic adolescents. *Anesthesiology Intensive Therapy* 46:137.

Furukawa Y, Shimizu H, Hiromoto K, Kanemori T, Masuyama T, and Ohyanagi M. 2006. Circadian variation of beat-to-beat QT interval variability in patients with prior myocardial infarction and the effect of beta-blocker therapy. *Pacing and Clinical Electrophysiology* 29:479–86.

Galetta F, Franzoni F, Prattichizzo F, Rolla M, Santoro G, and Pentimone F. 2003. Heart rate variability and left ventricular diastolic function in anorexia nervosa. *Journal of Adolescent Health* 32:416–21.

Grover CA, Robin JK, and Gharahbaghian L. 2012. Anorexia nervosa: A case report of a teenager presenting with bradycardia, general fatigue, and weakness. *Pediatric Emergency Care* 28:174–77.

Hon EH and Lee ST. 1963. Electronic evaluation of the fetal heart rate. VIII: Patterns preceding fetal death, further observations. *American Journal of Obstetrics and Gynecology* 87:814–26.

Isager T, Brinch M, Kreiner S, and Tolstrup K. 1985. Death and relapse in anorexia nervosa: Survival analysis of 151 cases. *Journal of Psychiatric Research* 19:515–21.

Isner JM, Roberts WC, Heymsfield SB, and Yager J. 1985. Anorexia nervosa and sudden death. *Annals of Internal Medicine* 102:49–52.

Ji J, Sundquist J, and Sundquist K. 2016. Association between anorexia nervosa and type 2 diabetes in Sweden: Etiological clue for the primary prevention of type 2 diabetes. *Endocrine Research* 23:1–7.

Kanbur NO, Goldberg E, Pinhas L, Hamilton RM, Clegg R, and Katzman DK. 2009. Second-degree atrioventricular block (Mobitz Type I) in an adolescent with anorexia nervosa: Intrinsic or acquired conduction abnormality. *International Journal of Eating Disorders* 42:575–78.

Kircher JN, Park MH, Cheezum MK, et al. 2012. Cardiac tamponade in association with anorexia nervosa: A case report and review of the literature. *Cardiology Journal* 19:635–38.

Kleiger RE, Miller JP, Bigger JT Jr, and Moss AJ. 1987. Decreased heart rate variability and its association with increased mortality after acute myocardial infarction. *American Journal of Cardiology* 59:25–262.

Koschke M, Boettger MK, Macholdt C, Schulz S, Yeragani VK, Voss A, and Bar KJ. 2010. Increased QT variability in patients with anorexia nervosa: An indicator for increased cardiac mortality? *International Journal of Eating Disorders.* 43(8): 743–50.

Kossaify A. 2010. Management of sinus node dysfunction with junctional escape rhythm in a case of anorexia nervosa. *Turk Kardiyoloji Dernegi Arsivi* 38:486–88.

Krantz MJ, Donahoo WT, Melanson EL, and Mehler PS. 2005. QT interval dispersion and resting metabolic rate in chronic anorexia nervosa. *International Journal of Eating Disorders* 37:166–70.

Krantz MJ, Gaudiani JL, Johnson VW, and Mehler PS. 2011. Exercise electrocardiography extinguishes persistent junctional rhythm in a patient with severe anorexia nervosa. *Cardiology* 120(4):217–20.

Krantz MJ and Mehler PS. 2004. Resting tachycardia, a warning sign in anorexia nervosa: Case report. *BMC Cardiovascular Disorders* 4:10.

Krantz MJ, Sabel AL, Sagar U, et al. 2012. Factors influencing QT prolongation in patients hospitalized with severe anorexia nervosa. *General Hospital Psychiatry* 34:173–77.

Lamzabi I, Syed S, Reddy VB, Jain R, Harbhajanka A, and Arunkumar P. 2015. Myocardial changes in a patient with anorexia nervosa: A case report and review of literature. *American Journal of Clinical Pathology* 143:734–37.

Mazurak N, Enck P, Muth E, Teufel M, and Zipfel S. 2011. Heart rate variability as a measure of cardiac autonomic function in anorexia nervosa: A review of the literature. *European Eating Disorders Review* 19:87–99.

Mehler PS, Lezotte D, and Eckel R. 1998. Lipid levels in anorexia nervosa. *International Journal of Eating Disorders* 24:217–21.

Melanson EL, Donahoo WT, Krantz MJ, Poirier P, and Mehler PS. 2004. Resting and ambulatory heart rate variability in chronic anorexia nervosa. *American Journal of Cardiology* 94:1217–20.

Mont L, Castro J, Herreros B, et al. 2003. Reversibility of cardiac abnormalities in adolescents with anorexia nervosa after weight recovery. *Journal of the American Academy of Child and Adolescent Psychiatry* 42:808–13.

Nakai Y, Fujita M, Nin K, Noma S, and Teramukai S. 2015. Relationship between duration of illness and cardiac autonomic nervous activity in anorexia nervosa. *Biopsychosocial Medicine* 9:12.

Oflaz S, Yucel B, Oz F, et al. 2013. Assessment of myocardial damage by cardiac MRI in patients with anorexia nervosa. *International Journal of Eating Disorders* 46: 862–66.

Rechlin T, Weis M, Ott C, Bleichner F, and Joraschky P. 1998. Alterations of autonomic cardiac control in anorexia nervosa. *Biological Psychiatry* 43:358–63.

Sachs KV, Harnke B, Krantz MJ, and Mehler PS. 2016. Cardiovascular complications of anorexia nervosa: A systematic review. *International Journal of Eating Disorders.* 49(3):238–48.

Shamim T, Golden NH, Arden M, Filiberto L, and Shenker IR. 2003. Resolution of vital sign instability: An objective measure of medical stability in anorexia nervosa. *Journal of Adolescent Health* 32:73–77.

Stone NJ, Robinson JG, Lichtenstein AH, et al. 2014. 2013 ACC/AHA guideline on the treatment of blood cholesterol to reduce atherosclerotic cardiovascular risk in adults: A report of the American College of Cardiology/American Heart Association Task Force on Practice Guidelines. *Circulation* 129(25 Suppl 2):S1–45.

Weinbrenner T, Zuger M, Jacoby GE, et al. 2004. Lipoprotein metabolism in patients with anorexia nervosa: A case-control study investigating the mechanisms leading to hypercholesterolaemia. *British Journal of Nutrition* 91:959–69.

8

Obstetric-Gynecologic Endocrinology and Osteoporosis

Philip S. Mehler, MD

Common Questions

What characteristic hypothalamic-gonadal hormonal alterations occur in patients with anorexia nervosa?

When does amenorrhea occur during the course of anorexia nervosa?

What is the relationship between weight loss and the onset of functional amenorrhea in anorexia nervosa?

What other hypothalamic hormonal responses occur in patients with anorexia nervosa? How are they similar to the hormonal responses of acute stress?

What therapeutic interventions may help treat the amenorrhea? Is such treatment important?

What body weight predicts the resumption of menses?

Do patients with a history of an eating disorder have long-term problems with pregnancy?

How common is osteoporosis in patients with eating disorders?

What are the clinical consequences of low bone mass in patients with eating disorders?

What features of eating disorders contribute to bone loss?

How is the diagnosis of osteoporosis and osteopenia made?

How is osteoporosis treated and monitored?

What therapeutic interventions are indicated to prevent bone loss and attenuate the risk of fracture?

Should all patients with anorexia nervosa who have osteoporosis be treated?

Case 1

H.M. was a 20-year-old female who presented with secondary amenorrhea. She had undergone normal puberty at age 12, initially having regular menstrual cycles. Secondary amenorrhea began at 18 years of age. Family members had typically undergone normal growth and sexual development. H.M. was "overweight" in grade school and in the first two years of high school. She expressed a dislike for obesity, as her mother and sister were "fat." Subsequently, she began markedly restricting her caloric intake and excessively exercising to achieve weight loss. In addition to the amenorrhea, she complained of cold intolerance, brittle hair, dry skin, and fatigue. H.M. weighed 100 pounds and was 5 feet 6 inches tall. Pubic hair and breast development were scant but normal. On careful questioning, she indicated that she was adhering to a strict 500-calorie-per-day diet. She exercised daily for 1–2 hours but denied self-induced vomiting. She had initiated her dieting at the age of 16; within the next 3 years, when her weight reached 104 pounds, her menstrual periods stopped. The diagnosis of anorexia nervosa was made, and she was referred to an internal medicine specialist for further evaluation.

Case 2

C.R., a 28-year-old female, was 5 feet 6 inches tall and weighed 98 pounds. She had a 12-year history of anorexia nervosa. She initially had weighed 164 pounds; after a 35% loss in body weight, she developed secondary amenorrhea. Over the course of her illness, she had lost 2 inches in height. She had recently been seen by her primary care provider for evaluation of low back pain. X-rays showed an L2 compression fracture, which a radiologist interpreted to be of recent onset. C.R. had never had a bone density test and was referred for evaluation of her medical status.

Background

People with anorexia nervosa may present with an extremely complex medical disorder resulting from the sociocultural pressures for thinness and attractiveness. The result is numerous psychoneuroendocrine-nutritional medical stresses as the patient relentlessly pursues thinness. Female patients with anorexia nervosa experience marked weight loss with resultant amenorrhea, which is defined as having missed at least three consecutive menstrual cycles.

Gynecologic Effects of Anorexia Nervosa

The Menstrual Cycle

The neuroendocrine regulation of normal female reproductive functions depends on a rhythm of nerve impulses generated within the medial basal hypothalamus, which governs the pulsatile release of gonadotropin-releasing hormone (GnRH) from nerve terminals. Pulsatile GnRH release is the central controller of pituitary luteinizing hormone (LH) and follicle-stimulating hormone (FSH) secretions, which determine the onset of normal menstrual function (Doufas and Mastorakos, 2000). At puberty, an increase in both the frequency and the amplitude of GnRH induces LH-FSH secretion. Patients with anorexia nervosa, however, have a characteristic "hypothalamic amenorrhea syndrome" with a variable reduction in pulsatile hypothalamic GnRH gonadostat signaling to the pituitary gland, resulting in a failure of ovulation. The degree of impairment varies among patients, but in general, the frequency and amplitude of the LH-FSH pulses are diminished in anorexia nervosa, with reversion to a prepubertal pattern and development of the commonly found amenorrheic state. Thus, this functional hypogonadotropic, hypogonadism-induced amenorrhea in anorexia nervosa reflects a temporary, reversible disturbance of hypothalamic-pituitary function (Singhal, Misra, and Klibanski, 2014). Moreover, most amenorrhea in patients with anorexia nervosa is of the secondary type, meaning that the individual previously had normal menstrual periods; this is in contrast to primary amenorrhea, in which there is no onset of menses.

Of female patients with anorexia nervosa, 20%–25% may experience amenorrhea before the onset of significant weight loss, and 60%–85% will experience amenorrhea during the course of dieting and its associated weight loss (El Ghoch, Bazzani, and Dalle Grave, 2014). Some patients experience amenorrhea only after more marked weight loss. This variability explains why amenorrhea was dropped as a criterion for the diagnosis of anorexia nervosa by DSM-5 (American Psychiatric Association, 2013). Menstrual irregularities are also common in bulimia nervosa, albeit much less severe and less prevalent than in anorexia nervosa (Gendall et al., 2000). On restoring weight toward normal, many patients will have resumption of their normal menstrual cycle. More than 40 years ago, Frisch and McArthur (1974) noted a critical relationship between body mass index (BMI), body fat, percentage of body weight loss, and the occurrence of amenorrhea. This relationship was confirmed more recently in a study demonstrating that menses can be expected to resume at a weight that exceeds 90%–93% of ideal body weight (Golden et al., 1997). Other studies have found the weight requirement for resumption of menses to be more variable and better predicted by the weight at which menstruation ceased (Swenne, 2004). A more recent cohort study of 56 adolescent females found a return of menses at a mean BMI percentile of 27 (Golden et al., 2008).

Despite these relationships, features other than weight loss may also be causing the amenorrhea. Given that the onset of amenorrhea can precede significant weight loss in about one-quarter of these women, that amenorrhea persists even after weight restoration in some women, and that menstruation resumes in some women despite a low body weight (Miller et al., 2004b), other factors may also promote this process. These factors include adaptive hormonal responses to sociocultural-psychic stress, excessive exercise, and chronic nutritional energy deficiency (Warren et al., 2002), along with reduced thyroid hormone and leptin levels. Stress, anxiety, exercise, smoking, and abnormal eating habits may contribute. As a result of the gonadotropin failure, however, individuals with anorexia nervosa have decreased blood levels of the sex hormones (estradiol, estrone, progesterone, and testosterone) (Miller et al., 2007). Consequently, women with anorexia nervosa may not always have withdrawal bleeding in response to a diagnostic progesterone challenge, which would indicate a more profound hypothalamic-pituitary gonadotropin deficiency state.

Thus, a critical weight may be necessary but not sufficient for menstrual function, and other factors may also be of importance (Gendall et al., 2006). The variation in patterns of menstrual disturbance with anorexia nervosa is in part the basis for removal of amenorrhea as a criterion for the diagnosis of anorexia nervosa, as noted above.

Treatment of Amenorrhea

Treating a patient with functional (hypothalamic) amenorrhea is not easy. The underlying cause of the amenorrhea, as it relates to sociocultural and environmental psychic stress, needs to be evaluated and primarily addressed. Assessment for clinical or subclinical depressive illness is warranted. Also important is a detailed history concerning parental relationships, self-image, social and environmental issues, stressors, sexuality, interpersonal relationships, and support systems. Spontaneous recovery of menstrual periods may occur with correction of the eating disorder and psychopathology and with weight restoration. The corollary of this, however, is that even with weight gain, menstruation may not resume if there is persistence of the abnormal eating behaviors or psychogenic factors that, in part, initiated the cessation of menses.

The progestin challenge test is sometimes used in the evaluation of amenorrhea. It may be of value to reassure the patient with an eating disorder who is working to recover that her reproductive system is in a semi-hibernation state but is functionally intact and ready to reactivate if she can restore her weight. The patient takes 10 mg of medroxyprogesterone (Provera) daily for 5 days. Withdrawal bleeding within 10 days of progesterone administration indicates adequate estrogen levels and is consistent with functional amenorrhea. Conversely, a lack of withdrawal bleeding connotes a state of profound estrogen deficiency or other gynecologic-endocrine problems. Estrogen-progesterone therapy might be considered, but only for patients who do not have withdrawal bleeding. A serum LH level below 5 mIU/mL is indicative of hypothalamic dysfunction in patients without withdrawal bleeding.

In the clinical setting of anorexia nervosa, however, especially with excessive weight loss, the progestin challenge test is not a crucial diagnostic exercise for evaluating the commonly found amenorrhea. Rather, efforts should be directed toward overall treatment of the eating disorder because there is little inherent value in administering female sex hormones to patients with anorexia nervosa. Although withdrawal bleeding can be calming, it may also promote a false sense of well-being and minimize the urgency for engaging in therapy for the eating disorder.

Pregnancy

The presence of an active eating disorder is thought to be a relative contraindication for pregnancy and infertility treatments. When pregnancy occurs, it is more often in individuals with bulimia nervosa who have near-normal body weight, although some women with anorexia nervosa do ovulate and become pregnant despite their amenorrhea. In fact, unplanned pregnancies are a significant problem in anorexia nervosa. During the course of the pregnancy, many patients subdue their binge eating and purging behaviors. However, many will return to these behaviors in the puerperium (Easter, Treasure, and Micali, 2011). If pregnancy does occur, both the pregnancy and lactation impose a tremendous stress on the maternal skeleton for mineralization of the fetal and newborn skeleton. Hence, it is important to provide vitamin D and calcium. Pregnancy in women with an eating disorder is associated with a greater incidence of premature birth, smaller head circumference, miscarriages, and low-birthweight infants, especially if the disease is active (Pasternak et al., 2012). If women with a recent history of an eating disorder want to become pregnant, it usually is advisable both to refer them to a reproductive endocrinologist for discussion of treatment options and to ensure that they have sufficient psychiatric support to help control their abnormal eating behaviors during the pregnancy.

Pregnancy for a woman with an eating disorder is a decision that should be made only after judicious deliberation. Referral to a multidisciplinary team is critical for all these patients so that the health of the mother and the fetus are preserved to promote the best possible outcome. In the long term, after a patient recovers from anorexia nervosa or bulimia, there seems to be no adverse effect on her ability to become pregnant. In the past, fertility was believed to be permanently impaired by a history of an eating disorder, but this is not accurate. Rather, these women simply tend to seek consultation with infertility specialists. However, both sexual dysfunction and postpartum depression are more common in patients with eating disorders.

Osteoporosis in Anorexia Nervosa

Osteoporosis is a disease characterized by low bone mass and deterioration of the microarchitectural structure of bone, resulting in bone fragility and the clinical syndrome of nontraumatic fractures as a direct result of the low bone mass. *Osteoporosis* is quantitatively defined by bone densitometry measurements, using dual-energy X-ray absorptiometry (DEXA), as a T-score of −2.5 standard deviations (SD) or less at the lumbar spine, femoral neck, and total hip. A loss of bone mass with a T-score of −1 to −2.5 SD is classified as *osteopenia* (Lorenzton and Cummings, 2015). Although there are other methods of assessing bone density, DEXA is preferred for patients with anorexia nervosa. Peak bone mass is defined as the highest level of bone mass achieved as a result of normal growth. Most skeletal bone growth occurs during childhood and adolescence. The timing of peak bone mass may vary but generally occurs between ages 17 and 22, a time that, unfortunately, frequently coincides with the onset of anorexia nervosa. Rapid bone loss, at an annual average rate of 2.5%, occurs in young women with anorexia nervosa. Osteoporosis is present in almost 40% of patients with anorexia nervosa, and osteopenia is present in 92% (Grinspoon et al., 2000). Trabecular bone, found in the lumbar spine and hips, is more affected than cortical bone (Faje et al., 2013). Of note, T-scores from DEXA scans should be used for adults, as opposed to Z-scores. The latter score is used for pediatric patients, for whom, due to the continuing growth in bone size, it is necessary to adjust bone mineral density according to the average values for age and sex. Also, the term *osteopenia* is best limited to adults.

Achieving an optimal peak bone mass depends on heredity and lifestyle factors. Lifestyle influences causing less than optimal peak bone mass may be nutritional, such as low calcium or low phosphate intake, a diet low in animal protein, excessive intake of carbonated dark soda-type drinks, a high-sodium diet, high caffeine intake, or a strictly vegetarian diet. Other lifestyle influences that have deleterious effects on bone mass include cigarette smoking, a low level of physical activity, and alcohol consumption. Weight-bearing exercise usually promotes skeletal development and an increase in bone mineral density through beneficial effects on skeletal microarchitecture, but when exercise is excessive—as in the athletic amenorrhea syndrome seen in female runners—and especially at low body weight, it may be associated with low bone mass and fractures. Weight-bearing exercise may be protective only if menstruation is preserved and only at normal body weight.

Factors Influencing Bone Remodeling

Whether an individual achieves peak adult bone mass depends on the time of onset, type, and duration of the eating disorder, the degree of nutritional depletion, changes in body composition, and the stress associated with anorexia nervosa. Bulimia nervosa per se is not a risk factor for low bone density. Once amenorrhea is present in anorexia nervosa, the estrogen-progesterone deficiency plays a role in arresting bone development and promoting deleterious bone resorption. The longer the duration of amenorrhea, the higher is the risk of osteoporosis (Baker, Roberts, and Towell, 2000).

Anorexia nervosa appears to be a low-turnover state characterized by both increased bone resorption and decreased bone formation, in contradistinction to postmenopausal osteoporosis. This imbalance or uncoupling contributes to the rapid and aggressive bone loss in individuals with anorexia nervosa. In addition to the hypothalamic hypogonadal state noted above, these patients have excess hydrocortisone secretion, low IGF-1 (insulin-like growth factor 1; somatomedin C) levels, and low androgen levels. Low levels of IGF-1 reduce the levels of osteocalcin and cause abnormalities in the osteoblasts, the bone-building cells. These low levels of IGF-1, despite increased growth hormone levels, are known to be a major correlate of low bone formation in anorexia nervosa, in contrast to the high levels of IGF-1 typically found in healthy adolescents. The elevated levels of cortisol are also inversely related to levels of osteocalcin (Misra et al., 2004). All of these factors, in addition to estrogen and androgen deficiency, are likely to promote the development of osteoporosis, and they render the osteoporosis associated with anorexia a unique clinical entity (Miller et al., 2007). Markers of bone resorption such as N-teleopeptide and deoxypyridinoline are higher in patients with anorexia nervosa, while markers of bone formation such as osteocalcin are not concomitantly elevated. This pattern is most closely analogous to steroid-induced osteoporosis. However, serum levels of calcium, vitamin D, and parathyroid hormone are all within the normal range. Body weight (especially fat cell mass) and muscle strength are positive predictors of bone mineral density in young women. Patients with anorexia nervosa have an altered body composition with depleted fat stores. In addition, in females, the fat cell is capable of independent estrogen synthesis from adrenal androgen precursors. A total body fat cell mass of at least 8% is generally needed for normal menstrual function. A lower BMI and longer duration of illness both predict lower bone mineral density (Misra, 2008).

Individuals with anorexia nervosa may be intensively involved in rigorous exercise programs, contributing to their secondary amenorrhea. Secondary amenorrhea is common in many young women who continually pursue high levels of physical activities such as running, ballet dancing, cycling, and swimming. The "female triad" seen in competitive female athletes is characterized by disordered eating, menstrual irregularity, and osteoporosis (Matzkin, Curry, and Whitlock, 2015). Osteoporosis and a tendency to develop stress fractures are also associated with menstrual irregularity in these women. Young estrogen-deficient women may lose bone mass at a rate as high as 3%–5% per year.

Diagnosis

An assessment of bone mineral density is easily obtained with a DEXA scan, which allows a reliable and highly precise measurement of skeletal bone mineral content in the lumbar spine and hip. For every 1 SD decrement in bone mineral content of the lumbar spine, the fracture risk of an individual is increased twofold. Likewise, for the hip, for every decrement in bone mineral content of 1 SD, the attributable fracture risk is elevated 2.5 times. Currently, DEXA is the gold standard for assessing bone mineral content, both in a screening mode and for monitoring bone density in patients with anorexia nervosa undergoing therapy for established osteoporosis. A DEXA scan should be obtained for all individuals with a 9- to 12-month history of anorexia nervosa. They should also have a follow-up DEXA scan every 2 years while the disease is active. Patients with bulimia nervosa do not require routine DEXA scans unless a past history of anorexia nervosa is elicited. Males with anorexia nervosa are also at increased risk for loss of bone density, and this elevated risk needs to be considered when treating this less common population of patients (Mehler, Sabel, and Andersen, 2008).

Onset of Bone Disease

Emerging evidence suggests that loss of bone mineral density is rapid and occurs relatively early in anorexia nervosa. Some studies suggest that an illness duration longer than 12 months predicts significant loss of bone mineral (Wong et al., 2001). In a study of 73 female patients with a mean age of 17.2 years, 20 months of amenorrhea was found to be the threshold above which the most severe osteopenia was seen (Audi et al., 2002). A longer duration of amenorrhea and later menarchal age both predict more extensive loss of bone mineral density (Maimoun et al., 2014).

Increased risk for future fracture in these young patients is a major concern, especially because fracture risk is known to double with each decrease of 1 SD in bone mineral density. Therefore, DEXA should be established as an important screening tool for all patients with disease duration greater than 9–12 months to determine the degree of reduction of bone mineral density. Moreover, there may be a psychotherapeutic benefit in providing individuals with their objective DEXA results as graphic visual evidence that they are at risk for serious medical problems due to their bone loss. Positive changes in unhealthy eating behaviors can perhaps be achieved by showing these patients that they have the same bone density as very old individuals, thus motivating them to more fully engage in treatment (Stoffman et al., 2005). However, there is a lack of definitive scientific evidence on when exactly to order the DEXA scan for patients with anorexia nervosa. Finally, although the value of repeating DEXA measurements 2 years after the initial scan for women with postmenopausal osteoporosis has been challenged, for individuals with anorexia nervosa, a repeat scan should be performed 2 years later—especially if the illness is ongoing or a therapeutic intervention for the bone density loss has been initiated or is being considered (Hillier et al., 2007).

Treatment

Both prevention and treatment of low bone density in anorexia nervosa are critical because, of all the potential medical complications of this eating disorder, this may be one that is never completely treatable. Moreover, young patients with osteoporosis resulting from anorexia nervosa have lifelong increased risks of fractures, in the range of 60% higher, even after their anorexia nervosa has been successfully treated. Weight gain, resumption of menses, and adequate calcium and vitamin D intake are the main focus for those who have either low normal bone density or osteopenia. More definitive treatment is reserved for osteoporosis.

HORMONAL THERAPY

Supplemental estrogen in the form of hormone replacement therapy or oral contraceptives is often prescribed in routine practice for female patients with anorexia nervosa, in an effort to minimize or ameliorate osteopenia or osteoporosis. Surveys indicate that this inappropriate practice is still common among practitioners caring for these patients. In reality, however, there is a distinct paucity of credible evidence supporting this practice (Mehler and MacKenzie, 2009). Early and small retrospective studies seemed to imply that oral contraceptives may attenuate loss of bone mineral density in anorexia nervosa, presumably by impeding osteoclast-mediated resorption of bone. However, there have been only two randomized controlled trials of estrogen therapy in anorexia nervosa. The first, a widely cited older study, demonstrated that estrogen treatment did not prevent a reduction in trabecular bone mineral density (Klibanski et al., 1995). A more recent prospective observational trial included 50 adolescents with anorexia nervosa. After 2 years of treatment, the group that received 35 mg of ethinyl estradiol, in addition to calcium supplementation, did not show any increase in bone mineral density compared with the group that received standard treatment. In this study, osteopenia was persistent, and in some cases was progressive despite estrogen therapy (Golden et al., 2002).

This lack of a beneficial effect from hormone therapy for bone mineral density in anorexia nervosa has been confirmed in other studies. An analytic survey including 130 women with anorexia nervosa examined four patient subgroups: (1) estrogen used in the past or the present, (2) estrogen never used, (3) estrogen currently used, and (4) estrogen used in the past but not currently. Spine and hip bone density was similar in all four subsets of women despite the differences in estrogen therapy (Grinspoon et al., 2000). An additional practical reason to refrain from using hormonal therapy is that it may cause resumption of menses, which may give the patient a false sense of being cured and reinforce denial in those who are still at a low weight.

Despite the clear evidence that hormonal therapy is effective in maintaining bone density in postmenopausal women by impairing osteoclast-mediated bone resorption, it is increasingly appreciated that health care providers should not continue to extrapolate from the therapeutic success in this patient group to patients with anorexia nervosa, for whom estrogen's effect on bone density has been disappointing. The postmenopausal and anorectic states are very different with regard to loss of bone density. The low estrogen levels that characterize the postmenopausal state and cause bone resorption can be effectively mitigated by the potent antiresorptive effects of estrogen replacement therapy. In contrast, the unique uncoupling of osteoblastic and osteoclastic functions in anorexia nervosa, which results in reduced bone formation concurrent with increased resorption, cannot be successfully treated with estrogen. Oral estrogen replacement therapy should not be viewed as evidence-based treatment at this time. Estrogen therapy may be necessary but seems to be insufficient to reverse the profound osteopenia or to promote adequate bone accretion for patients with malnutrition, low levels of circulating bone trophic factors such as IGF-I, excess cortisol, and decreased androgen production. More recently, there is some emerging evidence that transdermal estrogen with cyclic progesterone may be of utility in treating the osteoporosis of anorexia nervosa, but is probably not fully restorative.

Most approved therapies for osteoporosis inhibit bone resorption. Another approach is anabolic therapy, in which bone formation is directly stimulated. This seems prudent in anorexia nervosa, given that this illness is also characterized by decreased bone formation. DHEA (dehydroepiandrosterone) has not proved effective in improving bone mineral density, even though it is thought to function as an anabolic factor for bone by increasing levels of IGF-1 and by stimulating osteoblast function. Similarly, transdermal testosterone has not been shown to significantly increase markers of bone formation such as osteocalcin and bone-specific alkaline phosphatase in women with anorexia nervosa. There are no rigorous scientific trials providing data on other anabolic agents such as fluoride. However, the recently released synthetic parathyroid hormone medication teriparatide, which has desirable and unique anabolic properties, may become a treatment option, based on the promising results of a placebo-controlled trial. Caution should be exercised before using this medication for adolescents with open epiphyses or those with Paget's disease, due to a risk of osteosarcoma. Its other drawbacks are cost and the need for a daily injection.

BISPHOSPHONATES

In view of the less-than-favorable effects of commonly used therapeutic modalities for the bone disease of anorexia nervosa and the potential permanence of the low bone mineral density, there has been interest in the use of bisphosphonates. Past reticence to use these agents was predicated on concerns about their safety for women of reproductive age. Bisphosphonates, which inhibit bone remodeling, carry a category C rating for safety in pregnancy because they can persist in the body for many years after discontinuation of treatment, and there is only anecdotal information about their safety during fetal development. Thus, the long-term implications for women of childbearing age are of concern. Little information is available concerning infants born to mothers who regularly took bisphosphonates before pregnancy. On the other hand, the known effectiveness of bisphosphonates in decreasing bone resorption and increasing bone mineral density in postmenopausal women with osteopenia has raised interest in bisphosphonates as a treatment for patients with anorexia nervosa. Oral bisphosphonates, now available in generic form, are used in weekly or monthly doses. They cannot be taken by patients with renal insufficiency or patients with significant esophageal disease.

The first study to demonstrate the potential effectiveness of bisphosphonates was a closely monitored study of women with anorexia nervosa who received 5 mg of risedronate and had bone mineral density measurements at 6 and 9 months. Bone mineral density increased substantially in the spines of the patients who received risedronate (4.1% at 6 months), in contrast to bone loss in the controls despite weight gain (Miller et al., 2004a). A 5% increase in bone mass over a 3-year period is generally deemed clinically significant and is associated with a robust 25% reduction in fracture risk. No significant side effects were reported. The following year, a randomized, double-blind, placebo-controlled pilot study of alendronate was completed, including 32 patients with anorexia nervosa who had osteopenia. Mineral density in the spine and hip bone increased in both the treatment and the control groups, and the percentage increase did not differ significantly between groups (Golden et al., 2005). Markers of bone resorption and formation did not undergo significant change. Once again, the bisphosphonate was well tolerated. In fact, bisphosphonates have been used for years for adolescent patients with osteogenesis imperfecta to increase bone density, with no reports of significant adverse events.

Bisphosphonates should not be used casually for younger female patients with anorexia nervosa until further research defines their long-term safety and efficacy. There are also concerns about osteonecrosis of the jaw and atypical femur fractures with the use of these medications that need to be considered (Molvik and Kahn, 2015). However, they should be considered for more severe cases of osteoporosis, especially when the disease is unlikely to revert in the near future. They may also have a role for male patients with anorexia nervosa who have normal serum testosterone levels, given their known efficacy in osteoporosis in men, without the concern about teratogenesis (Ebeling, 2008). There are no credible studies using calcitonin or raloxifene for patients with anorexia nervosa.

WEIGHT GAIN

The cornerstone of treatment for individuals who have anorexia nervosa is weight restoration. Unfortunately, anorexia nervosa is often a protracted illness. Factors found to be predictive of a poor prognosis include a longer duration of illness, older age at onset, and weight loss that is persistent and is a higher percentage below ideal body weight (Winston, Alwazeer, and Bankart, 2008). The direct effect of weight gain on bone density is not as clearly beneficial. Studies have yielded conflicting results on the reversibility of the demineralization. Some earlier reports about recovery suggest that restoration of normal bone mass occurs with recovery from anorexia nervosa (Wentz et al., 2003). An annualized rate of increase of 3%–4% in bone mineral density, attributed solely to weight gain, was demonstrated in other studies of patients fully recovered from anorexia nervosa (Zipfel et al., 2001). Many studies, however, demonstrate that bone density may never be fully recoverable. One study confirms that despite weight gain, bone mineral density did not return to baseline after one year (Misra et al., 2004). This abnormal bone mineral accrual in patients who have recovered from anorexia nervosa may persist despite normalization of bone turnover markers and an increase in IGF-1 (Soyka et al., 2002). Of note, selective serotonin reuptake inhibitors might be associated with lower bone mineral density in anorexia nervosa.

OTHER MEDICAL THERAPIES

Denosumab is a recent addition to the medications for the treatment of osteoporosis. It is the first biologic therapy approved to treat osteoporosis and has a very distinct mechanism of action. While it may be of future utility, there are not yet any credible studies of its use for patients with anorexia nervosa—but it is an appealing treatment given the need to receive only one injection every 6 months. Similarly, there are no studies of testosterone use for males with anorexia nervosa, but it may be reasonable to try if the serum level is low, given the hormone's known anabolic effects.

CALCIUM

Current recommendations suggest that adults ingest 1,200 mg of calcium a day with 800 IU of vitamin D to achieve peak bone mass. Calcium requirements are known to increase during periods of rapid growth.

Dietary calcium and vitamin D deficiency are prevalent even in healthy adolescent girls and certainly in those with anorexia nervosa (Modan-Moses et al., 2015). Although necessary, however, calcium is not sufficient by itself to prevent loss of bone mineral density, nor are calcium and vitamin D major contributing factors to restoration of bone mineral content in anorexia nervosa.

EXERCISE

While weight-bearing exercises are known to be beneficial for older people to maintain healthy bones, this is not so for younger people during their anorexia nervosa illness. Aside from the predictable interference with desired weight gain, exercise may actually be deleterious to the microarchitecture of bone while a person is amenorrheic or still at low body weight.

Summary

Significant bone loss occurs among young patients with anorexia nervosa. Because body weight is the most important determinant of bone density, the optimal intervention is one that promotes weight restoration early in the course of the illness, before bone mineral loss has occurred. Once bone mineral is lost, the effect of weight restoration on bone density is variable. Moreover, most tested treatments for osteoporosis, including those such as estrogen therapy that are undeniably effective for postmenopausal women, have proved ineffective for individuals with anorexia nervosa. Because so few studies have been done on bisphosphonates, the possibility of effectiveness has not been excluded. More randomized clinical trials are needed to focus on combined anabolic/antiresorptive strategies, medications able to increase osteoblast function (including teriparatide), and bisphosphonates to prevent bone loss in young women with anorexia nervosa. But, because the bone quality is likely to be much better in a young patient with anorexia nervosa than in the postmenopausal population, judicious deliberation with patients is necessary as medications are considered. Because of the long-term increased risk of fracture in this young population of patients, there is a compelling need to define an effective and safe treatment to both prevent and reverse bone loss. Prevention, however, remains a key intervention. Therefore, identifying the patient who has anorexia and starting effective treatment before she has suffered irreparable loss of bone density are of utmost importance, while more research is performed to define the ideal treatment approach.

REFERENCES

American Psychiatric Association. 2013. *Diagnostic and Statistical Manual of Mental Disorders, 5th Edition: DSM-5*. Arlington, VA: American Psychiatric Association.

Audi L, Vargas DM, Gussinye M, Yeste D, Marti G, and Carrascosa A. 2002. Clinical and biochemical determinants of bone metabolism and bone mass in adolescent female patients with anorexia nervosa. *Pediatric Research* 51:497–504.

Baker D, Roberts R, and Towell T. 2000. Factors predictive of bone mineral density in eating-disordered women: A longitudinal study. *International Journal of Eating Disorders* 27:29–35.

Doufas AG and Mastorakos G. 2000. The hypothalamic-pituitary-thyroid axis and the female reproductive system. *Annals of the New York Academy of Science* 960:65–76.

Easter A, Treasure J, and Micali N. 2011. Fertility and perinatal attitudes towards pregnancy in women with eating disorders. *British Journal of Obstetrics and Gynecology* 118:1491–98.

Ebeling PR. 2008. Osteoporosis in men. *New England Journal of Medicine* 358:1474–82.

El Ghoch, Bazzani P, and Dalle Grave R. 2014. Management of ischiopubic stress fracture in patients with anorexia nervosa and excessive compulsive exercising. *BMJ Case Reports* Oct 9.

Faje AT, Karmin L, Taylor A, et al. 2013. Adolescent girls with anorexia nervosa have impaired cortical and trabecular microarchitecture and lower estimated bone strength at the distal radius. *Journal of Clinical Endocrinology and Metabolism* 98:1923–29.

Frisch RE and McArthur JW. 1974. Menstrual cycle: Fatness as a determinant of minimum weight for height necessary for maintenance or onset. *Science* 185:949–51.

Gendall KA, Bulik CM, Joyce PR, Mcintosh VV, and Carter FA. 2000. Menstrual cycle irregularity in bulimia nervosa. *Journal of Psychosomatic Research* 49:409–15.

Gendall KA, Joyce PR, Carter FA, Mcintosh VV, Jordan J, and Bulik CM. 2006. The psychobiology and diagnostic significance of amenorrhea in patients with anorexia nervosa. *Fertility and Sterility* 85:1531–35.

Golden NH, Jacobson MS, Schebendach J, Solanto MV, Hertz SM, and Shenker IR. 1997. Resumption of menses in anorexia nervosa. *Archives of Pediatrics and Adolescent Medicine* 151:16–21.

Golden NH, Lanzkowsky L, Schebendach J, Palestro CJ, Jacobson MS, and Shenker IR. 2002. The effect of estrogen-progestin treatment on bone mineral density in anorexia nervosa. *Journal of Pediatric and Adolescent Gynecology* 15:135–43.

Golden NH, Iglesias EA, Jacobson MS, et al. 2005. Alendronate for the treatment of osteopenia in anorexia nervosa: A randomized, double-blind, placebo-controlled trial. *Journal of Clinical Endocrinology and Metabolism* 90:3179–85.

Golden NH, Jacobson MS, Sterling WM, and Hertz J. 2008. Treatment goal weight in adolescents with anorexia nervosa: Use of BMI percentiles. *International Journal of Eating Disorders* 41:301–6.

Grinspoon S, Thomas E, Pitts S, et al. 2000. Prevalence and predictive factors for regional osteopenia in women with anorexia nervosa. *Annals of Internal Medicine* 133:790–94.

Hillier TZ, Stone KL, Bauer DC, et al. 2007. Evaluating the value of repeat bone mineral density measurement and prediction of fracture in older women. *Archives of Internal Medicine* 167:155–60.

Klibanski A, Biller BMK, Schoenfeld DA, Herzog DB, and Saxe VC. 1995. The effects of estrogen administration on trabecular bone loss in young women with anorexia nervosa. *Journal of Clinical Endocrinology and Metabolism* 80:898–904.

Lorenzton M and Cummings SR. 2015. Osteoporosis: The evolution of diagnosis. *Journal of Internal Medicine* 277:650–61.

Maimoun L, Guillaume S, Lefebvre P, et al. 2014. Role of sclerostin and dickkopf-1 in the dramatic alteration in bone mass acquisition in adolescents and young women with recent anorexia nervosa. *Journal of Clinical Endocrinology and Metabolism* 99:E582–90.

Matzkin E, Curry EJ, and Whitlock K. 2015. Female athlete triad: Past, present and future. *Journal of the American Academy of Orthopedic Surgeons* 23:424–32.

Mehler PS and MacKenzie TD. 2009. Treatment of osteopenia and osteoporosis in anorexia nervosa: A systematic review of the literature. *International Journal of Eating Disorders* 42:195–201.

Mehler PS, Sabel A, and Andersen AE. 2008. Male osteoporosis in anorexia nervosa. *International Journal of Eating Disorders* 41:666–72.

Miller K, Grieco KA, Mulder J, et al. 2004a. Effects of risedronate on bone density in anorexia nervosa. *Journal of Clinical Endocrinology and Metabolism* 89:3903–6.

Miller K, Grinspoon S, Gleysteen S, Grieco K, Ciampa J, and Breur J. 2004b. Preservation of neuroendocrine control of reproductive function despite severe under-nutrition. *Journal of Clinical Endocrinology and Metabolism* 89:4434–38.

Miller K, Lawson EA, Mathur V, et al. 2007. Androgens in women with anorexia nervosa and normal-weight women with hypothalamic amenorrhea. *Journal of Clinical Endocrinology and Metabolism* 92:1334–39.

Misra M. 2008. Long-term skeletal effects of eating disorders with onset in adolescence. *Annals of the New York Academy of Sciences* 1135:212–28.

Misra M, Miller K, Almazan C, et al. 2004. Alterations in cortisol secretory dynamics in adolescent girls with anorexia nervosa. *Journal of Clinical Endocrinology and Metabolism* 89:4972–80.

Modan-Moses D, Levy-Shraga Y, Pinhas-Hamiel O, et al. 2015. High prevalence of vitamin D deficiency and insufficiency in adolescent inpatients diagnosed with eating disorders. *International Journal of Eating Disorders* 48:607–14.

Molvik H and Kahn W. 2015. Bisphosphonates and their influence on fracture healing: A systematic review. *Osteoporosis International* 26:1251–60.

Pasternak Y, Weintraub AY, Shoham-Vard I, et al. 2012. Obstetric and perinatal outcome in women with eating disorders. *Journal of Women's Health* 21:61–65.

Singhal V, Misra M, and Klibanski A. 2014. Endocrinology of anorexia nervosa in young people: Recent insights. *Current Opinion in Endocrinology, Diabetes, and Obesity* 21:64–70.

Soyka LA, Misra M, Frenchman A, et al. 2002. Abnormal bone mineral accrual in adolescent girls with anorexia nervosa. *Journal of Clinical Endocrinology and Metabolism* 87:4177–85.

Stoffman N, Schwartz B, Austin SB, Grace E, and Gordon CM. 2005. Influence of bone density results on adolescents with anorexia nervosa. *International Journal of Eating Disorders* 37:250–55.

Swenne I. 2004. Weight requirements for return of menstruation in teenage girls with eating disorders, weight loss and secondary amenorrhea. *Acta Paediatrica* 93:1449–55.

Warren MP, Brooks-Gunn J, Jox RP, Holderness CC, Hyle EP, and Hamilton WG. 2002. Osteopenia in exercise-induced amenorrhea using ballet dancers as a model: A longitudinal study. *Journal of Clinical Endocrinology and Metabolism* 87:3162–68.

Wentz E, Mellstrom D, Gillberg C, Sundh V, Gillberg IC, and Rastam M. 2003. Bone density 11 years after anorexia nervosa onset in a controlled study of 39 cases. *International Journal of Eating Disorders* 34:314–18.

Winston AP, Alwazeer AEF, and Bankart MJG. 2008. Screening for osteoporosis in anorexia nervosa: Prevalence and predictors of reduced bone density. *International Journal of Eating Disorders* 41:284–87.

Wong JC, Lewindon P, Mortimer R, and Shepherd R. 2001. Bone mineral density in adolescent females with recently diagnosed anorexia nervosa. *International Journal of Eating Disorders* 29:11–16.

Zipfel S, Seibel MJ, Lowe B, Beumont PJ, Kasperk C, and Herzog W. 2001. Osteoporosis in eating disorders: A follow-up study of patients with anorexia and bulimia nervosa. *Journal of Clinical Endocrinology and Metabolism* 86:5227–33.

9

General Endocrinology

Philip S. Mehler, MD

Common Questions

Are there routine endocrine blood tests that should be ordered in the initial assessment of patients with eating disorders?

Why are some thyroid hormone levels often low in patients with anorexia nervosa?

What is the significance of a low fasting blood sugar in patients with anorexia nervosa?

What is the etiology and significance of hypercortisolism (elevated cortisol levels) in patients with anorexia nervosa?

Is there a role for growth hormone in the treatment of anorexia nervosa?

What are the levels of appetite hormones in anorexia nervosa?

Case

G.L. was a 30-year-old woman with anorexia nervosa. At an earlier assessment, in 2010, when she reported constipation, her thyroid-stimulating hormone (TSH) level was 2.5 mIU/L; in 2011, when she reported fatigue, it was 3.5 mIU/L. Both are in the normal range (0.27–4.2 mIU/L). A repeated TSH measurement in 2012, when she reported a family history of "thyroid problems," was slightly elevated (5.8 mIU/L). In 2013, she reported fatigue; her TSH level (5.9 mIU/L) was similar to the 2012 measurement, and her free thyroxine (T4) was normal (0.93 ng/dL). Given the stability of her TSH level, treatment was not initiated. More recently, she reported intermittent constipation and persistent fatigue.

At a recent periodic health examination, G.L.'s blood pressure was 136/79 mm Hg and her heart rate was 57 beats per minute. Her weight had increased by 9 pounds, to 100 pounds (BMI 15.7). Findings on her thyroid examination were normal. A repeated TSH measurement was 6.5 mIU/mL, and free T4 was 1.0 ng/dL. She wondered whether she should begin thyroid replacement therapy to help her metabolism as she continued her attempts at weight restoration.

Background

People with anorexia nervosa have a number of abnormalities in neuroendocrine function. The hypothalamic amenorrhea that almost universally accompanies this disorder (see chapter 8) represents one common manifestation of hypothalamic dysfunction (Miller, 2013). Another is that, although secretion rates of cortisol (an adrenal gland steroid) are generally normal, metabolic clearance rates are decreased in anorexia nervosa, with the result that the half-life of cortisol may be prolonged in malnourished individuals. The normal circadian rhythm of cortisol and pituitary adrenocorticotropic hormone secretion is not disrupted in anorexia, but serum cortisol levels are not suppressed after the administration of dexamethasone as would normally be expected. Recent studies suggest that hypercortisolism develops in individuals with anorexia nervosa because of hypersecretion of corticotrophin-releasing hormone from the hypothalamus. The pituitary seems to respond normally to regular feedback from glucocorticoids, suggesting a defect at or above the hypothalamus that causes the elevated cortisol levels. The clinical significance of this elevated cortisol is unknown, but it may play an adverse role in the aggressive loss of bone density noted in anorexia nervosa, and it may facilitate the physiologic stress response to chronic starvation (Usdan, Khaodhiar, and Apovian, 2008). However, these patients do not develop signs of Cushing's syndrome, given their low baseline levels of adipose tissue.

Hormonal Abnormalities

Growth Hormone

Alterations in growth hormone (GH), insulin-like growth factor 1 (IGF-1), and growth hormone binding protein (GHBP) are not as well understood as the abnormalities in the hypothalamic-pituitary-adrenal axis. Levels of IGF-1 are decreased in anorexia and improve with weight recovery

(Golden et al., 1994). Yet, fasting GH levels in anorexia may be normal or elevated, while serum GHBP is low, indicative of GH resistance due to starvation. Serum GHBP levels correlate well with body mass index, suggesting that nutritional deprivation may downregulate the GH receptor causing this resistance and that this effect is reversible with refeeding. Administration of IGF-1 to patients with anorexia has been shown to increase markers of bone turnover, but the effect of chronic administration on weight gain or bone metabolism has not been tested (Grinspoon et al., 2002). Thus, IGF-1 does not currently have a role in the treatment of anorexia nervosa, nor does GH, even for arrested linear growth and short stature in young patients with anorexia nervosa. There is no reason, then, for regularly measuring GH or IGF-1 levels.

Thyroid

The thyroid abnormalities in individuals with anorexia nervosa resemble those of the euthyroid sick syndrome, in which total thyroxine (T4) and triiodothyronine (T3) levels are low. The key, however, is that in euthyroid sick syndrome TSH usually remains in the normal range (LeFevre, 2015). Levels of T3 usually decrease in proportion to the degree of weight loss. Total T4 levels are low because T4 is preferentially converted to a biologically inactive reverse T3. These changes reduce the metabolic rate and conserve limited resources in the starved state. As is true for the euthyroid sick syndrome, thyroid hormone replacement is not beneficial and is actually contraindicated. Only when a high TSH and a low T4 persist after several weeks of weight restoration should thyroid hormone replacement be prescribed. It is important to avoid unnecessary and potentially dangerous thyroid hormone for low-weight patients with anorexia nervosa when the thyroid function tests are most consistent with euthyroid sick syndrome, as these typically normalize with just nutritional rehabilitation. The risk of unnecessary thyroid hormone therapy is especially prominent because of its deleterious effect on bone mineral density in a population of patients who are already at risk for severe osteoporosis (Abrahamsen et al., 2015). For a summary of general endocrine changes in anorexia nervosa, see table 9.1.

Subclinical hypothyroidism is a related condition wherein the TSH levels are slightly greater than 4.5 mIU/L with normal T4 levels. Antithyroid antibody tests may often be positive in subclinical hypothyroidism, but not

Table 9.1. Summary of endocrine changes in anorexia nervosa

Hormonal or metabolic change	Alteration	Cause
Cortisol (hypothalamic-pituitary-adrenal axis)	Increased plasma	Increased corticotrophin-releasing hormone from hypothalamus; decreased metabolic clearance; normal pituitary response
Growth hormone	Decreased IGF-1; increased or normal fasting GH; decreased serum GHBP	Downregulation of GH receptor by nutritional deprivation
Thyroid hormones	Euthyroid sick syndrome: 1. Low or low normal T4 and T3 2. Normal TSH 3. Increased reverse T3	T4 decreased due to conversion to inactive reverse T3
Glucose	Fasting hypoglycemia present with severe anorexia nervosa	Depleted liver glycogen stores; disrupted gluconeogenesis
Serum leptin	Decreased	Unknown, possibly low fat mass
Cholesterol (total)	May be increased due to increased HDL	Possible changes in thyroid, estrogen, and glucocorticoids
Gonadal hormones	Decreased estrogen in females; decreased testosterone in males	Central hypothalamic hypogonadism resulting from low weight associated with inappropriately low pituitary LH and FSH levels

in euthyroid sick syndrome. The treatment of subclinical hypothyroidism with low-dose levothyroxine is controversial (Burns et al., 2016). However, treating these patients with low-dose thyroid hormone does not appear to cause further weight loss if closely monitored to prevent overtreatment.

Glucose and Other Hormones

Dietary restriction accompanied by weight loss and excessive exercise leads to depletion of hepatic glycogen stores and disruption of hepatic gluconeogenesis, resulting in abnormalities of glucose metabolism. In early, milder cases of anorexia, hypoglycemia rarely causes symptoms. In contrast, individuals with advanced anorexia nervosa and persistent severe hypoglycemia have a poor prognosis; severe hypoglycemia has been associated with sudden death because it indicates liver failure and a depletion of substrate to maintain safe blood glucose levels (Rich et al., 1990). In the presence of hypoglycemia, insulin levels are appropriately decreased, and insulin sensitivity is normal in most individuals with eating disorders. Documented hypoglycemia should simply imply an urgent need for weight restoration and close monitoring of blood glucose levels at an inpatient level of care.

Adrenal androgens in women with eating disorders are usually normal to low-normal, while men with eating disorders usually have low testosterone levels, similar to the low estrogen levels consistently noted in females with anorexia nervosa. These low sex hormone levels probably account for the low sexual functionality found in those with anorexia nervosa (Gonidakis, Kravvariti, and Vandarsou, 2014). Low testosterone levels may be associated with the osteoporosis seen in males with anorexia nervosa. Although there is no definite therapeutic role for testosterone replacement therapy for their bone disease (Miller, Grieco, and Klibanski, 2005), it is reasonable to offer testosterone replacement to male patients older than 20 as it may help attenuate their loss of bone mineral density. Serum prolactin is generally normal in both men and women.

Leptin is a hormone that is secreted by adipose tissue and normally plays a role in satiety and energy balance as an anorexigenic adipokine. Leptin levels are appropriately reduced in patients with anorexia and correlate well with weight, percentage of body fat, and IGF-1 (Mehler, Eckel, and Donahoo, 1999). The exact clinical significance of this is unknown, but as weight approaches ideal body weight, leptin levels revert to normal (Modan-Moses et al., 2007). Ghrelin, produced by the stomach and also known as orexigenic gut peptide, normally increases appetite. It is increased in anorexia nervosa (Dostolova and Haluzik, 2009). Although some reports suggest abnormalities of vasopressin secretion, polyuria, and diabetes insipidus in anorexia nervosa, overall these are uncommon.

As many as 50% of patients with anorexia have been reported to have hypercholesterolemia (Ohwada et al., 2006). It is often due to a high level of cardioprotective HDL but insignificant elevations in LDL levels (Mehler, Lezotte, and Eckel, 1998). The reason for the elevated HDL is not well understood, but presumably it reflects excessive exercise and weight loss. Abnormalities in estrogen, thyroid hormone, and glucocorticoids may explain the mildly elevated LDL-lipid levels, which should not be treated with lipid-lowering agents during the active phase of anorexia nervosa unless there is clear evidence of a significant elevated risk of vascular disease. Vitamin D levels are commonly found to be low in anorexia nervosa and should be augmented if less than 20 IU/mL (Veronese et al., 2015).

Symptoms and Signs of Endocrine Disorders

Abnormalities found on physical examination that might suggest endocrine dysfunction in patients with eating disorders include hypotension (low blood pressure), cold intolerance, and hypothermia. Only rarely will the hypotension represent adrenal hypofunction, and the characteristic findings of primary adrenal insufficiency (decreased serum sodium levels, increased serum potassium levels, and hyperpigmentation) are generally absent. Cold intolerance, low heart rate, and hypothermia are all consistent with hypothyroidism, while weight loss could be exacerbated by overactive thyroid function. Other findings that might suggest endocrine dysfunction are hair loss, easy bruisability, light-headedness, and dizziness. It is not surprising that the patient who has anorexia nervosa, especially occult anorexia with denial of dieting, may be referred to an endocrinologist for initial evaluation before the diagnosis of anorexia nervosa has been made.

Despite the high serum and urine cortisol levels that may accompany anorexia nervosa, the striae, hyperglycemia, hypertension, and skin atrophy seen with cortisol excess (Cushing's syndrome) are not present. The lack of symptoms related to cortisol excess suggests that tissues may be resistant to glucocorticoids. It is widely assumed that the hypercortisolism contributes to the osteopenia of anorexia, although patients with eating disorders do not have elevated urine calcium excretion, which should occur in the presence of hypercortisolemia.

Endocrine Testing

At times, a battery of endocrine tests may be necessary to define the accurate diagnosis (table 9.2). On initial evaluation, thyroid function should be tested and is best assessed by measuring free T4 and TSH levels. It is not necessary to measure T3 and reverse T3 to confirm the diagnosis of euthyroid sick syndrome, because the diagnosis can be made clinically and

Table 9.2. Suggested hormone and hormone-related metabolic testing
for patients with eating disorders

1. TSH and free T4 (anorexia nervosa)
2. Fasting glucose
3. Testosterone (males with anorexia nervosa)

neither measurement will affect therapy. If the TSH level is normal, thyroid hormone replacement is not indicated. Very low or suppressed levels of TSH suggest hyperthyroidism, hypopituitarism, or the effects of malnutrition and need to be interpreted carefully, in conjunction with measurements of free T4 and T3, in the setting of the clinical picture. However, a patient with anorexia nervosa who has a low free T4 and an elevated TSH has primary hypothyroidism and should receive low doses of thyroid hormone, with careful monitoring in view of the low body weight and likely need for smaller doses of thyroid replacement. A dose of 0.025–0.05 mg of levothyroxine is a good starting point. TSH level should be rechecked 2–3 months after therapy begins, with a goal level of 0.4–4.5 mg/dL.

There is little advantage in measuring GH or IGF-1 levels in individuals with anorexia, as replacement therapy is not likely to be of therapeutic utility. Stimulation tests of pituitary function are also rarely helpful. For an individual who has anorexia and an expected low T4 but an unexpected low TSH level and symptoms of pituitary dysfunction, a thyroid-releasing factor (TRF) stimulation test could be employed. This will be difficult to interpret, however, as malnutrition and depressive illness may affect TSH responsiveness to TRF. Referral to an endocrinologist may be prudent for some of these more complicated scenarios.

Summary

People who have eating disorders may present to endocrinologists with symptoms caused by their eating disorder but suggestive of possible adrenal, pituitary, thyroid, pancreatic, or reproductive hormone abnormalities. Most endocrine changes are secondary to weight loss, nutritional alteration, and purging behavior. It is best to diagnose an eating disorder by history and mental status examination, not by first "ruling out" all possible medical causes. Most of the endocrine complications of eating disorders revert to normal with early diagnosis and successful treatment of the eating disorder, but normalization may lag behind weight restoration.

Consider treating hypothyroidism in patients with anorexia nervosa only if their free or total T4 is decreased and TSH is also increased. Further evaluation of pituitary function should also be considered if atypical, non-starvation-related endocrine findings are present.

REFERENCES

Abrahamsen B, Jorgensen HL, Lauland AS, et al. 2015. The excess risk of major osteoporotic fractures in hypothyroidism is driven by cumulative hyperthyroid as opposed to hypothyroid time: An observational register-based time-resolved cohort analysis. *Journal of Bone and Mineral Research* 30:898–905.

Burns RB, Bates CK, Hartzband P, and Smetana GW. 2016. Should we treat for subclinical hypothyroidism? Grand rounds discussion from Beth Israel Medical Center. *Annals of Internal Medicine* 164:764–70.

Dostolova I and Haluzik M. 2009. The role of ghrelin in the regulation of food intake in patients with obesity and anorexia nervosa. *Physiology Research* 58:159–70.

Golden NH, Kreitzer P, Jacobson MS, et al. 1994. Disturbances in growth hormone secretion and action in adolescents with anorexia nervosa. *Journal of Pediatrics* 125:655–60.

Gonidakis F, Kravvariti V, and Varsou E. 2014. Sexual function of women with anorexia nervosa and bulimia nervosa. *Journal of Sex and Marital Therapy* 41:368–78.

Grinspoon S, Thomas L, Miller K, Herzog D, and Klibanski A. 2002. Effects of recombinant human IGF-1 and oral contraceptive administration on bone density in anorexia nervosa. *Journal of Clinical Endocrinology and Metabolism* 87:2883–91.

LeFevre ML 2015. Screening for thyroid dysfunction: U.S. Preventive Services Task Force recommendation statement. *Annals of Internal Medicine* 162:641–50.

Mehler PS, Eckel R, and Donahoo WT. 1999. Leptin levels in restricting and purging anorectics. *International Journal of Eating Disorders* 26:189–94.

Mehler PS, Lezotte D, and Eckel R. 1998. Lipid levels in anorexia nervosa. *International Journal of Eating Disorders* 24:217–21.

Miller KK. 2013. Endocrine effects of anorexia nervosa. *Endocrinology and Metabolism Clinics of North America* 42:515–28.

Miller KK, Grieco KA, and Klibanski A. 2005. Testosterone administration in women with anorexia nervosa. *Journal of Clinical Endocrinology and Metabolism* 90:428–33.

Modan-Moses D, Stein D, Pariente C, et al. 2007. Modulation of leptin during refeeding of female anorexia nervosa patients. *Journal of Clinical Endocrinology and Metabolism* 92:1843–47.

Ohwada R, Hotta M, Oikawa S, and Takano K. 2006. Etiology of hypercholesterolemia in patients with anorexia nervosa. *International Journal of Eating Disorders* 39:598–601.

Rich LM, Caine MR, Findling JW, and Shaker JL. 1990. Hypoglycemic coma in anorexia nervosa. *Archives of Internal Medicine* 150:894–95.

Usdan LS, Khaodhiar L, and Apovian CM. 2008. The endocrinopathies of anorexia nervosa. *Endocrine Practice* 14:1055–63.

Veronese N, Solmi M, Rizza W, et al. 2015. Vitamin D status in anorexia nervosa: A meta-analysis. *International Journal of Eating Disorders* 48:803–13.

10

The Dual Diagnosis of Eating Disorder and Diabetes Mellitus

Ovidio Bermudez, MD, and Philip S. Mehler, MD

Common Questions

Is diabetes mellitus type 1 a risk factor for the development of eating disorders?

What is the definition of the dual diagnosis of eating disorder and type 1 diabetes mellitus?

How does insulin omission or underdosing affect weight?

How can patients with diabetes disable their insulin? Why would they do so?

To what extent are patients with eating pathologies and type 1 diabetes typically aware of the diabetes complications that can arise from insulin manipulation?

When do patients diagnosed with diabetes make the connection that insulin deficiency leads to weight loss?

How common is intentional insulin manipulation by individuals with type 1 diabetes?

Is insulin omission or underdosing an effective way of inducing weight loss?

Why is a comprehensive medical and psychiatric assessment imperative for safe management in cases of combined eating pathology and type 1 diabetes?

What do "permissive hyperglycemia" and "relative hypoglycemia" mean?

Why is an "assume then resume" stance in the care of patients with eating pathologies and type 1 diabetes a core principle of treatment?

How does eating pathology combined with type 1 diabetes compare with other eating disorders with respect to mortality risk?

Case

S.M. was a 20-year-old female with a 12-year history of type 1 diabetes mellitus. At age 15, after using insulin injections for 7 years, she had an insulin pump inserted. Although she continued to have good blood sugar control for the subsequent 3 years, at age 18 she was admitted to hospital for treatment of diabetic ketoacidosis (DKA). Her hemoglobin A1c level was noted to be markedly elevated at 13%. Upon further inquiry, she shared with the diabetes educator that she had become frustrated with her weight gain and the constant badgering about her diet. Therefore, she had begun to manipulate her pump settings to reduce her insulin infusion, with resultant hyperglycemia and associated osmotic diuresis. However, this also resulted in overall poor sugar control, albeit with desired weight loss.

Background

From a historical perspective, there is no reason to believe that eating disorders and diabetes mellitus would coincide. Both disease entities have a long and rich clinical history. Diabetes was first described by Aretaeus de Cappadocia in the first century AD as "the melting down of flesh and limbs into the urine," conveying the weight loss associated with insulin deficiency. Nearly two millennia later, in 1921, Frederick Banting discovered insulin, and in 1959, the two types of diabetes—insulin-deficient, or type 1, and insulin-resistant, or type 2—were described. In 1963, the insulin pump was invented by Arnold Kadish.

For eating disorders, the first cases that can be identified forensically date back to the 1300s; Catherine of Sienna (1347–1380) may have suffered from anorexia nervosa. In 1689, Richard Morton described the illness as "ptisis nervosa." In 1873, Charles Lasègue and William Gull nearly simultaneously coined the term *anorexia nervosa*. It was not until 1979 that Gerald Russell described bulimia nervosa. The incidence and prevalence of both types of diabetes and of eating disorders have increased worldwide over several decades, but not until recent decades did the complicated relationship between these two illnesses become better understood. Individuals with type 1 diabetes can manipulate their insulin injections, either to induce weight loss or to avoid weight gain after eating excessively or binge eating, by "purging" the calories through a self-induced insulin deficiency. The lay media have dubbed this syndrome *diabulimia* (Davidson, 2014). A better and more descriptive term is "the dual diagnosis of eating disorder and diabetes mellitus type 1" (ED-DMT1). The other possible association is that of an eating pathology and type 2 diabetes (ED-DMT2), in which individuals gain weight related to excessive eating or binge eating and thus increase their risk of developing insulin resistance and, potentially, type 2 diabetes.

Thus, the relationship between diabetes and eating pathology is different for the two types of diabetes. Type 1 diabetes is a risk factor for the development of eating disorders. In contrast, any eating disorder that has associated weight gain is a risk factor for development of type 2 diabetes (Peterson, Fischer, and Young-Hyman, 2015). Still, today there are individuals with type 1 or type 2 diabetes who also develop an eating disorder and in whom these two entities coexist but do not interact, as they do in ED-DMT1 or ED-DMT2. To clarify, a case in which a person with diabetes develops an eating disorder so that the two illnesses coexist, but the diabetes is not used to intentionally serve the eating disorder mentality, is quite different from the case in which the diabetes is intentionally manipulated to serve the eating disorder. The differentiation is critical for understanding and appropriately addressing the comorbidity. This chapter focuses on ED-DMT1.

Definition

When individuals with type 1 diabetes develop an eating disorder, they may intentionally misuse insulin for the purpose of weight control. This may happen by strategically delaying the dosing, by underdosing, or by omitting insulin altogether. These patients may (1) not use insulin adequately and restrict their caloric intake, or (2) eat normally, or (3) not cover their intake with insulin for binge episodes. In the first two instances, weight loss is likely to ensue. In the third instance, there may be weight loss, weight maintenance, or weight gain. However, the intent of the patient is to avoid weight gain or induce weight loss (Colton et al., 2009).

Pathophysiology

When carbohydrates are normally ingested and digested, blood glucose rises. If insulin is available, glucose can be taken up by cells and utilized for energy. When insulin is deficient or absent, the glucose cannot be transported across cell membranes and thus the cells can become starved. Cellular starvation leads to weight loss. When blood glucose exceeds the renal absorptive threshold, glucose is spilled in the urine. The diuretic effect of glucosuria can lead to dehydration and weight loss. As cells starve, they resort to alternative metabolic pathways for energy, which can lead to production and accumulation of ketone bodies, ketonuria, and metabolic acidosis. This triggers a cascade of events that lead to short-term and long-term complications of insulin deficiency. The short-term complications include hyperglycemia, glucosuria, ketosis, ketonuria, dehydration, and metabolic acidosis. These may culminate in an episode of diabetic ketoacidosis, which can lead to shock, end-organ failure, cerebral edema, or death. The long-term complications are related to long-standing hyperglycemia and microvascular disease and include diabetic retinopathy, nephropathy, cardiomyopathy, and peripheral neuropathy. In addition, any individual who experiences significant weight loss can suffer from the medical complications described in other chapters. In these cases, the compounding effects of the complications of the eating disorder related to weight loss and those of the poorly managed diabetes lead to increased medical morbidity and mortality risk. In addition, these patients can suffer from psychiatric comorbidities, including the increased risk for suicide for any patient with an eating disorder.

Mechanisms of Insulin Manipulation

The ways in which insulin can be manipulated are growing in sophistication, and there are some commonalties and some differences between manipulations by patients using subcutaneous insulin injections and those using an insulin pump. In either case, the intended consequence in the mindset of the patient is to influence body weight. The unintended consequences, the risks of which are often well understood by the patient, are the complications discussed later in this chapter. The notion that patients understand the risk involved is important, in that simply reeducating patients about the risks of poorly managed diabetes and the subsequent persistent hyperglycemia is unlikely to alter or stop their behaviors once they have crossed the line into a mental illness such as an eating disorder.

The hallmark of mental illness is a loss of perspective that often relates to risk-taking behaviors. From the point of view of the patient, these behaviors are a calculated risk in which the value of avoidance of weight gain or induction of weight loss outweighs the known risks of complications. This is clearly present in other eating disorders but is more difficult for clinicians and families to grasp in the context of ED-DMT1. Thus, the mechanisms of insulin manipulation are intended to achieve the weight control that patients seek, avoid complications to the extent possible, and mask the insulin misuse so that they are not suspected of it. Like patients with anorexia nervosa, those with ED-DMT1 often rationalize their risk taking by saying to themselves and others, "If I feel well, I must be well."

Dr. Morton, in 1689, noticed and referred to this notion as "an intellectual perversion," and he considered it pathognomonic of the "ptisis nervosa" he was describing. The associated temperamental characteristics of an individual may lead to specific patterns of insulin manipulation. For example, a patient who tends to consistently restrict calories may more consistently underdose insulin, whereas a patient with binge and purge behaviors may more impulsively not cover binges or may go into spells of insulin omission, yet at other times attempt to manage the diabetes well. As in other eating disorder–related behaviors, for some of these patients this pattern may be lifelong, while for others it is variable or intermittent.

Management of the diabetes for those with type 1 diabetes mellitus involves blood glucose monitoring and insulin administration. Blood glucose is most frequently measured by pricking the fingers to draw blood ("finger stick") and placing a drop of blood on the test strip of a glucometer. Another alternative is to use a continuous glucose monitoring device in which a catheter placed in the skin measures the blood glucose in the interstitial fluid. Both types of glucose measuring devices keep records that can be reviewed.

Injectable insulin comes in short-acting and long-acting forms. The time to onset of action, peak of action, and duration of action for the different types of insulin currently available in the United States can be found on several Internet sites. Some formulations combine short- and long-acting insulin in an effort to minimize the number of injections required, but these are not likely to be used by patients with ED-DMT1 because they would be more difficult to manipulate.

The short-acting insulin must be injected subcutaneously before each ingestion of carbohydrates, the dose calculated as number of insulin units per gram of carbohydrate to be ingested (e.g., 1 unit of insulin for every 12 grams of carbohydrate to be ingested, or "1:12 grams"; this is called the *coverage ratio*). The long-acting insulin is also injected subcutaneously, once or twice daily depending on the half-life of the formulation of insulin used, as number of units per injection (e.g., "22 units before dinner," called *long-acting insulin dose*). Some patients may divide the long-acting insulin into two daily doses for better blood glucose control. Short- and long-acting insulin can be combined in a syringe to decrease the number of injections required daily. Short-acting insulin is also used to correct for elevated blood glucose levels, as number of units of insulin per milligram per deciliter of measured blood glucose above a certain level of blood glucose (e.g., 1 unit of insulin for every 50 mg/dL of measured blood glucose above 150 mg/dL, or "1:50 above 150"; this is called a *correction factor*).

Insulin pumps use only short-acting insulin, which is drawn from a storage chamber, passes through a plastic tube into the pump itself, and then passes through another tube into the catheter placed under the skin. The patient programs the pump by dialing in a basal rate, which can be the same or different for different periods of time throughout the day, and by dialing in a coverage ratio for grams of carbohydrate ingested at each meal or snack. If the blood sugar is elevated, then the pump, if provided with that information, suggests an amount of insulin to be infused according to the correction factor programmed into it.

The basal rate is continuously delivered as programmed into the pump. In contrast, insulin for the coverage ratio for meals and snacks and for the correction factor when insulin is elevated is delivered only after ingestion of carbohydrates or when the blood sugar is elevated and the hyperglycemia needs be corrected, respectively. Subcutaneous insulin is most effective and is usually administered before eating, given the pharmacokinetics of currently available insulin. This leads to better blood glucose management. On the other hand, once insulin is injected subcutaneously or delivered by the pump, undereating or refusal to eat can lead to hypoglycemia. This is one reason that diabetics learn to eat and complete meals based on the external cue of insulin administration rather than internal cues of hunger and satiety.

In the case of ED-DMT1 in patients with a history of caloric restriction, we should consider the possibility that the patient may refuse a meal or snack after the insulin has been delivered. In this case, it is safer to administer the insulin after meals or snacks to avoid the risk of hypoglycemia, until the patient has demonstrated that she or he is able and willing to complete each meal and snack.

Another aspect of insulin delivery is to rotate injection sites or catheter insertion sites. Areas that get overused are likely to develop inflammation and scarring that may interfere with insulin absorption.

Finally, health care providers can better understand how well a patient's blood glucose has been managed by testing for glycosylated hemoglobin, or hemoglobin A1c (HbA1c, or simply A1c), which measures the percentage of total hemoglobin that is glycosylated. The higher the percentage of A1c, the higher is the estimated average blood glucose (eAG) over the preceding 8–12 weeks. The different percentages of A1c correlate with published eAG values. For example, an A1c of 6% correlates with an eAG of 126 mg/dL, and an A1c of 10% correlates with an eAG of 240 mg/dL, in the preceding 2–3 months.

Patients can use several different mechanisms of insulin manipulation.

1. *Sustained insulin omission* for a person with type 1 diabetes who has no residual endogenous insulin production is incompatible with life. People with type 1 diabetes are taught this. So total omission is short-lived (1–3 days). Intermittent omission of insulin is practiced by some patients, including those who monitor for ketonuria and resume insulin use when they notice increasing ketones in the urine. For those who use injectable insulin, this implies not injecting. For those who use an insulin pump, it implies wearing the pump and turning it off (there is really no reason for an insulin pump to be turned off under normal circumstances) or not wearing it at all. Either of these methods would be reflected in the pump record and therefore difficult to justify, so pump users are likely to resort to other means such as wearing the pump but not inserting the catheter in the skin (thus "wasting" the insulin) or filling the insulin chamber with water or saline solution (in which case, pump records will reflect "adequate" insulin delivery).

2. *Underdosing insulin* can avoid some short-term complications and still lead to hyperglycemia and weight loss. Underdosing can look different from patient to patient and for those who use subcutaneous injections versus an insulin pump.

a. Those who use subcutaneous insulin may use the prescribed amount of long-acting insulin once or twice daily, but may either decrease the units of short-acting insulin injected per gram of carbohydrate to be ingested or use the correct amount of short-acting insulin but underdose or omit the long-acting insulin. For others, it may mean underdosing insulin only on certain days (usually related to subjectively or objectively overeating, experiencing worse body image, not exercising, or experiencing greater emotional distress).

b. Those who use an insulin pump may lower or omit the basal rate, lower the number of units per gram of carbohydrate to be ingested, or undercorrect for hyperglycemia.

c. Another important mechanism of insulin underdosing is to use insulin as prescribed when eating normally but not use insulin to cover binges. In this instance, this becomes more of a purging mechanism—hence the popularization of the term *diabulimia*.

3. *Disabling insulin* is an effective way to conceal the insulin manipulation even from a close observer. This includes replacing the insulin in a vial or storage chamber of the pump with an inert liquid such as water or saline, or diluting the insulin with water or saline, or heating the insulin vial to render it ineffective (microwaving for just a few seconds can achieve this). All of these maneuvers apply to both subcutaneous insulin and pump users. Insulin pens can also be heated to disable the insulin.

4. *Delays in insulin administration* is another way in which insulin availability can be altered as carbohydrates ingested are digested and cellular glucose uptake is impaired. Patients with type 1 diabetes generally understand that optimal dosing time for insulin is shortly before a meal and that delays in administration can serve as a weight control maneuver. However, patients often report that when they achieve a modest sense of weight control or weight loss, their tendency is to "speed it up" and advance the severity of insulin misuse.

5. *Impairing the absorption of insulin* is usually an effort by the patient to conceal insulin misuse. This may include injecting or inserting the catheter repeatedly in an indurated, scarred, or atrophied site on the skin (referred to as "dead spots"), which leads to malabsorption or erratic absorption of insulin. Another way is to "leak the shots" by

pushing the plunger of the insulin syringe too early (the insulin is lost on its way to the subcutaneous space) or too late (the insulin is lost intradermally or on the skin). The magician's expression "the hand is quicker than the eye" is apt in this context: even an experienced observer may not perceive this.

6. *Falsifying blood glucose records* is another way in which a patient may attempt to conceal insulin manipulation. It is a more common practice for patients using finger sticks for blood glucose monitoring. Diluting blood samples or using non-blood substances with a predictable glucose content are the main mechanisms. The diluting agents can be water, saline, or alcohol. Non-blood substances include diluted fruit juices, ketchup, and others. Glucometers use a control solution for calibration, and these solutions can be used to "make blood glucose records look good." It is more difficult to falsify blood glucose records with continuous blood glucose measurement devices. Patients tend to suspend the use of the device in periods when they would like to conceal their blood glucose levels.

Pathogenesis

Published models for the pathogenesis of ED-DMT1 start from the stance that the management goals of type 1 diabetes mellitus imply that patients must constantly deal with efforts to maintain near-normal glycemia, must count carbohydrates to calculate coverage doses of short-acting insulin, and must practice portion control and variable degrees of dietary restraint. This can lead to frustration with less-than-optimal blood glucose control, given patients' baseline perfectionistic tendencies and frustrations with weight gain, and/or a sense of nutritional deprivation, which can lead to subjective binges (they feel they overate) or objective binges (they actually overate). These factors can result in weight gain. In addition, negative feelings about body size and weight and symptoms of depression can lead to further efforts at dietary restraint or purging behaviors and can thus contribute to the risk of weight gain or fears of weight gain. This sets the stage for the option of insulin manipulation to avoid weight gain or induce weight loss, in spite of the risks.

Like most gateway behaviors for eating disorders, such as dieting and exercise, once insulin manipulation is practiced, it can be intermittent or can cross a threshold into a compulsion. This may push the behaviors into greater frequency and intensity, despite the patient's understanding of the risks, and may foster the usually false belief that "I can keep it under check" or "the complications will not happen to me." This mentality represents not only a loss of perspective but also a fairly adolescent developmental stance of not internalizing the personal risk that may come with a behavior (Treasure et al., 2015).

Risk Factors

Diabetes education by the American Diabetes Association has been highly successful, due to its consistency and scalability. One drawback is that it emphasizes "control of the diabetes," and with that comes a focus on a patient's consistency, numbers, "good control," dietary restraint, adequate portioning, carbohydrate counting, insulin calculation, timely administration of insulin, eating in response to external cues such as having administered insulin, and exercise as an aid in blood glucose control. At the onset of type 1 diabetes mellitus, patients usually experience increased hunger and thirst, excessive urination, and weight loss. With the implementation of insulin therapy, these symptoms subside and the lost weight is regained. In a weight-vigilant cultural environment, even young patients tend not to miss this association: weight loss with insulin deficiency; weight gain with appropriate insulin administration. In addition, over time, patients with type 1 diabetes tend to have higher BMIs than their peers without diabetes (Meltzer et al., 2001) and also experience more symptoms of depression (Colton et al., 2013). Some studies have demonstrated twice the incidence of clinical depression among individuals with type 1 diabetes compared with the general population. Being educated about and living with type 1 diabetes in a westernized cultural environment that values thinness is a risk factor for the development of eating-related pathology, including an eating disorder. Insulin restriction and/or disordered eating have been documented for 1 in 3 females and 1 in 6 males with early-onset type 1 diabetes after an average of 10 years of living with the diabetes (Wisting et al., 2013).

Some studies have found predictive factors for those with type 1 diabetes who are at higher risk of developing ED-DMT1. Some of these factors are related to clinical characteristics or behaviors that individuals may already show or may develop. These include disordered eating behaviors such as caloric restriction, binge eating, purging behaviors, or excessive exercise; a prior history of insulin restriction or manipulation; poor management of diabetes, especially if associated with elevated A1c levels, repeated episodes of ketoacidosis or presence of microvascular complications; and recurrent episodes of hypoglycemia. Other researchers have cited psychological or demographic features, including lower socioeconomic status; less cohesive family structure; perfectionism, with a focus on numbers; and a higher sense of emotional distress (Neumark-Sztainer et al., 2002). However, *every* individual with type 1 diabetes is at risk for engaging in insulin manipulation.

Epidemiology

Several authors have looked at the incidence and prevalence of insulin manipulation in patients with type 1 diabetes. Some of their findings are as follows:

1. Partial and full syndrome eating disorders are twice as common in females with type 1 diabetes than in their peers without diabetes: full syndrome eating disorder in 10% of those with diabetes versus 4.5% in controls; partial syndrome eating disorder in 14% versus 8% in controls (Jones et al., 2000).

2. Increased risk of disturbed eating behaviors was found in preteen girls (ages 9–13) with type 1 diabetes: full or partial syndrome eating disorder in 8% of those with diabetes versus 1% in controls (Colton et al., 2004).

3. Deliberate insulin omission is the most common form of purging for girls with type 1 diabetes; it starts early and increases through the teenage years: about 2% for preteens, 11%–15% for mid-teens, and 30%–39% for late teens and in the early adult years.

4. A study of disordered eating habits in 87 females with type 1 diabetes between the ages of 11 and 25, using a semistructured interview, found that about 25% had disordered eating or weight control behaviors and 36% reported intentional insulin dose reduction or omission; there was a significant relationship among disordered eating habits, insulin misuse, and microvascular complications of diabetes (Peveler et al., 2005).

Epidemiologic conclusions can be summarized as follows: In females with type 1 diabetes, the risk of an eating disorder (by intentional insulin misuse) is greater than in peers without diabetes, and this can start at young ages and increases with age until young adulthood. Therefore, individuals of both genders (although current data support this more clearly for females) with type 1 diabetes should be considered at risk for the development of disordered eating behaviors and eating disorders. This implies that for health care professionals who oversee diabetic care in young patients, educating them with the goal of increasing their index of suspicion and promoting greater surveillance is imperative for early recognition and timely intervention in ED-DMT1.

Clinical Presentation

Children diagnosed with diabetes at a young age are likely to begin insulin therapy and blood glucose monitoring under parental or caretaker supervision. When diagnosed later in childhood, this is less likely to be the case. As young people mature while living with diabetes, there is a transfer of responsibility from caretaker to patient. For different families this happens at different ages and stages of developmental readiness, and happens more gradually or more suddenly. Once young people have significant autonomy in the management of their type 1 diabetes, they have the option to intentionally misuse their insulin. When insulin misuse happens in such a manner as to avoid noticeable weight loss or measurable derangement in blood glucose control, the misuse may be difficult to detect. Adolescence is a time when patients with type 1 diabetes may experience less tight control of their glycemia, for reasons related to rebelliousness, competing demands, sense of invincibility, or resentment at having to live with diabetes as, with their growing autonomy, they revisit grief and loss issues. Adolescence and puberty in themselves may challenge the tight management of diabetes; these shifts in blood glucose management are expected and identifiable in the developmental context. Both psychological and biological factors may make the management of diabetes more difficult during adolescence. Nevertheless, deteriorations in blood glucose management, especially if accompanied by weight changes, should raise the index of suspicion for the possibility of insulin manipulation. Significant weight loss in a patient with type 1 diabetes should be a concern unless actively sought with a health care provider's endorsement, and it should be considered abnormal.

Patients with type 1 diabetes who engage in insulin manipulation can present with weight loss, poor blood glucose control, elevated levels of A1c, repeated episodes of ketoacidosis, and early onset or rapid advancement of microvascular complications of diabetes (Criego et al., 2009). This is especially true when these changes are unexpected, given how long the diabetes has been diagnosed (Rydall et al., 1997). In addition, as with any other clinical presentations of an eating disorder, if these patients are verbalizing body dissatisfaction or concerns about body weight, size, or shape, are making negative comments about their appearance, are changing their eating or exercise habits, or are suspected of purging behaviors, the index of suspicion should be even higher.

There are some data to support the notion that once individuals with ED-DMT1 understand the impact of insulin manipulation on weight loss, they may stop using other purging modalities. In a 4-year follow-up study of girls between the ages of 12 and 18 years living with type 1 diabetes for an average duration of 7 years, at baseline, 38% were dieting, 45% were binge eating, 14% were engaging in insulin omission, and 8% were self-inducing vomiting. Four years later, 50% were dieting, 50% were binge eating, and 33% were omitting insulin. Of note, at the follow-up, none of the girls were self-inducing vomiting. This is probably due to the effectiveness of insulin manipulation in inducing weight loss in a group of patients whose focus on quick results may trump their concern for the risk of complications of their diabetes.

Other important clinical considerations include the increased diabetic morbidity and overall increased mortality faced by patients with ED-DMT1. Anorexia nervosa has the highest mortality rate of any psychiatric illness. Its medical morbidity correlates with the degree of underweight and malnutrition. Some studies have looked at the high morbidity related to early onset or rapid advancement of diabetic complications in ED-DMT1, but none have looked at the increased morbidity risk of the complications of malnutrition, per se, in this population. It is logical to assume that a patient who develops severe malnutrition related to an eating-related pathology and whose survival physiology also has to contend with preexisting metabolic challenges such as diabetes is less resilient to the effects of malnutrition (Goebel-Fabbri et al., 2008). Such data may be lacking as related to morbidity, but not to mortality. The association of an eating disorder that leads to an underweight state (as in anorexia nervosa) and type 1 diabetes carries a heightened mortality risk that far surpasses that of diabetes alone or anorexia alone.

In a 1997 study that prospectively followed 91 patients with type 1 diabetes for 4 years, those who at baseline were identified as engaging in disturbed eating behaviors, including insulin manipulation, had three times the rate of retinopathy 4 years later (Rydall et al., 1997). These findings suggest that for patients with type 1 diabetes, the association with eating-disordered behaviors was more predictive of retinopathy than was the duration of diabetes. As to mortality, a 2002 publication reported increased risk for individuals with ED-DMT1 compared with those with diabetes alone or anorexia alone (Nielsen, 2002). This was a 10-year retrospective study based on a Scandinavian mortality registry per 1,000 person-years. There were 2.2 deaths per 1,000 person-years for those with type 1 diabetes alone, 7.3 deaths for those with anorexia nervosa alone, and 34.6 deaths for those with ED-DMT1 Thus, the mortality risk of ED-DMT1 is the highest of any psychiatric illness, surpassing that of anorexia nervosa alone. Another way of stating this is that ED-DMT1 is the eating disorder with the highest mortality rate. In either case, this makes a strong case for clinicians to maintain a high index of suspicion to facilitate early recognition. Screening in primary care settings and endocrinology clinics can be made more efficient by using a screening tool. The SCOFF questionnaire is a five-question tool validated to screen for eating disorders. It has been modified as the mSCOFF to screen for ED-DMT1 (Zuijdwijk et al., 2014). Once the diagnosis is made, rapid and effective interventions are essential to improve mortality and morbidity risk. Finally, maintaining surveillance once patients have achieved recovery may prevent relapses, which carry a high cost for these patients.

Management

Because of the high associated morbidity and mortality risk, when a patient with type 1 diabetes mellitus is diagnosed with an eating disorder that includes intentional manipulation of insulin, initial hospitalization—medically, psychiatrically, or in an eating disorder treatment facility with expertise in the management of ED-DMT1—should be considered (Bermudez et al., 2009). This is especially true when the patient is in denial of the risks, has already experienced severe acute complications such as ketoacidosis, or has low motivation for change. A protracted assessment period or outpatient management efforts that prove unsuccessful may give the patient time to continue or increase these behaviors, and serious deterioration can follow.

Management should begin with a comprehensive assessment. This includes evaluation for medical risk related to diabetes (both short- and long-term complications discussed above) and the eating disorder (may include weight loss, malnutrition, and the consequences of purging behaviors by various modalities, binge eating, or excessive exercise). Assessment also includes evaluation for psychiatric risk involving self-injurious behaviors, suicidality, impulsivity and risk taking, psychosis, unstable mood, depression, anxiety, panic, obsessive compulsive features, and use/abuse of alcohol or drugs. It is also important to understand the patient's motivation for change, since this may influence treatment decisions such as outpatient versus inpatient and required level of care. If a referral is made to a facility that the patient would need to travel to, then consideration should be given to the risk of travel: either stabilize the patient locally first (as long as experienced care is available) or plan for adequate, secure travel services, medically or psychiatrically. Finally, once the dual diagnosis of ED-DMT1 is made, the patient and family should be informed and educated about the diagnosis, current state of understanding, risks, and recommendations for management. It is unfortunate when, due to lack of understanding, patients and families may not fully grasp what this diagnosis entails and continue to focus solely on managing the diabetes. Like other eating disorders, ED-DMT1 is a serious mental illness, and patients are best served when it is conceptualized as such and managed accordingly.

The principles that guide treatment and the goals of interventions are similar for different levels of severity at the time of presentation and at any level of care. The goals are to support and supervise the patient to the degree required to achieve the full interruption of insulin manipulation and all eating-disordered behaviors; to reestablish consistent, appropriate insulin use; to establish gradual and consistent weight recovery, when indicated, while avoiding refeeding complications; to establish weight maintenance at target where the patient is back to a normal weight; to normalize glycemia and A1c; and to ensure the patient demonstrates the ability and willingness to sustain those changes. If the patient has engaged in other purging behaviors, full interruption of those is imperative. When applicable, the clinician should diagnose and treat to remission any psychiatric comorbidities. Thus, the level of care required depends on the possibility for these changes to start right away in the least restrictive care environment, but clearly prioritizing effecting immediate behavior change.

The patient must have ongoing supervision and accountability. When the care is implemented in an outpatient setting, very close and consistent follow-up with accountability to a support system (usually family or a school health clinic) (Hasken et al., 2010) should be in place and closely monitored (Goebel-Fabbri et al., 2009). This is true for an intensive outpatient program or partial hospitalization program, in which the program offers some structure but the patient is responsible for self-monitoring outside the structure of the program. For patients with more severe findings on presentation, 24-hour care is indicated to start with, and the severity of blood sugar abnormalities, other medical findings, and psychiatric concerns will probably determine whether inpatient or residential care is needed. When 24-hour care is required, it is critical that the program has expertise, or at least experience, both medically and psychiatrically, in managing ED-DMT1. This includes having protocols in place for consistent blood glucose monitoring and insulin administration and the interruption of other eating-disordered behaviors, and the ability to manage decompensation of diabetes, including hypoglycemia, hyperglycemia, fluid and acid-base abnormalities, and psychiatric decompensation. Achievement of this requires a well-trained staff across all disciplines to be in place: professionals who have developed a significant level of comfort working with this specific pathology and have established clear pathways of communication and role definition.

At Eating Recovery Center, in Denver, Colorado, we have developed a highly specialized treatment protocol for ED-DMT1 (as detailed in the next section). This protocol is guided by several principles. First, start from an "assume then resume" stance toward managements of the diabetes. This means that the staff initially assumes responsibility for all aspects of diabetes care, then works with the patient so that she or he gradually resumes the responsibility by demonstrating the ability and willingness to effectively and consistently manage the diabetes. This is usually achieved in three phases.

In phase 1, the care is assumed fully by the staff. In phase 2, the care is shared by staff and patient with strict staff supervision. In phase 3, the patient resumes responsibility for care, with gradual weaning from staff supervision until she or he can successfully practice full self-care. Phases 1 and 2 often include removal of the insulin pump if one has been in use. Patients and families may become concerned about losing the pump because they have learned that, when used adequately, a pump has advantages over subcutaneous insulin injections for glycemic control. However, the patient's ability to manipulate the pump even under close staff supervision makes this too risky a practice. Once the clinician carefully explains this and reassures them that interruption of pump use can be a temporary measure, patients and families are more likely to understand and accept this.

The second principle is the requirement for consistency on the part of all staff interacting with the patient. In the treatment of eating-related pathology, often when a patient feels able to get away with a behavior, this opens the door for constant testing of boundaries and attempts to practice such behaviors—and this is so for a patient with ED-DMT1. Having protocols in place that are consistently followed 24 hours per day and by all staff is essential. In addition, one must remain vigilant to detect new behaviors, since the patient may struggle with challenges often seen when individuals with eating disorders are in a group setting. These include contagion (they may learn things from each other), comparison (they notice how others manifest their eating pathology, or who is thinner, or who has lost weight more rapidly), and competition (they may think they have to "enhance their efforts" if they feel they are not "the sickest person there"). For patients with ED-DMT1, another aspect of their experience in treatment may be their sense of alienation from others with more traditional presentations of eating pathology. Comments such as "I do not restrict what I eat or make myself vomit so I am not like these other people" imply that a patient may be questioning whether she or he truly has an eating disorder. Educating patients about the similarities among eating-related pathologies, regardless of size or shape, is important. Helping patients connect through the similarities in their plights may help them integrate and make better use of the treatment experience.

The third principle is to approach improvement in glycemic control gradually. It is medically unwise to try to go rapidly from poor glycemic control to normalization of blood glucose. Such attempts may increase the risk of hypoglycemia, both subjectively and objectively, and may exacerbate the patient's focus on glucose management rather than addressing all aspects of the eating disorder. It is best to aim to improve glycemic control gradually, even if it means transiently accepting blood glucose levels higher than normal; this has been called "permissive hyperglycemia" (Brown and Mehler, 2014). To achieve this, it is important to discuss the principle with the patient and the family at admittance and again as needed thereafter, especially because many of these patients, even though aware of how they have elected to induce hyperglycemia, become obsessive about "excellent diabetes management" as they enter treatment. This is particularly true as patients experience weight recovery. Normoglycemia is difficult to achieve as a patient is gaining weight, amid the metabolic shift of refeeding and concomitant changes is insulin requirements. So, preparing patients to accept episodes of hyperglycemia and hypoglycemia is important. Also important is to monitor and record blood sugars in a format in which the trends are clear. In our experience, a graph format gives a clear visual clue of trends, which is helpful for all involved to track.

The fourth principle involves other ways to prepare the patient and family and set realistic expectations for the treatment experience. Preparation of the patient and family should also address the notion of "relative or subjective hypoglycemia." Some of these patients have become accustomed to experiencing near constant hyperglycemia. As blood sugars trend downward, they may experience symptoms of hypoglycemia even at abnormally high blood glucose levels. These events should not be treated as true hypoglycemia because that would exacerbate the persistence of hyperglycemia. In addition, the patient needs to expect that with normalization of insulin management, some weight gain is likely. When the patient has become underweight and weight restoration is indicated, this is usually difficult but expected. There are other circumstances in which a patient with ED-DMT1 may present at normal weight or overweight. In this case, accepting weight gain tends to become more emotionally distressing. Patients who were significantly overweight when their eating disorder started and then lost weight may particularly fear losing control as they gain weight and returning to the former overweight state. This scenario can cause significant distress and should be proactively addressed in treatment.

Our program does not view any foods as unacceptable for those with diabetes. So, in preparing the patient and family, rather than focusing on abstinence from "bad foods" we focus on moderation and appropriate insulin management—including for foods with higher carbohydrate or caloric content.

One more issue to address is the role of exercise. For many individuals with type 1 diabetes, physical activity can support normalization of blood glucose. Some with "exercise sensitivity" may need to incorporate regular physical activity to manage their glycemia adequately. However, physical activity may need to be curtailed or interrupted for those who are underweight, including while they are refeeding. Patients with ED-DMT1 may feel that this could cause difficult-to-control blood sugars during the refeeding period. Although this may be partially true, the risk-benefit ratio of including physical activity during the refeeding and weight recovery phase of treatment has to be taken into account. At least for some patients, they will need to forgo physical activity until their cardiovascular and metabolic status improves.

Lastly, some degree of retraining in diabetes management is imperative, or at least verification that the patient is able to fully understand the principles and implement appropriate diabetes self-care. Some patients are resistant to this; they may feel they are the ones who have lived with their diabetes and better understand it. However, they sometimes become so accustomed to intentionally mismanaging their diabetes that getting them reacquainted with what they were trained to do when they were first diagnosed with diabetes or started to use an insulin pump is by far in their best interest.

These management principles make it evident that a multidisciplinary team approach in which each discipline contributes its individual expertise is necessary. Understanding role definition and role integration is critical to a well-functioning clinical team. The dietician in the team has a particularly active role in preparing the meal plan, carbohydrate counting, tracking completion of the meal plan and the timely and appropriate use of insulin, and making sense of blood glucose trends in the light of carbohydrate intake, level of activity, weight recovery trend or weight stability, and the patient's overall progress.

Eating Recovery Center's Management Approach

At the Eating Recovery Center, we begin by carefully vetting potential admissions to the program. The intake team completes a comprehensive telephone assessment with the patient, family, or referring professional (as the situation requires or allows). The team also gathers pertinent medical records, including a detailed history of the management of the diabetes and, specifically, recent endocrinology records, including A1c results and insulin orders. This information is reviewed by the admissions team, which may request further information, refer the patient to a more appropriate setting, or accept the patient for admission. When necessary, one or more members of the clinical team may communicate with the patient and/or family to clarify expectations and begin to shape the treatment plan. This rigorous process is necessary to ensure that the patient meets our admission criteria, that there are no exclusion criteria, and that our approach is a good fit for the needs of the patient.

On the day of admission, members of the clinical team work to understand the role of their particular discipline. After a nursing assessment that includes measuring vital signs, height, and weight and doing initial blood work, the clinical team meets with the patient and the family (if available) to complete the interdisciplinary admission assessment. Each discipline has a specific role in preparation for the admission and on the day of admission.

1. Role of the physician (pediatrician, family practitioner, internist)
   a. Identify medical complications of the diabetes or the eating disorder that require urgent attention, including vital sign abnormalities and severity of malnutrition. Some patients may need to be diverted temporarily to a different facility for intensive care services, medical stabilization, or psychiatric stabilization.
   b. Review blood glucose trends and adjust insulin orders as necessary.
   c. Establish a plan for the management of hypoglycemia and hyperglycemia.
2. Role of nursing
   a. Implement orders related to blood glucose testing, administration of insulin, and all other medications.

  b. Document blood glucose values and insulin administered.

  c. Manage hypoglycemia or hyperglycemia as per order.

  d. Communicate to the rest of the team the patient's extent of compliance or resistance.

3. Role of the dietician

  a. Plan meals and snacks for the day of admission and complete carbohydrate counts for each meal and snack, using the "macronutrient spreadsheet."

  b. Review available data to determine insulin-to-carbohydrate (I/C) ratios for meals and snacks.

  c. Discuss I/C ratios and plan for insulin administration with MD and RN (e.g., is insulin to be administered before each meal and each snack or administered before each meal only but dosed to cover the subsequent snack also? Is insulin going to be administered before eating or after eating?).

  d. Initiate and update the "diabetes management sheet" and the glucose graph.

  e. Report on these values in team meetings.

4. Role of the psychiatrist

  a. Assess for psychiatric safety.

  b. Explore psychiatric comorbidity diagnoses and establish a plan for addressing them.

  c. Monitor the patient for safety as treatment progresses.

  d. Prescribe and adjust psychotropic medications as required.

5. Role of the psychotherapist

  a. Asses for motivation for change.

  b. Establish a therapeutic alliance.

  c. Maintain communication with the family.

  d. Implement psychotherapeutic efforts.

All patients then progress through the steps of the Blood Glucose Management Level System, which has six levels. The first is the evaluation phase; all patients admitted start at this level. They can then progress through levels A through E.

1. Evaluation phase: Expectations and level system are clarified and communicated to the patient and family. All care is assumed by the staff.

2. Level A: At least 24–48 hours of collaboration from the patient is achieved; staff is doing all blood glucose checks, insulin dose calculations, and insulin administration. Insulin is administered after meals.

3. Level B: At least 48–72 hours of collaboration from the patient is achieved; staff is doing all blood glucose checks, insulin dose calculations, and insulin administration. Insulin is administered before meals because the patient has demonstrated that he or she can complete meals or use oral liquid supplementation if unable to fully complete the meal or snack.

4. Level C: Collaboration from the patient is ongoing, including improving trend in blood glucose levels and establishing weight recovery, if applicable. Blood glucose checks, carbohydrate count calculation, and insulin administration done by the patient, with strict staff supervision. Insulin dose is still calculated by staff. There is no minimum or maximum time at this level.

5. Level D: Patient demonstrates the ability to adhere to the treatment plan, achieves blood glucose normalization, has continuing or completed weight recovery, and demonstrates competency in counting carbohydrates, calculating insulin dose required, and administering insulin with limited (and gradually less strict) staff supervision. At this level the patient may request to resume the use of an insulin pump.

6. Level E: Patient is managing all aspects of diabetes care independently and reports to the team, as she or he would to the endocrinology service as an outpatient.

Levels A to C are usually used in 24-hour care settings. Patients often step down to a partial hospitalization program level of care on level C, and also tend to start at this level if admitted directly to the partial hospitalization program.

Some patients who have interrupted the use of an insulin pump may not wish to return to that right away, and we usually support this decision until they feel ready. Others may wish to resume using the pump sooner, and for those we offer a process of "applying" to resume pump use. The reason for the cautious approach is that the time when patients reach level D often coincides with their reaching a weight close to their target weight, and this tends to raise the distress that they experience—including worsening of negative body image. So it is important not to resume pump use casually at a time when the lure of weight loss through insulin manipulation can pose a significant challenge to successful completion of treatment. Thus, patients request to resume pump use through the application process. This is vetted by their clinical team and also often by their peers, and finally the clinical team signs off on the application form approving the request. Heightened vigilance is suggested during this transition period. Core components of the discharge and aftercare plan are clear expectations about continued appropriate diabetes management, weight maintenance according to the team's recommendations, consistent completion of the prescribed meal plan, adherence to any prescribed medications including psychotropic medications, and close follow-up by a multidisciplinary team with expertise or experience in managing both eating disorders and diabetes.

Other Important Considerations

Varied clinical presentations of eating disorders are on the rise. Terms such as *orthorexia*, *pregorexia*, *brideorexia*, and *drunkorexia*, popularized by the lay press, describe new or atypical presentations of eating pathology that most clinicians see in their practices, and all can carry serious consequences both physically and psychologically. In addition, we are seeing "new" medical comorbidities and eating-related pathologies beyond ED-DMT1, and a high index of suspicion for these should be maintained. Some of these are also related to diabetes. These include a syndrome of self-imposed hypoglycemia in patients with type 1 diabetes, which involves intentional overuse of insulin sometimes coupled with excessive exercise to maintain a low body weight (Moosavi, Kreisman, and Hall, 2015). It turns out that chronic hypoglycemia also leads to weight loss or maintenance of an abnormally low body weight. We have also seen patients with type 1 diabetes who have used diabetic supplies or paraphernalia for self-injury (such as cutting themselves with lancets or stabbing themselves repeatedly with insulin needles). To my knowledge, these specific modes of self-harm have not been reported.

Other "new" medical comorbidities involve not diabetes but other medical illness in which intentional manipulation of the treatment or the illness itself can lead to weight loss or avoid weight gain. Examples are:

1. Patients with hypothyroidism who take excessive doses of the prescribed thyroid hormone to induce a hyperthyroid state and thus lose weight or maintain a low body weight.
2. Patient with hyperthyroidism who strategically underdose medications prescribed to downregulate thyroid hormone production and thus "allow" the hyperthyroid state to persist for the purpose of weight reduction.
3. Patients with inflammatory bowel disease who strategically underdose or omit their antiinflammatory medications to allow enough bowel inflammation to impair absorption of nutrients and thus favor weight control.
4. Patients with cystic fibrosis who underdose or omit their digestive enzymes to impair absorption of nutrients.

Given the readily available sharing of information on the Internet, it is likely that we will see more of these types of manipulation of medical diagnosis as part of the repertoire of manifestations of eating pathology.

Summary

Type 1 diabetes mellitus is a risk factor for the development of eating disorders. Insulin manipulation is prevalent in this patient population and warrants a high level of vigilance on the part of any health care professional interacting with these patients. Intentional insulin manipulation should be considered in any individual with type 1 diabetes whose management of her or his diabetes deteriorates. Early recognition and timely intervention for patients with ED-DMT1 can prevent the high morbidity and mortality associated with this presentation of eating-related pathology. Care should be offered by clinicians with expertise or experience in the care of patients with ED-DMT1 and in settings where a multidisciplinary approach brings to bear the necessary medical, endocrine, psychological, dietetic, and psychiatric know-how to meet the needs and clinical complexity of these patients. We should reexamine how diabetes care education is imparted to see whether more creative approaches can be less triggering to vulnerable individuals with type 1 diabetes and thus at risk for insulin manipulation.

REFERENCES

Bermudez O, Gallivan H, Jahraus JP, Lesser J, Meier M, and Parkin C. 2009. Inpatient management of eating disorders in type 1 diabetes. *Diabetes Spectrum* 22:153–58.

Brown CA and Mehler PS. 2014. Anorexia nervosa complicated by diabetes mellitus: The case for permissive hyperglycemia. *International Journal of Eating Disorders* 47:671–74.

Colton PA, Olmsted MP, Daneman D, Rydall AC, and Rodin G. 2004. Disturbed eating behavior and eating disorders in preteen and early teenage girls with type 1 diabetes: A case-controlled study. *Diabetes Care* 27:1654–59.

Colton PA, Rodin G, Bergenstal R, and Parkin C. 2009. Eating disorders and diabetes: Introduction and overview. *Diabetes Spectrum* 22:138–42.

Colton PA, Olmsted MP, Daneman D, and Rodin G. 2013. Depression, disturbed eating behavior, and metabolic control in teenage girls with type 1 diabetes. *Pediatric Diabetes* 14:372–76.

Criego A, Crow SJ, Goebel-Fabbri AE, Kendall D, and Parkin C. 2009. Eating disorders and diabetes: Screening and detection. *Diabetes Spectrum* 22:143–46.

Davidson J. 2014. Diabulimia: How eating disorders can affect adolescents with diabetes. *Nursing Standard* 29:44–49.

Goebel-Fabbri AE, Fikkan J, Franko DL, Pearson K, Anderson BJ, and Weinger K. 2008. Insulin restriction and associated morbidity and mortality in women with type 1 diabetes. *Diabetes Care* 31:415–19.

Goebel-Fabbri AE, Uplinger N, Gerken S, Mangham D, Criego A, and Parkin C. 2009. Outpatient management of eating disorders in type 1 diabetes. *Diabetes Spectrum* 22:147–52.

Hasken J, Kresl L, Nydegger T, and Temme M. 2010. Diabulimia and the role of school health personnel. *Journal of School Health* 80:465–69.

Jones JM, Lawson ML, Daneman D, Olmstead MP, and Rodin G. 2000. Eating disorders in adolescent females with and without type 1 diabetes: Cross sectional study. *BMJ* 320:1563–66.

Meltzer LJ, Johnson SB, Prine JM, Banks RA, Desrosiers PM, and Silverstein JH. 2001. Disordered eating, body mass, and glycemic control in adolescents with type 1 diabetes. *Diabetes Care* 24:678–82.

Moosavi M, Kreisman S, and Hall L. 2015. Intentional hypoglycemia to control bingeing in a patient with type 1 diabetes and bulimia nervosa. *Canadian Journal of Diabetes* 39:16–17.

Neumark-Sztainer D, Patterson J, Mellin A, Ackard DM, Utter J, Story M, and Sockalosky J. 2002. Weight control practices and disordered eating behaviors among adolescent females and males with type 1 diabetes: Associations with sociodemographics, weight concerns, familial factors, and metabolic outcomes. *Diabetes Care* 25:1289–96.

Nielsen S. 2002. Eating disorders in females with type 1 diabetes: An update of a meta-analysis. *European Eating Disorders Review* 10:241–54.

Peterson CM, Fischer S, and Young-Hyman DL. 2015. Topical review: A comprehensive risk model for disordered eating in youth with type 1 diabetes. *Journal of Pediatric Psychology* 40:385–90.

Peveler RC, Bryden KS, Neil HW, Fairburn CG, Mayou RA, Dunger DB, and Turner H. 2005. The relationship of disordered eating habits and attitudes to clinical outcomes in young adult females with type 1 diabetes. *Diabetes Care* 28:84–88.

Rydall A, Rodin G, Olmsted M, Devenyi R, and Daneman D. 1997. Disordered eating behavior and microvascular complications in young women with insulin-dependent diabetes mellitus. *New England Journal of Medicine* 336:1849–54.

Treasure J, Kan C, Stephenson L, Warren E, Smith E, Heller S, and Ismail K. 2015. Developing a theoretical maintenance model for disordered eating in type 1 diabetes. *Diabetic Medicine* 32:1541–45.

Wisting L, Froisland DH, Skrivarhaug T, Dahl-Jorgensen K, and Rø Ø. 2013. Disturbed eating behavior and omission of insulin in adolescents receiving intensified insulin treatment: A nationwide population-based study. *Diabetes Care* 36:3382–87.

Zuijdwijk CS, Pardy SA, Dowden JJ, Dominic AM, Bridger T, and Newhook LA. 2014. The mSCOFF for screening disordered eating in pediatric type 1 diabetes. *Diabetes Care* 37:e26–27.

11

Oral, Dental, Ear, and Eye Complications

Carrie Brown, MD, and Philip S. Mehler, MD

Common Questions

What dental findings are consistent with purging through self-induced vomiting?

What effect does bulimia nervosa have on the salivary glands? When does it usually occur?

What are the treatment options for swelling of the salivary glands (parotid hypertrophy)?

What should you recommend as oral care for a patient who has bulimia nervosa and engages in self-induced vomiting?

What is the significance of the amylase level in a patient who has bulimia and purges by means of self-induced vomiting?

What effects do eating disorders have on the eyes and ears?

Case

S.B., a 25-year-old female, had a 5-year history of bulimia and admitted to intermittently vomiting five to seven times per day. She presented to her internist complaining of painless swelling on both sides of her face in the area of the mandible. Although she was working with a therapist, she admitted that she had lapsed into a binge and purge episode of several days' duration. She stopped the behavior 4 days prior to the visit to her internist.

On physical examination, S.B. had obvious enlargement of her parotid glands bilaterally, which were soft and not very tender to palpation. Oral examination revealed erosion of the enamel on the lingual surfaces of her maxillary teeth and a reddened posterior pharynx. Laboratory blood work results demonstrated a total serum amylase of 220 U/L (normal 16–90). Her serum lipase, bicarbonate, and potassium levels were normal.

The internist recommended that S.B. suck on tart candies to induce excessive salivation, apply warm compresses to the swollen area multiple times per day, and increase her visits with her therapist. On a follow-up visit 2 weeks later, she reported no further purging episodes, and the parotid swelling had completely resolved.

Six months later, S.B. returned with more severe bilateral parotid swelling, as well as submandibular gland enlargement. This time, her parotid glands were tender and painful. She had not seen her therapist in more than 2 months and reported numerous self-induced vomiting episodes, but none in the last 2 weeks. Although she had tried warm compresses and tart candies, there was no decrease in the size of her glands. She was frustrated that the swelling seemed to develop a few days after she had decided to stop purging but was not present during her bouts of excessive vomiting.

Over the next 2 years, S.B. had four episodes of parotid swelling, which once required the use of pilocarpine (while she was hospitalized for electrolyte abnormalities, and under close observation with cardiac telemetry). Generally, her parotid swelling resolved with conservative care. She had a job as a receptionist in a large firm and was concerned about the cosmetic appearance of the swollen glands. The option of having a surgical procedure to remove her parotid glands was raised, but given the potential morbidity and facial scarring, S.B. opted to continue to use the standard treatments of warm compresses, antiinflammatory medication, and tart candies.

Background

Oral complications are common among individuals who have bulimia nervosa. These complications are primarily related to the chronic regurgitation of acidic gastric contents with self-induced vomiting. Oral complications may be the first and only clue to an underlying eating disorder, and up to 25% of patients are first diagnosed with bulimia during a dental appointment (Douglas, 2015). The main oral-facial complications of self-induced vomiting include angular cheilosis (sores in the angles of the lips), loss of enamel and dentin on the lingual surface of the teeth (perimylolysis), pharyngeal soreness, gingivitis, and hypertrophy of the salivary

Table 11.1. Oral complications associated with bulimia nervosa and self-induced vomiting

Oral finding	History and physical findings	Proportion of patients
Cheilosis	Erythematous, dry, painful fissures at angles of lips	Uncommon (<10%)
Erosion of the enamel and dentin of teeth (perimylolysis)	Erosion primarily of the lingual and occlusal surfaces of the anterior maxillary teeth; sensitivity to hot and cold foods	Up to 40%
Gingivitis	Painful, erythematous gums	Uncommon (<10%)
Salivary gland enlargement (parotid hypertrophy)	Bilateral enlargement of the parotid (less often submandibular) glands; generally painless	10%–66%
Sialadenosis	Painful parotid gland swelling	Uncommon (<10%)
Hyperamylasemia	None	10%–66% of patients with sialadenosis

glands (table 11.1). Focusing the history and physical examination on these possible complications can alert a health care provider to an underlying eating disorder. Dentists and dental hygienists can therefore play a crucial role in the secondary prevention of bulimia nervosa, through timely identification of the oral and physical manifestations of this disorder and referral of the individual to an eating disorder professional. Early identification is especially useful for individuals with bulimia, who often maintain normal body weight and are better able to hide the severity of their illness than individuals who have anorexia. Subconjunctival hemorrhages and patulous eustachian tube dysfunction are eye- and ear-specific complications that may be noted in patients with anorexia nervosa.

Oral and Dental Complications
Oral Soft Tissue Findings
Oral complications among patients with eating disorders may be related to dry mouth, or xerostomia; these complications include gingivitis, tooth decay, cheilosis, and cracked lips. Dehydration and medications such as antidepressants may contribute to the xerostomia. Patients with

eating disorders report a significantly increased frequency of dry or cracked lips compared with controls (Johansson et al., 2012). Angular cheilosis is a form of stomatitis (inflammation of the mucous membranes of the mouth) seen in patients with eating disorders, characterized by pallor and maceration of the mucosal lining at the corners of the mouth. The lesions are due to the direct caustic effects of the acidic content of the vomitus. In severe cases, linear fissures can leave scars after healing. The lesions are typically painful and should be distinguished from herpes simplex vesicles, which are more often unilateral and in the middle of the lips, away from the corners of the mouth. Herpetic lesions are also different in that they have a prodrome of mild pain and itching a few days before the lesions appear. Cheilosis may represent an underlying deficiency in B vitamins, zinc, or iron. It may be prudent to check serum levels of these nutrients and to prescribe supplements if levels prove to be low (Park, Brodell, and Helms, 2011). Topical petroleum jelly following gentle washing with warm water can assist in healing of these sores. Keeping the area clean and dry is the main way to hasten resolution (table 11.2). When examining the oropharynx of patients with bulimia, the clinician may note traumatic lesions and, in severe cases, ulcerations on the palate and oropharynx resulting from the repeated use of a finger or other object to induce vomiting (Douglas, 2015; Solomon et al., 2007).

Tooth Erosion (Perimylolysis)

Perimylolysis, or erosion of the enamel and dentin of the teeth, is the most specific manifestation of bulimia nervosa. Perimylolysis has been

Table 11.2. Treatment of oral complications associated with bulimia nervosa

Oral finding	Treatment
Cheilosis	B complex multivitamins; topical petroleum jelly
Enamel erosion (perimylolysis)	Dental consultation; rinsing of mouth with baking soda solution (1 teaspoon in 1 quart of water); consider brushing gently after vomiting
Gingivitis	Mouth rinses; flossing
Salivary gland enlargement (sialadenosis)	Hot compresses, sialagogues (tart candies), and pilocarpine in recalcitrant cases

Note: The primary goal of treatment is the cessation of self-induced vomiting.

reported to occur in up to 64% of people who have bulimia and purge by means of self-induced vomiting (Conviser, Fisher, and Mitchel, 2014). Chronic contact with gastric contents leads to loss of superficial tooth enamel and the dentin that lies underneath the enamel. The average pH of vomitus is 3.8, which is quite acidic, and this may contribute to tooth erosion. Proteolytic enzymes present in saliva after purging, such as pepsin and trypsin, may also play a role in perimylolysis (Schlueter et al., 2012). Finally, consumption of acidic or sweetened foods has also been linked to more severe perimylolysis (Otsu et al., 2014). The dental areas affected first are primarily the lingual surfaces of the upper anterior teeth, followed by the palatal and posterior occlusal surfaces of the maxillary teeth. By contrast, other causes of enamel erosion, such as eating a highly acidic diet (e.g., lemons), first affect the facial teeth surfaces and spare the lingual surfaces. Early perimylolysis is characterized by a smooth, glossy appearance (Aranha, Eduardo, and Cordas, 2008). As erosion continues, the teeth appear shortened in length and have dull enamel surfaces with irregular incisal edges. In severe cases, there may be loss of enamel on incisal edges of the anterior teeth and, finally, involvement of the posterior teeth. If a tooth with a previous restoration is involved, a characteristic prominence is created when loss of enamel leads to projection of the amalgam restoration above the tooth's surface.

If destruction of the enamel is visible, the care provider can assume that the patient has experienced at least 6 months to 2 years of regular and excessive vomiting. Other factors that influence the severity and rate of enamel loss include the types of food consumed, the quality of tooth structure, and overall oral hygiene, including oral care after purging episodes. Patients with severe cases will complain of excessive tooth sensitivity to hot and cold food due to exposed dentin, along with chipping of the edges of the teeth.

Cavities (Caries)

Bulimia, per se, does not put individuals at increased risk of dental caries (Johansson et al., 2012). It may be that people who binge on sweet, high-carbohydrate foods are more likely to develop caries. On the other hand, some people with eating disorders are fastidious in their dental care and have healthy teeth. Other factors also are important in the development of caries, such as the use of fluoridated water, oral hygiene, type of diet, and genetic predisposition.

Gingivitis

Gum disease (gingivitis) is a result of chronic irritation from the low-pH (acidic) gastric contents and is associated with pain and erythematous gums. Gingivitis has also been attributed to xerostomia, which can occur as a result of dehydration due to chronic purging or reduced salivary flow in patients with eating disorders, or as a side effect of certain medications (Steinberg, 2014). Although patients with eating disorders appear to have an increased incidence of gingivitis, they do not seem to be predisposed to progressive periodontitis. Sometimes associated with gingivitis are throat erythema and soreness, which can also be a manifestation of gastroesophageal reflux disease (discussed in chapter 6).

Dental Hygiene

Prevention of perimylolysis, dental caries, and gingivitis among patients with bulimia requires meticulous oral hygiene and dental care. Thus, it is extremely important that patients with oral complications of eating disorders establish care with a knowledgeable and understanding dentist. The most beneficial means of preventing and treating dental complications is to stop the self-induced vomiting. Because success in this effort takes time, care providers need to counsel patients on what to do if they are still engaging in self-induced vomiting. Typically, it is recommended that patients undergo fluoride treatments, both in the dentist's office and at home. Artificial saliva can be used to mediate the effects of xerostomia. Rinsing one's mouth with water or a slightly basic solution containing baking soda or sodium fluoride after vomiting may help to neutralize acid and protect tooth surfaces (Steinberg, 2014). A mouth guard for use during vomiting episodes may also be considered to protect the teeth from vomitus. The optimal tooth brushing practice for patients with bulimia remains controversial as there is concern that the abrasive mechanical action of brushing after vomiting may accelerate enamel erosion (Schlueter et al., 2012). Most clinicians recommend gentle brushing, given the lack of evidence that tooth brushing, per se, contributes to erosion. Crowns or restorative dental work are typically delayed until bulimic behaviors are controlled and recovery is imminent. Palliative treatments for pain or temporary cosmetic procedures may be considered for patients who are not yet in recovery from their eating disorder (Steinberg, 2014).

Enlargement of Salivary Glands

Parotid hypertrophy is common in patients with bulimia, occurring in up to 66% of patients (Mandel and Surattanont, 2002). The diagnosis of bulimia should be considered for any young person with persistent, bilateral enlargement of the parotid glands without another apparent cause. Other causes of salivary gland enlargement are obstruction of the ducts, local infection, Sjögren's syndrome, diabetes mellitus, alcoholism, cirrhosis, hypothyroidism, and hypovitaminosis A. In patients who have bulimia, the swelling is usually painless, bilateral, and readily apparent on physical examination, with the parotid salivary glands being enlarged to two to five times their normal size. The severity of parotid hypertrophy is directly related to the frequency of vomiting. Further, patients with parotid swelling seem to be more likely to also have enamel erosion. The submandibular glands, too, are occasionally involved. In some cases, acute, severe swelling begins 2–3 days *after* a purging episode, which can be disconcerting for the patient with bulimia who has finally decided to cease purging. An acute increase in parotid gland size, which is often painful, is termed sialadenosis (Gaudiani and Mehler, 2016).

The exact pathophysiology of parotid hypertrophy is undetermined; however, one theory implicates dysregulation of the autonomic nervous system, which controls salivary gland function. It has been hypothesized that intracellular secretory zymogen granules begin to accumulate as a result of dysregulation of the acinar cells' sympathetic nerve supply, thus leading to the enlargement of individual parenchymal cells (Mandel, 2014). Biopsies of the parotid glands often show only normal cells but may demonstrate increased acinar size and increased numbers of secretion granules without inflammatory cells (Aframian, 2005).

Autonomic dysregulation may occur as a result of chronic regurgitation of stomach contents, leading to increased cholinergic nerve stimulus. Alternatively, the stimulation of lingual taste receptors by pancreatic proteolytic enzymes, which come in contact with the oral mucosa during vomiting, may lead to autonomic dysregulation. Another proposed hypothesis is that of "work hypertrophy," in which the glands enlarge due to their extra work in providing saliva during normal eating as well as during the regurgitation of gastric contents.

Treatment of sialadenosis depends on the severity of the swelling and the patient's concern over his or her cosmetic appearance. Abstinence from vomiting alone will lead to the resolution of swelling in most cases. In addition, hot compresses, nonsteroidal antiinflammatory medication (such as ibuprofen), and sialagogues (tart candies) can aid in the resolution of swelling. More severe cases have been successfully treated with pilocarpine tablets (5.0 mg three times per day). Pilocarpine is a cholimimetic parasympathomimetic agent that works by causing increased salivation and resultant decompression of the glands (Mehler and Wallace, 1993). The main side effects of pilocarpine are transient blurring of the vision, lacrimation, sweating, a lowering of heart rate, and dizziness due to a lowering of blood pressure. Patients with significant cardiovascular disease may be unable to compensate for the transient changes in blood pressure and pulse induced by pilocarpine, and this medication should initially be administered to patients with bulimia only under observation with cardiac telemetry.

Recalcitrant cases of parotid hypertrophy have been treated with the surgical procedure of parotidectomy. Unfortunately, parotidectomy can lead to facial scarring and disfigurement, which can be particularly troublesome to these patients who already are extremely fixated on their self-image. Additional morbidity from the surgery, such as dry mouth and salivary fistulae, can also be problematic. Finally, patients who revert to self-induced vomiting after parotidectomy risk recurrence of salivary gland enlargement (Wilson and Price, 2003).

Hyperamylasemia

Ten to 66 percent of patients with parotid hypertrophy also have an elevated serum amylase level. Amylase is an enzyme found in saliva, but it is also present in pancreatic fluid and aids in digestion of carbohydrates. Elevated blood amylase level is a known indicator of bulimia. There is some research to suggest that amylase is more commonly increased in patients who binge and purge than in those who induce vomiting without binge eating (Wolfe et al., 2011). Since elevated amylase levels may be of pancreatic or salivary origin, ordering laboratory tests for both salivary isoamylase and pancreatic isoamylase will aid in confirming the source: only the salivary fraction is elevated in bulimia. Another way to differentiate salivary from pancreatic hyperamylasemia is to test for concurrent lipase level. Normal lipase in the presence of the elevated amylase indicates a salivary gland source rather than a pancreatic source. As is the case with salivary gland enlargement, elevated amylase levels are more common in patients who have more frequent binge eating and vomiting. Salivary amylase level should be considered helpful but not definitive in the diagnosis of self-induced vomiting. Some patients who engage in self-induced vomiting have a normal amylase level, and salivary amylase may be increased secondary to other conditions such as hyperemesis gravidarum of pregnancy. In addition, the amylase level does not necessarily correlate with severity of symptoms (Wolfe et al., 2011). If cessation of binge eating and purging is successful, the amylase levels return to normal within a few days to weeks.

Conditions Affecting the Ears and Eyes

Problems with sensory organs only add to the many discomforts associated with eating disorders (table 11.3). Patients may report bothersome changes in hearing, including, "I can hear my own voice very loudly in my head," a symptom termed autophony; or, "I can hear myself breathing very loudly." Patulous eustachian tubes might be the cause of hearing complaints (Godbole and Key, 2010). Under normal physiologic conditions, the eustachian tubes, which track between the inner ear and posterior oropharynx, are closed. Yawning, chewing, or swallowing temporarily opens the tubes and allows pressure equalization, such as when descending in an airplane. It is hypothesized that rapid weight loss may cause loss of the tissue, or "fat pad," that aids in keeping the eustachian tubes closed, resulting in perpetually open (patulous) eustachian tubes and the associated

Table 11.3. Eye and ear complications associated with anorexia nervosa

Sensory organ finding	History and physical findings	Proportion of patients	Treatment
Patulous eustachian tubes	Autophony, hearing one's own voice and breathing very loudly	Uncommon (<10%)	Weight restoration; referral to an otolaryngologist
Lagophthalmos	Dry, irritated eyes	Uncommon (<10%)	Artificial tears; ophthalmic ointment at night; rehydration; weight restoration

autophony. On otoscopic examination, movement of the tympanic membrane in concert with breathing is a reliable indicator of a patulous eustachian tube. Weight gain is the most effective method of resolving symptomatic patulous eustachian tubes among patients with anorexia nervosa (Gaudiani and Mehler, 2016). If the patient is unsuccessful with weight restoration goals, and if the autophony symptoms do not subside, referral to an otolaryngologist is necessary.

Dry eyes are another common complaint among patients with eating disorders. Specifically, patients with severe anorexia nervosa who are dehydrated and extremely underweight may develop enophthalmos, or sunken eyes, thereby disrupting the normal physiology of eyelid movement so that they may not close completely. Lagophthalmos, the inability to completely close the eyelids, is diagnosed when part of the eyeball is still visible after the patient closes his or her eyes. Without treatment, the patient risks developing corneal abrasions due to lack of normal lubrication and excessive exposure to air. Treatment of lagophthalmos consists of frequent use of artificial tears and use of ophthalmic ointment at night. One may consider taping the eyes closed at night as well. Finally, volume repletion, either with intravenous fluids or with nutrition alone, and weight restoration ultimately work to alleviate the enophthalmos and associated dry eyes (Gaudiani et al., 2012). Usually symptoms resolve within 2 weeks in the treatment center setting.

Rarely, subconjunctival hemorrhage, or bleeding under the clear outer layer of the eyeball, may occur in patients with self-induced vomiting. Retching causes an acute increase in pressure in the eye that may cause the fragile blood vessels under the conjunctiva to rupture. Subconjunctival hemorrhage causes the white part of the eye to turn bright red. Fortunately, the condition is benign and typically resolves without intervention within 2 weeks.

Summary

Oral, dental, eye, and ear complications are easily overlooked but important indicators of the presence of anorexia nervosa and bulimia nervosa. Individuals with suspected eating disorders should be asked about mouth, teeth, eye, and ear symptoms and have a thorough examination of the oral cavity and eyes. Health care providers should ask about a history of posterior throat pain, thermal sensitivity of the teeth, problems with the gums, sores at the angles of the mouth, dry eyes, and changes in hearing. Likewise, the physical examination should focus on detecting cheilosis, perimylolysis, posterior pharyngitis, swelling of the parotid glands, and lagophthalmos. If the history or physical findings are consistent with an eating disorder, then a more complete general history and physical are warranted to look for other manifestations and complications associated with eating disorders. Ultimately, alleviation of oral, eye, and ear complications hinges on concerted and coordinated efforts directed at resolving or improving the underlying eating disorder.

REFERENCES

Aframian DJ. 2005. Comment on anorexia/bulimia-related sialadenosis of palatal minor salivary glands. *Journal of Oral Pathology and Medicine* 34:383–84.

Aranha AC, Eduardo CdeP, and Cordas TA. 2008. Eating disorders, part I: Psychiatric diagnosis and dental implications. *Journal of Contemporary Dental Practice* 9(6):73–81.

Conviser JH, Fisher SD, and Mitchel KB. 2014. Oral care behavior after purging in a sample of women with bulimia nervosa. *Journal of the American Dental Association* 145(4):352–54.

Douglas L. 2015. Caring for dental patients with eating disorders. *BDJ Team* 1, no. 15009.

Gaudiani JL, Braverman JM, Mascolo M, and Mehler PS. 2012. Ophthalmic changes in severe anorexia nervosa: A case series. *International Journal of Eating Disorders* 45:719–21.

Gaudiani JL and Mehler PS. 2016. Rare medical manifestations of severe restricting and purging: "Zebras," missed diagnoses, and best practices. *International Journal of Eating Disorders* 49:331–44.

Godbole M and Key A. 2010. Autophonia in anorexia nervosa. *International Journal of Eating Disorders* 43:480–82.

Johansson AK, Norring C, Unell L, and Johansson A. 2012. Eating disorders and oral health: A matched case-control study. *European Journal of Oral Sciences* 120:61–68.

Mandel L. 2014. Salivary gland disorders. *Medical Clinics of North America* 98(6):1407–99.

Mandel L and Surattanont F. 2002. Bilateral parotid swelling: A review. *Oral Surgery, Oral Medicine, Oral Pathology, Oral Radiology, and Endodontology* 93(3):221–37.

Mehler PS and Wallace JA. 1993. Sialadenosis in bulimia: A new treatment. *Archives of Otolaryngology: Head and Neck Surgery* 119:757–88.

Otsu M, Hamura A, Ishikawa Y, Karibe H, Ichijyo T, and Yoshinaga Y. 2014. Factors affecting the dental erosion severity of patients with eating disorders. *Biopsychosocial Medicine* 8:25.

Park KK, Brodell RT, and Helms SE. 2011. Angular cheilitis, part 2: Nutritional, systemic, and drug-related causes and treatment. *Cutis* 88:27–32.

Schlueter N, Ganss C, Potschke S, Klimek J, and Hannig C. 2012. Enzyme activities in the oral fluids of patients suffering from bulimia: A controlled clinical trial. *Caries Research* 46:130–39.

Solomon LWW, Merzianu M, Sullivan M, and Rigual NR. 2007. Necrotizing sialometa-plasia associated with bulimia: Case report and literature review. *Oral Surgery, Oral Medicine, Oral Pathology, Oral Radiology, and Endodontology* 103(2):e39–42.

Steinberg BJ. 2014. Medical and dental implications of eating disorders. *Journal of Dental Hygiene* 88:156–59.

Wilson T and Price T. 2003. Revisiting a controversial surgical technique in the treatment of bulimic parotid hypertrophy. *Americal Journal of Otolaryngology* 24:85–88.

Wolfe BE, Jimerson DC, Smith A, and Keel PK. 2011. Serum amylase in bulimia nervosa and purging disorder: Differentiating the association with binge eating versus purging behavior. *Physiology and Behavior* 104:684–86.

12

Athletes and Eating Disorders

Arnold E. Andersen, MD

Common Questions

Does participation in athletics predispose to or protect from eating disorders?

Which sports tend to increase eating disorders in females?

What does the term "relative energy deficiency in sport" (RED-S) mean?

Which sports tend to increase eating disorders in males?

What are some vulnerabilities that predispose particular athletes to developing eating disorders?

When does a sport become unhealthy in relation to development of eating disorders?

How can physicians, mental health professionals, coaches, and dieticians work together?

How do you approach an athlete who raises your concern about disordered eating?

Can athletes who have eating disorders return to their sport after treatment?

Do preventive efforts work in sports?

How does muscle/body dysmorphia relate to eating disorders?

How risky are performance-enhancing drugs in relation to the symptomatology of eating disorders?

What role do primary and secondary schools play?

Does losing weight increase performance?

What do overactive, underfed rats teach us?

Case 1

A.B. was a 19-year-old female long-distance runner whose eating disorder began at age 12. Shortly after she entered puberty, she lost weight by dieting because she disliked the changes in her body shape, and menses stopped. She responded to outpatient treatment with limited insight but a 10-pound increase in weight. At age 14, she began to challenge herself with endurance running, a sport in which she excelled, winning many championships. She maintained her weight at an improved, but still low-for-age level; by age 16, she weighed 115 pounds, at 5 feet 7 inches tall (BMI 18). Menses did not return, due to a combination of low weight and strenuous exercise. In addition to chronic restricted eating, at age 15 she developed a pattern of small binge episodes followed by purging, which led to chronic gastroesophageal reflux; at times, unwanted food spontaneously came up into her mouth. At 16, she began taking metoclopramide 1 hour before meals, but this was of limited help. In addition to diagnosing and treating her gastroesophageal reflux disease, her primary care physician referred her to orthopedics for evaluation of chronic knee and hip pain. The more she ran, the more painful her symptoms became, but she did not disclose her discomfort until her physician found knee pain on palpation.

The orthopedist noted hamstring tendonitis with pes anserine bursitis. Upon examination, A.B. experienced tenderness along the semitendinosus tendon of the pes anserine bursa. With resisted flexion of the knee, she had significant pain. The bursitis was treated with injection into the bursa of 1% lidocaine (Xylocaine) and 2 mL of injectable betamethasone. She obtained complete relief, but would agree to rest for only 1 day before running 5,000 meters the second day after treatment. The DEXA scan of bone mineral density showed a deficiency of $T = -2.5$ standard deviations in the left hip and $T = -2.0$ in the lumbar spine.

Because of significant anxiety, A.B. was started on escitalopram, titrating up to 20 mg per day, with partial relief. She continued to be preoccupied with staying thin and continued to be very competitive. Secondary amenorrhea continued. She started taking Ortho-Novum 1/35 (norethindrone and ethinyl estradiol) to restore menses artificially. At age 17, she complained of feeling tired, out of energy, and drained. She began falling asleep in classes, a new problem, and started to take naps—something she previously disdained as a sign of weakness. Laboratory work revealed total serum iron of 35 µg/dL (normal 72–130). Iron saturation was 7% (normal

27–44). Hemoglobin was 11.0 g/dL (normal 11.9–15). Weight was stable. The night before track competitions, she experienced high anxiety as well as an increase in regurgitation, and she induced vomiting multiple times. At the examination, for the first time, she had a weepy affect and scratched herself to obtain relief. Escitalopram was increased to 30 mg per day.

At the end of her eighteenth year, she began college. Menses were regular while on birth control pills but only 3 days in duration. She took a break from competitive running, working as a library assistant for her freshman year. Her anxiety decreased; she felt "stronger and healthier." Hemoglobin increased to 12.5 g/dL. Weight increased to 120 pounds. She was considered to have improved but to still meet the diagnostic criteria for the female athletic triad because of her continued amenorrhea without oral contraceptive, continued low weight resulting from disordered eating with fear of fatness, and deficient bone mineral density.

At age 19, in the fall of her second year, A.B. resumed running, working up to 60–80 miles per week, with several runs of more than 10 miles. Her gastroesophageal reflux was improved. Anxiety had lessened over her year of abstention from competitive running. She still had joint pain but continued to override it with a "runner's high." Only the future will tell whether she will remain healthy enough to run competitively without serious medical complications. She said she planned on a career as an orthopedic surgeon.

Case 2

C.D. was a 16-year-old male high school sophomore who was referred by his parents for evaluation of abnormal eating and weight fluctuation. In the eighth grade, at 5 feet 8 inches, he had weighed 185 pounds (BMI 28.2). He became winded while running across the football field. When a teammate called him "fat ass," he stopped drinking soda pop and cut out snack food. He reduced his weight to 140 pounds over 18 months, but by then had grown to 6 feet 3 inches tall (BMI 17.5). He felt cold compared with others, felt weak, and was mentally preoccupied with his body much of the day.

C.D. decided to develop his body through bodybuilding, eating six meals a day that consisted only of fruits, vegetables, whole grains, chicken, skim milk, and yogurt. He consumed five 2-pound containers of soy protein in short periods of time, causing distress to his parents. He insisted on eating every 90 minutes and consumed a gallon of soy milk and a gallon of water daily. When, on New Year's Day, the fitness club was closed, he went up to the door and pounded on it to no avail; then he went home and used his weights in the basement. He underwent cycles of weight increase and bulking, followed by cutting weight with running. His goal was to win a bodybuilding contest at age 17. He stated, "I don't care what I weigh, as long as I keep getting bigger, get well-defined, and have 'cut' muscles with no body fat."

His BMI at the time he was seen in clinic was 22.3 (178.2 pounds, 6 feet 3 inches tall). C.D. looked in every mirror he passed, as well as at his reflection in shop windows. He said his self-esteem depended on his body size and shape. He met the criteria for muscle dysmorphic disorder with a past history of anorexia nervosa. His "emergency weights" went with him whenever he left home. He would not answer questions about steroid abuse. He agreed to therapy with a psychologist experienced with athletes who was located close to his home.

Case 3

E.F. was a 21-year-old female junior who transferred from an East Coast university and self-referred for continuation of treatment for an eating disorder. She had been diagnosed with an eating disorder in her sophomore year of high school. Despite having had surgery on her knee, she decided to lose weight because her coach told her to get thinner. She went from 140 pounds at 5 feet 8 inches tall (BMI 21.2) to 105 pounds (BMI 16.8), eating 300 calories a day. E.F. realized she was too thin, decided to increase her lean muscle weight by weightlifting, and restored to 130 pounds (BMI 19.8), with body fat of 13%. Her menses stopped. She switched to basketball, again restricted, and began to binge-eat and induce vomiting before each game. A stress fracture was diagnosed hen she reported foot pain. At 135 pounds (BMI 20.6) she reported to volleyball summer camp. The coach said she needed to lose "quite a bit of weight" if she wanted a college athletic scholarship. She reduced to 105 pounds again, the weight at which she reported to college.

In college, she could not stop throwing up spontaneously and lost weight to 95 pounds (BMI 14.5). She required treatment in an emergency department for dehydration. A shoulder tear required surgery, and her weight increased during convalescence. At the soonest possible time after surgery, she returned to working out, exercising 8–10 hours per day, and reduced her weight to 93 pounds (BMI 14.2). Her binge-purge cycles, throwing up 20 times a night, required repeated emergency room treatments with IV fluids. She often had EKG abnormalities. The school restricted her athletic training and forbade volleyball practice. When she tried to restore weight using weightlifting, a trainer threw her out of the training room because she did not officially belong to a team any more.

When E.F. began to work out informally with the tennis team, the coach said he wanted to "break her," and the trainer kept asking her if she had "had enough yet." She continued to binge and purge two or three times a day, with binges now triggered by any "crummy feeling" rather than hunger. She continued to work out for 4–5 hours per day, despite stress fractures, engaging in running and weightlifting. She met the criteria for anorexia nervosa, binge-purge subtype, and obsessive compulsive disorder.

A year later, E.F. presented herself to the eating disorder diagnostic clinic, weighing 169 pounds (BMI 25.7). By that time her illness had migrated to a diagnosis of bulimia nervosa, purging subtype. She complained of a sore throat and hoarseness and had significant parotid swelling. Despite being at a higher weight, she did not regain menses. She used six laxatives a day, felt cold, and was constantly preoccupied with thoughts of food and weight. Her mood was low, and the perfectionist aspects of her temperament were apparent. She agreed to treatment, but having concealed her disorder from college officials, she required that they not be told. Her future was unclear. This case illustrates, again, the complex course of an eating disorder in an athlete driven to put sports ahead of health.

Background

Participation in sports may either predispose to the development of eating disorders or be a strongly protective factor. The literature differs widely in its findings. One study, for example, found that the prevalence of eating disorders was higher in non-athletes than in athletes (Wollenberg, Shriver, and Gates, 2015), as also reported by Fortes et al., 2014. Other studies have found the opposite (Martinsen and Sundgot-Borgen, 2013). Much depends on the nature of the sport, the gender of the athlete, the motivation and temperament of the athlete, and the actions of the coaching staff, especially for elite athletes. For the majority of the population, sports serve as recreation, as stress release, as a contribution to identity, and as a bonding experience from childhood throughout life, in addition to providing well-documented health benefits, both physical and psychological.

For elite athletes—those on school varsity teams, in competition for the Olympics, in training for competitive sports such as the Boston Marathon—and for professionals, the pressures to succeed in sports are greater. Powers and Johnson (1996) distinguished between thinness for performance goals and thinness for appearance goals in sports as separate risk factors. The combination of the two, as in girls' gymnastics, appears to pose a greater risk than either one alone. Since delineation of these variables, additional studies have noted the predisposition to eating disorders, primarily in males, when the sport requires substantial muscle development, as is increasingly common in professional sports (football, baseball) and in competitive nonprofessional sports such as weightlifting and varsity football.

A comparison of photos of Joe DiMaggio, a great baseball player of the past, and of Barry Bonds or José Canseco in games of several years ago shows the difference in body bulk that has become almost normative. A report on a university football team defensive line documented an increase in average body weight of approximately a pound a year for the past 100 years. Compulsive running and gym workouts by non-athletes who are in the process of developing eating disorders represent secondary overexercise syndromes, rather than predisposing factors. Table 12.1 summarizes, by gender, sports emphasizing thinness or muscle bulk alone and those emphasizing thinness or muscle bulk plus the added pressure of weight-related appearance norms for adjudicated performances.

Prevalence of Eating Disorders in Athletes

The prevalence of eating disorders and eating disordered behaviors differs greatly from one sport to another. In a large study of 1,445 student varsity athletes in all sports, surveyed from Division 1 schools (Johnson, Powers, and Dick, 1999), almost 3% of females had a clinically significant problem with anorexia nervosa, compared with 0% of males; 11% of females reported binge eating at least weekly, compared with 13% of males Thirty-one percent of women versus 5% of men had BMIs of 20 or lower. Women desired a body with 13% fat, while men desired 8.6%. Norms for

Table 12.1. Body norms or requirements, by gender, of some of the most common sports

Body norm/requirement	Sport	
	Females	Males
Slimness for performance	Cross-country and marathon running	Low-weight crew (rowing), cross-country and marathon running, horse racing (jockey), low-weight wrestling, rock climbing, cycling
Slimness and appearance for adjudicated sports	Ballet, gymnastics, figure skating, diving	Diving, figure skating
Increased muscularity for performance	Sprinting, basketball, softball, weightlifting	Football, baseball, basketball, hockey, sprinting, weightlifting
Increased muscularity and appearance for adjudicated sports	Bodybuilding	Gymnastics, bodybuilding

body fat content for people of college age are 19%–23% for women and 10%–15% for men. The study authors estimated that 34.75% of women were at risk for anorexia nervosa, compared with 9.5% of men. For bulimic disorders, 38% of both females and males were at risk. These were conservative estimates, given the nature of the survey criteria.

More recently, Giel et al. (2016) compared adolescent athletes participating in technical sports, endurance sports, aesthetic sports, weight-dependent sports, ball games, and power sports. They confirmed that the frequency of positive findings on SCOFF screening was twice as high for female as for male athletes. Constant dieting was highest in females in aesthetic sports (e.g., synchronized swimming); the large majority of both males (76.5%) and females (80.4%) in weight-dependent sports used compensatory behaviors (dehydration, vomiting, laxatives, diuretics).

Diagnosis and Evaluation

In sports that encourage thinness for excellence, several issues are involved. Thinness is probably overrated despite the almost unquestioned iconic status given to a skeletal body in some sports. Powers (1999)

Table 12.2. Other terms for eating disorders and weight disorders in athletes

Obligatory running	Weight cycling
Anorexia athletica	"Reverse" anorexia
Pathogenic weight control	Exercise dependence
Activity-induced anorexia	Cutting weight
Female athletic triad	Manorexia

noted that "athletes think being thinner, no matter what, improves performance. There is good evidence that this is not the case." How much thinness is too much? No easy answer can be given because the weight-performance relationship varies from sport to sport, but a few guidelines may be helpful. One obvious measure of too much is a decrease in performance. A more subtle measure is when, despite improved performance, thinness becomes an all-consuming goal in cognition and behaviors. In such cases the athlete pays excessive attention to limiting calories, weighs frequently, and exhibits the psychological features of starvation, such as decreased mental concentration, lowered mood outside of competitive situations, and obsessive fear of becoming fat. Table 12.2 lists synonyms for anorexia-like syndromes in athletes.

A diagnosis of anorexia nervosa is made—when a clinical interview is possible—with the same criteria noted in chapter 1. These criteria are primarily an overvaluation of the benefits of thinness, self-induced starvation to a degree producing medical or psychological symptomatology, a morbid fear of becoming fat, and, often, overestimation of body size despite obvious thinness. For bulimia nervosa, symptoms are frequent episodes of binge eating that lead to guilt, regret, or medical discomfort, followed by compensation by purging (80%) or nonpurging methods such as stricter dieting or increased exercise (20%). Screening questionnaires are useful for identifying eating disorders, but there is a tendency for athletes to "fake normal" to avoid limitations in sports activities. Additionally, some less ethical coaches may limit health professionals' access to athletes. Or, more benign in intent but no less damaging in consequence, coaches may simply ignore or be unaware of eating disorder symptomatology in the face of a "win at all costs" attitude. Bulimia in athletes is not as obvious as the publicly visible body of an athlete with anorexia, but athletes with bulimia have similar preoccupations with weight at less thin levels. Binge-eating disorder is seldom present in sports that mandate thinness.

Eating disorders often go undiagnosed due to a lack of screening or the athlete's fear of shame or embarrassment.

Predisposing Factors

An array of factors may predispose athletes to the development of eating disorders (table 12.3). The nature of the sport is a major factor, but an unresolved question is whether more-predisposed individuals are more attracted to certain sports, such as endurance running. Some sports, such as girls' gymnastics with its requirement of thinness for both perfor-mance and appearance standards, seem to try to maintain girls at a prepubertal weight with minimal breast development and continued open epiphyses for longer bones. This presents ethical problems that are some-times overlooked by trainers and coaches. There are exceptions, thankfully, as seen in the performance of some normal-weight world-class female athletes competing in gymnastics.

Ballet is in many ways an athletic activity, requiring increasing degrees of athleticism in modern dance. In preprofessional schools of ballet, a high percentage of girls (50% in one study) experience amenorrhea, and there is a sevenfold increase in cases of anorexia nervosa compared with the gen-eral population. Anorexia nervosa is as correct a diagnosis when there is a failure to increase in weight proportional to increases in height and age as when there is a loss of weight through dieting and excess exercise.

Psychological factors play a major role in predisposition to eating dis-orders in athletes. An external locus of control—psychological terminology

Table 12.3. Psychological and behavioral characteristics that predispose athletes to eating disorders

Perfectionism	Emotional immaturity relative to age
Low self-esteem	All-or-none reasoning: winning or failure
Sports injury limiting participation	seen as only outcome
Rejection sensitivity	Pressure from coaches
History of childhood/preadolescent	Excess parental pressure
obesity	External locus of control
History of abuse	Participation in sports to please others
Body/muscle dysmorphia	Body weight dissatisfaction
Social isolation	Chronic dieting, frequent weighing
Family history of mood or eating	Anxious or depressive illness or traits
disorders	

for basing self-esteem primarily on approval from others—mandates continued winning in athletics at all costs, a fragile basis for self-esteem. An external locus of control predisposes an athlete to be excessively sensitive to comments from coaches and peers. Perfectionism is associated with all-or-none thinking: not winning equals losing and being a failure. An added burden is rejection sensitivity, with the perception that anything less than first place is a rejection. Performance anxiety may be so severe that an eating disorder comes to be an alternative strategy for relief from anxious participation in sports.

A sports injury may represent an annoyance or a major tragedy in the mind of an athlete. For those with little identity outside of athletics, an injury that requires a time of healing away from the sport—or, more traumatic, discontinuation of the sport in which the athlete has shown excellence—can be devastating. During time away from the sport, an injured athlete may overcompensate for reduced energy output by excessive restriction of food intake, predisposing him or her to anorexia nervosa. In addition, for those with an almost exclusive focus on sport for identity, depression, demoralization, and a perception that life has passed them by may ensue. Overuse injuries represent an imbalance between activity and recuperative forces, fostered by drivenness in athletics. The number of women participating in sports has increased dramatically as a result of both cultural factors and governmental requirements for gender parity in college sports (Hilibrand et al., 2015), leading to an increase in the number of female athletes with eating disorders and sports-related injuries.

Risk by Gender and Sport

Gender-Neutral Sports

Numerous studies have evaluated symptoms of eating disorders in athletes who participate in endurance running and triathlons, which are gender-neutral sports. Thompson (2007) found that 19.4% of female cross-country runners had previous or current eating disorders, 23% had irregular or absent menses, and 29.1% had inadequate calcium intake. Low bone mineral density of the lumbar spine was found in both male and female endurance runners (Hind, Truscott, and Evans, 2006). A majority of female triathletes with a healthy BMI wished to be smaller, in contrast to a minority (19.3%) of males (DiGioacchino DeBate, Wethington, and Sargent, 2002). High dietary restraint, a prelude to an eating disorder, has been documented in adolescent female endurance runners (Barrack et al., 2008). A Scandinavian study found that a high proportion (46.7%) of athletes in leanness sports had clinical eating disorders, compared with 19.8% in non-leanness sports (Torstveit, Rosenvinge, and Sundgot-Borgen, 2008). Disordered eating and eating disorders in aquatic sports ranged from 18% to 45% in female athletes, compared with 0% to 28% in male athletes.

Female-Related Sports

The term *relative energy deficiency in sport* (RED-S) has been proposed as a broader label to include the commonly used *female athletic triad*, a construct referring to the combination of an eating disorder, amenorrhea, and osteoporosis that can develop in young female athletes who have achieved a low body weight (Sundgot-Borgen, 1994). The "Authors' 2015 Additions to the IOC Statement" (Mountjoy et al., 2015) describes RED-S as a gender-neutral condition in sports that includes impaired physiologic functioning caused by relative energy deficiency, combining such features as cardiovascular health, protein synthesis, bone health, and metabolic rate. In one study, most distance-running young women with amenorrhea had a family member with a mood disorder and/or an eating disorder, whereas no relatives were affected with an eating disorder or a mood disorder in a comparison group of eumenorrheic runners (Gadpaille, Sanborn, and Wagner, 1987). A family history of mood or eating disorders predisposes female athletes to seek low body weight.

Women's gymnastics contrasts markedly with men's gymnastics. The ideal female performer is often very young, often prepubertal in endocrine development. Pubertal changes may diminish flexibility and competitive performance in complex gymnastic maneuvers. Female gymnasts accepted into college on sports scholarships may find that development of an adult body endangers their performance and their scholarship status. In contrast, male gymnasts often do not reach their peak until the end of their college years or shortly thereafter, with developmental body changes along with strenuous training improving their performance. In one study, more than 60% of elite female athletes in sports demanding leanness reported pressure from coaches regarding body shape (Kong and Harris, 2015).

Only a few female sports require increased muscularity and weight. These sports, such as female bodybuilding, are somewhat anomalous for most young women. Lean muscularity is more normative in female sprinters. In both of these categories, women may be at risk for anabolic steroid abuse, more common in male athletes.

Male-Related Sports

In male athletes, dieting and disordered eating occur primarily in the male-related sports in which leanness improves performance or aesthetic judgments are involved (Goltz, Stenzel, and Schneider, 2013). Thinness for performance as a risk factor for eating disordered behavior in men has been documented in lightweight rowers compared with heavyweight rowers (Pietrowsky and Straub, 2008), with lightweight rowers scoring very high on restrained eating and body dissatisfaction. Thinness for performance as a risk factor has also been documented in low-weight wrestlers (Thiel, Gottfried, and Hesse, 1993), as well as in male racing jockeys (King and Mezey, 1987), young rock climbers (Morrison and Schöffl, 2007), and male cyclists (Riebl et al., 2007).

Many primarily male sports require increased muscle bulk, usually accompanied by striving for extremely low body fat. The more professional the level of participation in the major sports (football, baseball, basketball, hockey), the more muscularity is valued—with a few exceptions, such as the quarterback in football, who may maintain slim muscularity in place of bulky muscularity. For male sports requiring both greatly defined muscularity and low body fat, such as bodybuilding, the dark side of competitiveness enters with the abuse of anabolic steroids, often at heroic doses (Piacentino et al., 2015; Pope and Kanayama, 2004). These athletes may have "reverse anorexia," which is characterized by perceptual distortion of the opposite kind seen in female anorexia nervosa: never being large enough or muscular enough, being insufficiently "cut" and too fat, even at very low percentages of body fat. Binge eating is common.

Some of the health hazards of anabolic steroid abuse, in both genders, include excessive weight increase, abnormal liver function, increased hemoglobin (predisposing to strokes, blood clots), and abnormal functioning of reproductive hormones. The quest for performance and winning gold, unfortunately, overrides rational consideration of the health hazards of anabolic steroids (table 12.4). In males, especially, the areas of the brain primarily involved in judgment and decision making are located mostly in the prefrontal cortex, which develops later than in females—but, one

Table 12.4. Medical and psychological problems associated with abuse
of anabolic steroids

Males	Females	Both genders
Atrophy of testes	Facial hair	Acne
Reduced sperm count	Irregular or absent menses	Abnormal liver function,
Impotence	Clitoral enlargement	jaundice
Baldness	Deepened voice	Reduced HDL ("good")
Gynecomastia (enlarged	Reduced breast size	cholesterol
breasts)	Laryngeal enlargement	Increased chance of
Premature prostate		injury to tendons,
enlargement		ligaments
Increased rage and lack		Edema, fluid retention,
of anger control in		Increased body weight,
predisposed males		Increased hemoglobin
		(blood clots, strokes)

hopes, by the mid-twenties; the robust, less well-regulated, earlier developing impulsivity centers in the amygdala are highly active during the teenage years. The catchphrase "Get big or die" is, unfortunately, too often promoted. "Get big and live—by healthy means" is a rational choice, but less appealing before full psychosocial maturity.

Treatment Recommendations

How can a concerned sports-related person approach an athlete with a possible eating disorder? This is the first question asked by worried peers, teachers, coaches, and parents. A nonjudgmental expression of concern is the beginning. When several concerned individuals, such as peers and a coach, together approach the athlete and recommend to him or her a specific expert in eating disorders who is familiar with athletes, the athlete will often accept a confidential referral. A period of absence from a sport until improvement occurs is often necessary, so the long-term goal of coming back as an even better athlete needs to be stressed. Occasionally, an athlete is simply not suited to a particular sport. For example, a larger-boned woman who wants to compete with low-BMI endurance runners may do better in another sport. Similarly, a larger male who wants to row in lightweight crew is at increased risk for an eating disorder.

The core of eating disorders, of course, has little to do with weight, shape, or food. Eating disorders are strategies for dealing with deeper issues in life, such as peer approval, self-esteem, perfectionism, lack of balance, developmental arrests, mood regulation, and relationship conflicts. Activities therapy experts in an experienced eating disorder team can guide the athlete back into a slowly graded increase in athleticism as the eating disorder improves. A significantly lowered bone density, probably less than −2 standard deviations from norms, suggests that high-impact sports should be avoided. Specific advice about participation in a sport should be geared toward individual differences. Early intervention in the female athletic triad benefits the long-term health of girls and women (Lebrun, 2007).

The injured athlete presents a challenge, especially when that person's identity is largely centered on excellence in sports. Early intervention for injuries, rather than after repeated trauma to joints, ligaments, and tendons ("Let me complete the season"), is essential.

Inappropriate dietary restraint is unhealthy, whereas abstention from "junk foods" high in trans fats or concentrated sweets is healthy. Excess dietary restriction limits calcium, an essential component of improved bone mineral density. Up to 95% of bone density is completed by the late teen years. Lowered calcium intake during those years has long-term consequences for building strong bones that will last a lifetime. Garner, Rosen, and Barry (1998) summarized recommendations for intervention and treatment for eating disordered behaviors in athletes.

Typically, a team approach to treatment of the athlete with an eating disorder works best, with the coach and the trainer being involved in nonconfidential aspects of the treatment. No specific psychopharmacologic agents have proved to be of benefit in the treatment of anorexia nervosa, but specific antidepressants may be individually prescribed, especially for comorbid depression and anxiety. For bulimia nervosa, cognitive behavioral therapy is still the gold standard, but here, too, antidepressants may be of use as minority partners in treatment.

The Role of Coaches in Promoting or Preventing Eating Disorders

Coaches either can promote eating disorders or can be essential partners in their treatment by supporting the clinician and encouraging the athlete to seek full remission of the eating disorder rather than a small amount of improvement. Coaching style clearly affects an athlete's vulnerability to an eating disorder. There are important ethical issues in coaching. Placing the long-term welfare of the athlete first is crucial. The "winning at all cost" philosophy is unethical, certainly from grade school through college. Professional athletes may choose to play when injured, being of reasonable age to make such a choice even though it may still be an unwise decision that leads to early career drop-out due to injury. Young athletes who are still developing are not always sufficiently mature to make choices in their best interest, despite what they think, and may be overly influenced by pressure from coaches to place performance above all else. Good coaches are among the most influential and admired persons in an athlete's life. One study found that 67% of athletes with eating disorders reported that they were dieting on advice from their coach (Sundgot-Borgen, 1994). Sherman et al. (2005) summarized the role of coaches in 23 sports in identifying and managing athletes who had disordered eating, noting that "athletic trainers, teammates, and coaches are frequently involved in identification." A modified version of a team approach to the athlete with an eating disorder is shown in figure 12.1 (Joy, Kussman, and Nattiv, 2016). Martinsen, Sherman, et al. (2015) document a sevenfold improvement in coaches' knowledge after an interventional teaching program about nutrition, weight regulation, and eating disorders.

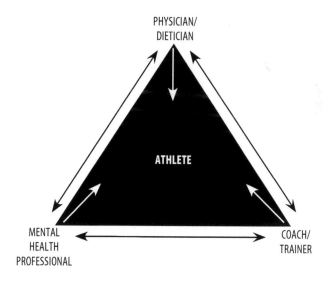

Figure 12.1. Multidisciplinary care of athletes with eating disorders.

The Role of Schools in Healthy Athleticism

Schools, by their action or inaction, promote or hinder healthy athleticism. School policies and practices can promote healthy sports (table 12.5). A 2013 report by Sundgot-Borgen (a long-term leader in the field of sports and eating disorders) and coauthors summarizes how to minimize the health risks to athletes who compete in weight-sensitive sports. The ruthless decimation of sports programs for average students during the school years leads to more obesity and, in later years, more heart disease—major public health issues. It is said that World War II was won on the playing fields of Eton, in terms of building character and fitness. Likewise, many of the lifelong health hazards of adulthood in modern society might be prevented or lessened on the nation's playing fields—now often unavailable—by the participation of all students in sports of some kind, and certainly in daily physical activity of 45 minutes, five times a week. The contribution of regular participation in an aerobic sport, as well as in strength training, to "mens sana in corpore sano" (a healthy mind in a healthy body) is supported by many evidence-based studies. Regular exercise can be as effective as antidepressants in nonpsychotic depression and in anxiety states.

In the United States, there is a too frequent division of students at about the middle school level into elite athletes, for whom facilities are provided for intense participation in sports, and the large majority of students for whom athletics is neglected but who would benefit from encouragement to participate in sports that could carry over for a lifetime of better health. The rise of electronic games and social media has contributed to obesity and physical passivity for many students. Electronic sports games provide an illusion of participation. School board decisions as well as busy parents govern these practices of inattention to sports for the average student and the neglect of physical activity. While political advocacy is not the usual focus of an academic physician, this author strongly supports the use of tax monies for construction of facilities for mandatory daily physical education in schools and the participation of all students in some level of sports—with financial support for the teachers and coaches of these activities as assured as the funds for teaching English and mathematics. Unfortunately, most families cannot afford the expensive preparatory schools that almost always implement this kind of balanced education.

Table 12.5. School policies and practices to promote fitness and prevent eating disorders

- Involve all students in athletics: cardiopulmonary, strength, flexibility, team sports.
- Stop limiting athletics to elite athletes, as is currently done beginning in junior high school.
- Regulate the body fat and recent weight loss allowed in wrestlers, cross-country and endurance runners, and gymnasts.
- Identify eating disorders early and refer students for treatment.
- Involve coaches in designing a program balance between promoting competitiveness and preventing eating disordered and weight disordered behaviors.
- Monitor in particular all sports requiring leanness and/or aesthetic appearance (girls' gymnastics, cross-country, ballet, etc.).
- Involve parents with coaches in program balance.
- Include judges of adjudicated sports in the loop with health professionals, coaches, and parents for a role in discouraging excess/rapid weight loss for participation in sports.
- Emphasize fitness in place of thinness.
- Make nutritional education and school lunches both fun and healthy (as in France and Scandinavia).
- Remove soda machines.
- Provide individualized sports/exercise programs for students for the school year.
- Provide psychological counseling for injured athletes unable to participate.
- Promote a functional view of the body for girls and young women rather than an objectification of body size and shape that leads to critical judging of worth by self and others.
- Emphasize lifetime "carry-over" sports and fitness patterns for during and after the school years.
- Emphasize participation by students with disabilities.

Possibilities for Prevention

Whether measures for the prevention of eating disorders and RED-S in athletes are possible is a subject debated among eating disorders experts and approached in different ways by different nations. Some would argue for primary prevention (Martinsen, Bahr, et al., 2014), while others recommend secondary prevention (early intervention). Norway, for example, encourages primary prevention. It designates a nurse clinician in each district who is trained to intervene early for athletes who might have an eating disorder. The United Kingdom and the United States tend to wait until eating disorders are more fully entrenched, or to ignore their existence in the service of winning performances. Powers and Johnson (1996) addressed "small victories" occurring in the prevention of eating disorders in athletes. Oppliger et al. (1995) reported on states such as Wisconsin that have instituted mandatory standards to limit unhealthy dieting among student wrestlers. Limiting the amount of weight that may be lost to participate in endurance running or ballet can sometimes turn around a potential eating disorder before it reaches the point of having no voluntary component.

More indirect, long-term preventive efforts include changing the culture in which women's bodies are objectified. Young women need to learn to view their bodies from a stance of functional instrumentality (i.e., having a healthy body to *do* things), not as something to be objectified and judged by peers or oneself in terms of thinness and appearance norms. Skepticism of the media is healthy, as is replacing magazines that promote thinness with healthy role models. "Normative cultural distress"—giving lip service to the need to diet a little, but having that dessert anyway—is healthy; a total unconcern about weight is unrealistic. Building "body armor" by encouraging a balance between sports participation and academics for girls will allow them to increase their self-esteem by internalizing skills in athletics during developmentally critical years.

Dieting is the crucial behavior that promotes a transition from an athlete with a culturally healthy concern about weight to one with an eating disorder. The United States is both an underfit and an overfat nation. If every parent required each student to present a sweat-stained T-shirt before allowing him or her to use a computer or play video games, there would be less adolescent obesity and less need or desire to diet. *Diet* is, after all, a four-letter word.

Basic Science Research: What Can Rats Teach Us?

In laboratory studies on rats, scientists have reproduced conditions similar to those faced by athletes: unrestricted access to an activity wheel and restricted food intake. This combination of hyperactivity plus "dieting," very common in athletes, leads to a vicious circle of losing more weight and eating less food, despite the availability of adequate calories. Activity-based anorexia is facilitated by neuropeptide Y (Nergårdh et al., 2007) and suppressed by leptin (Exner et al., 2000), suggesting that in this model of anorexia nervosa, hyperactivity and self-starvation are regulated in the hypothalamus and other areas of the limbic system, areas in which neuro-peptide Y and leptin interact.

The basic science model of anorexia, of course, cannot duplicate the overvaluation of thinness, but it does strongly suggest that biological factors may lock in anorexia nervosa in the presence of conditions similar to those under which athletes compete. Obligatory runners and other compulsive exercisers often feel dysphoric when not allowed to run. Eating disorders may be initiated by choice, but then sustained past a certain point by brain peptides.

Summary

Eating disorders are a major concern in athletics. The emphasis on thinness for performance and for appearance increases the probability of developing an eating disorder. The participation of predisposed young athletes, those with a number of risk factors, in thinness-mandating or aesthetic sports leads to the highest prevalence of eating disorders. Clinicians need to be knowledgeable about the healthy and unhealthy aspects of sports and to work closely with coaches, trainers, and sports educators. Success in detecting eating disorders by requiring athletes to respond to questionnaires is limited by several factors, including an athlete's wish to appear healthy and fit and not be excluded from sports participation. A well-educated, ethical coach, as well as a programmatic school-based approach to healthy eating and activity, can identity and treat or, even better, prevent eating disorders. The preponderance of evidence supports the encouragement of life-time athletic participation for all persons, including those with disabilities. Whether elite athletes are more likely to develop eating disorders than the average non-elite athlete or nonparticipatory student remains controversial. In the meantime, it is important to identify and treat the subset of athletes who do develop eating disorders, recognizing certain sports as posing a higher risk.

REFERENCES

Barrack MT, Rauh MJ, Barkai HS, and Nichols JF. 2008. Dietary restraint and low bone mass in female adolescent endurance runners. *American Journal of Clinical Nutrition* 87(1):36–43.

DiGioacchino DeBate R, Wethington H, and Sargent R. 2002. Body size dissatisfaction among male and female triathletes. *Eating and Weight Disorders* 7:316–23.

Exner C, Hebebrand J, Remschmidt H, et al. 2000. Leptin suppresses semi-starvation induced hyperactivity in rats: Implications for anorexia nervosa. *Molecular Psychiatry* 5(5):476–81.

Fortes LdeS, Kakeshita IS, Almeida SS, et al. 2014. Eating behaviours in youths: A comparison between female and male athletes and non-athletes. *Scandinavian Journal of Medicine and Science in Sports* 24:e62–68.

Gadpaille WJ, Sanborn CF, and Wagner WW. 1987. Athletic amenorrhea, major affective disorders and eating disorders. *American Journal of Psychiatry* 144:939–42.

Garner DM, Rosen LW, and Barry D. 1998. Eating disorders among athletes: Research and recommendations. *Child and Adolescent Psychiatric Clinics of North America* 7:839–57.

Giel KD, Hermann-Werner A, Mayer J, et al. 2016. Eating disorder pathology in elite adolescent athletes. *International Journal of Eating Disorders* doi: 10.1002/eat.2251.

Goltz FR, Stenzel LM, and Schneider CD. 2013. Disordered eating behaviors and body image in male athletes. *Revista Brasileira de Psiquiatria* 35:237–42.

Hilibrand MJ, Hammoud S, Bishop M, et al. 2015. Common injuries and ailments of the female athlete; pathophysiology, treatment, and prevention. *Physician and Sportsmedicine* 43:403–11.

Hind K, Truscott JG, and Evans JA. 2006. Low lumbar spine bone mineral density in both male and female endurance runners. *Bone* 39(4):880–85.

Johnson C, Powers PS, and Dick R. 1999. Athletes and eating disorders: The National Collegiate Athletic Association study. *International Journal of Eating Disorders* 26:179–88.

Joy E, Kussman A, and Nattiv A. 2016. 2016 update on eating disorders in athletes: A comprehensive narrative review with a focus on clinical assessment and management. *British Journal of Sports Medicine* 50:154–62.

King MB and Mezey G. 1987. Eating behaviour of male racing jockeys. *Psychological Medicine* 17:249–53.

Kong P and Harris LM. 2015. The sporting body: Body image and eating disorder symptomatology among female athletes from leanness focused and nonleanness focused sports. *Journal of Psychology* 149:141–60.

Lebrun CM. 2007. The female athletic triad: What's a doctor to do? *Current Sports Medicine Reports* 6:397–404.

Martinsen M and Sundgot-Borgen J. 2013. Higher prevalence of eating disorders among adolescent elite athletes than controls. *Medicine and Science in Sports and Exercise* 45:1188–97.

Martinsen M, Bahr R, Børresen R, et al. 2014. Preventing eating disorders among young elite athletes: A randomized controlled trial. *Medicine and Science in Sports and Exercise* 46:435–47.

Martinsen M, Sherman RT, Thompson RA, et al. 2015. Coaches' knowledge and management of eating disorders: A randomized controlled trial. *Medicine and Science in Sports and Exercise* 47:1070–78.

Morrison AB and Schöffl VR. 2007. Physiological responses to rock climbing in young climbers. *British Journal of Sports Medicine* 41(12):852–61; discussion 886i.

Mountjoy M, Sundgot-Borgen J, Burke L, et al. 2015. Authors' 2015 additions to the IOC consensus statement: Relative energy deficiency in sport (RED-S). *British Journal of Sports Medicine* 49:417–20.

Nergård R, Ammar A, Brodin U, Bergström J, Scheurink A, and Södersten P. 2007. Neuro-peptide Y facilitates activity-based-anorexia. *Psychoneuroendocrinology* 32(5):493–502.

Oppliger RA, Harms RD, Herrmann DE, Streich CM, and Clark RR. 1995. Grappling with weight cutting: The Wisconsin wrestling minimum weight project. *Physician and Sportsmedicine* 23(3):69–78.

Piacentino D, Kotzalidis GD, del Casale A, et al. 2015. Anabolic-androgenic steroid use and psychopathology in athletes. A systematic review. *Current Neuropharmacology* 13:101–21.

Pietrowsky R and Straub K. 2008. Body dissatisfaction and restrained eating in male juvenile and adult athletes. *Eating and Weight Disorders* 13(1):14–21.

Pope HG Jr and Kanayama G. 2004. Bodybuilding's dark side: Clues to anabolic steroid use. *Current Psychiatry* 3(12):12–20.

Powers PS. 1999. Athletes and eating disorders: Some ramifications of the NCAA study. *Eating Disorders Reviews* 10(6):1–3.

Powers PS and Johnson C. 1996. Small victories: Prevention of eating disorders among athletes. *Eating Disorders* 4(4):364–77.

Riebl SK, Subudhi AW, Broker JP, Schenck K, and Berning JR. 2007. The prevalence of subclinical eating disorders among male cyclists. *Journal of the American Dietetic Association* 107(7):1214–17.

Sherman RT, Thompson RA, Dehass D, and Wilfert M. 2005. NCAA coaches survey: The role of the coach in identifying and managing athletes with disordered eating. *Eating Disorders* 13:447–66.

Sundgot-Borgen J. 1994. Risk and trigger factors for the development of eating disorders in female elite athletes. *Medicine and Science in Sports and Exercise* 26:414–19.

Sundgot-Borgen J, Meyer NL, Lohman TG, et al. 2013. How to minimise the health risks to athletes who compete in weight-sensitive sports review and position statement on behalf of the Ad Hoc Research Working Group on Body Composition, Health and Per-formance, under the auspices of the IOC Medical Commission. *British Journal of Sports Medicine* 47(16):1012–22.

Thiel A, Gottfried H, and Hesse FW. 1993. Subclinical eating disorders in male athletes: A study of the low weight category in rowers and wrestlers. *Acta Psychiatrica Scandinavica* 88:259–65.

Thompson SH. 2007. Characteristics of the female athlete triad in collegiate cross-country runners. *Journal of American College Health* 56(2):129–36.

Torstveit MK, Rosenvinge JH, and Sundgot-Borgen J. 2008. Prevalence of eating disor-ders and the predictive power of risk models in female elite athletes: A controlled study. *Scandinavian Journal of Medicine and Science in Sports* 18(1):108–18.

Wollenberg G, Shriver LH, and Gates GE. 2015. Comparison of disordered eating symp-toms and emotional regulation difficulties between female college athletes and non-athletes. *Eating Behaviors* 18:1–6

13

Males with Eating Disorders

Arnold E. Andersen, MD

Common Questions

How is the "manscape" evolving today?

What is the most common ideal body physique for men?

What is "physique anxiety"?

What economic forces are involved in male body dissatisfaction?

How common are eating disorders in boys and men?

Why are there fewer males than females with eating disorders?

Is the diagnosis of eating disorders in males different from that in females?

Has *DSM-5* changed the diagnosis of eating disorders for male patients?

How do eating disorders differ from muscle dysmorphia?

What do the terms "macromusculophilia" and "microsomatophobia" mean?

Which males are more likely to develop eating disorders?

Are eating disorders and muscle dysmorphic disorders forms of addiction?

What is "reverse" anorexia nervosa?

What are the medical needs of male patients with eating disorders?

How can male patients with anorexia nervosa achieve a desired body shape and be less likely to return to dieting after weight restoration?

Do males with eating disorders develop osteoporosis?

What are the most common comorbid psychiatric disorders in
   male patients?

How do you determine a target weight for male patients with
   anorexia nervosa?

How do you treat binge-eating disorder in a male patient who is
   obese?

Can males with eating disordered behaviors return to intensive
   sports activities?

How common is a gay orientation in males with eating disorders?

Why are male military personnel and prisoners at risk for eating
   disorders?

How can boys and teens with eating disorders relate better to their
   fathers?

Can eating disorders in males be prevented?

Case 1

D.J. was an 18-year-old male admitted for treatment of anorexia nervosa, binge-purge subtype. As a preteenager, he had been teased for having
a "gut." At age 14, at 170 pounds and 5 feet 6 inches tall (BMI 27.5), he dieted to improve his performance in wrestling. In the spring of each year,
he dieted more intensively to improve his cross-country running. By age
16, he weighed 115 pounds at 5 feet 8 inches (BMI 17.5) and began to experience regular binge-purge episodes, with purges increasing to three times a
day before admission to treatment. His weight increased to 125 pounds
while he was in outpatient therapy, but his binge-purge episodes did not
decrease.

D.J.'s childhood had been marked by his father's verbal abuse of him
and his mother when the father was drunk, leading to a divorce when D.J.
was 10. He had only occasional contact with his biological father thereafter, unknown to his mother, who was protective of the patient and did not
allow contact with the father. In the year before admission, D.J. had experienced depressed mood.

As his weight declined, he was no longer able to participate in sports
because of weakness. His testosterone decreased to 200 ng/dL (normal
340–800). His sexual drive diminished, but he continued to "hang out"
with his girlfriend. TSH and T4 levels were normal. Potassium was slightly
low at 3.3 meq/L. During treatment, his weight improved; he gained skills

in cognitive behavioral therapy to challenge his overvaluation of the benefits of obtaining better athletic performance through dieting. Sertraline, titrated up to 100 mg per day, was prescribed for his depression. In men's group, D.J. began to open up and discuss his emotions; he was challenged to practice response inhibition when he felt urges to purge. He decided against joining the Marine Corps as a way to "grow up." Instead, he began courses at a community college toward an AA degree. His testosterone levels increased to normal range after 2 months at his target weight range of 143–147 pounds. He gradually returned to recreational sports.

Case 2

L.S. was a 31-year-old medical student referred by his father, a social worker, who was concerned that his son might be suffering from anorexia nervosa or depression. The patient was about 135 pounds in college, at 5 feet 6 inches tall (slim normal). In the context of competing in triathlons and the Iron Man competition, he compulsively exercised to increase speed in the three areas of competition: swimming, biking, and running. His weight decreased over several years of competition until he fluctuated between 100 and 105 pounds. Despite feeling cold and lacking in appetite, when confronted by his physician for being too thin he said, "I don't see it." L.S.'s primary goal was increased athletic skill. He did not initially desire to decrease his weight. Only after his weight fell into the clearly anorexic weight category did he develop a fear of eating normally and becoming fat. He began to experience binges at night without any purging, but engaged in compensatory starvation the following day and increased his exercise program despite extreme fatigue (anorexia nervosa, binge subtype with other compensation). "I started feeling fat. I'm sure my weight is controllable. I feel some shame about the overeating. I don't think I'm too thin." He had impossibly high standards of excellence in work as well as in athletics. On mental status examination, he was not depressed and did not meet criteria for OCD. He did have a morbid fear of fatness and a relentless drive to remain at his anorexic weight.

After motivational interviewing, L.S. was given psychoeducation about the nature of anorexia nervosa, the risks of continued underweight, and a summary of the steps in treatment. He was informed about the genetic predisposition to eating disorders and noted that his mother was an extremely anxious person with whom he could not discuss anything. He was referred to a local psychiatrist experienced in the treatment of eating disorders but declined to meet. His was a case of inadvertent onset of anorexia nervosa, not initially wanting to lose weight or perceiving himself as being too fat. Only after he had lost a considerable amount of weight did he develop a distorted perception of his body size as being too big along with a fear of eating too much and becoming fat.

L.S. consulted with several additional mental health professionals to determine whether there was consensus that he needed treatment. After several months of his weight continuing in the anorexic range, and despite his honest and non-delusional belief that he was not too thin, he cautiously began outpatient therapy with an experienced psychiatrist. After failing to restore weight as an outpatient, he reluctantly accepted a referral to the day hospital, where his treatment is ongoing.

The Evolving "Manscape"

Chi (2015) used the term *manscape* to describe the evolving sociocultural milieu concerning body weight and body shape in which men live today. Galen said that men did not withstand fasting as well as women. Western societies have been less preoccupied with promoting thinness in men compared with the relentless sociocultural pressures promoting weight loss directed at women (Zhang, 2014). But throughout most of western history, men have been vitally concerned about body shape, with records from Sparta in ancient Greece documenting the demand for an athletic physique. Today, half of all males wish to increase weight, while almost half wish to decrease weight. Overriding such weight-change goals, however, for males from the preteen years onward, are increasing demands to attain the "holy grail" of lean muscularity as the only acceptable body physique. David Beckham, Tom Brady, and Brad Pitt are examples of lean muscularity. Higher weight is acceptable if associated with large muscle mass and low body fat. A minority desire the boney thinness of Mick Jagger. Soto Ruiz et al. (2015) summarize the current social milieu regarding gender-specific body goals as follows: "Current models of beauty represent an extreme thinness in the women and a muscular body in the men . . . In general women saw themselves as being fatter than [they] really were while men saw themselves as being thinner than they really were."

Strong economic forces present boys and men with images of impossibly fit males showing "washboard abs" as ideals, resulting in negative self-comparisons in consumers of the media (Hobza et al., 2007; Pritchard and Cramblitt, 2014). The economic goal is to create a negative self-image in all males that can be remedied only by purchasing health-, appearance-, weight-, and shape-improving consumer products. Compared with girls and women, who most often desire only thinness, boys and men seek a plurality of body physique goals, although lean muscularity is the most vigorously promoted image. The three body image ideals for males with eating disorders are shown in figures 13.1, 13.2, and 13.3: the very thin, the lean muscular (most common), and the extremely muscled bodybuilder ideal. "Physique anxiety" in otherwise healthy boys and men is common if not pervasive. The ideal of lean muscularity becomes a source of envy (fig. 13.4).

In the social learning process, boys learn to perceive themselves as fat, on average, at weights slightly above population norms, whereas women perceive themselves as fat at more than 15%–18% below population norms. This early social learning process takes place largely between the first and fifth grades. After that time, there is a continuing and increasing perception of body fatness in 40%–75% of school-aged girls (Schreiber et al., 1996). The prevalence of actual obesity in grade-school children is lower than that of perceived overweight, despite recent increases in average weights. Adolescent males who go on to develop an eating disorder are most likely to begin their dieting at two or more standard deviations above population weight norms (Welch, Ghaderi, and Swenne, 2015).

Because there is less general cultural endorsement for boys to diet, they tend to do so only when they are objectively heavier than average and usually in response to one of four specific provocations: (1) to avoid being teased again as they were for childhood obesity; (2) to increase sports performance; (3) to avoid developing weight-related medical illnesses that they have seen in their fathers; and (4) to improve a gay relationship. More than half of male patients with eating disorders at the University of Iowa began dieting for one of these reasons, in contrast to approximately 10% of female patients. Males with eating disorders fall into three age categories: those with childhood onset before 12 years of age; adolescents, from preteens through the early twenties; and young adults and more mature adults. There is increasing recognition of eating disorders in men at midlife and beyond (Reas and Stedal, 2015). The issues prompting dieting in these three groups differ significantly: very young boys often express

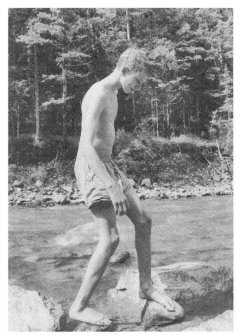

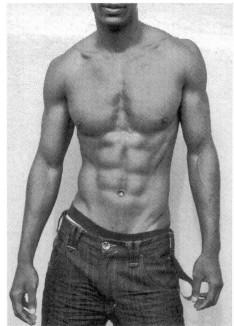

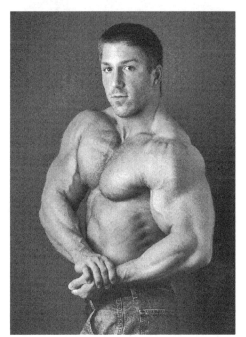

Figure 13.1, *top left.* **Thin ideal.**
istockphoto.com.

Figure 13.2, *top right.* **Lean muscular ideal.** istockphoto.com.

Figure 13.3, *bottom left.* **Extreme muscular ideal.** istockphoto.com.

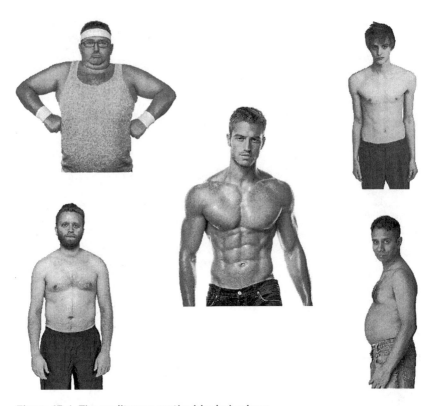

Figure 13.4. The reality versus the ideal physique

family conflict or changes in location or family composition; adolescent males struggle with attaining an individual identity, wanting to develop confidence in sports, dating, and peer recognition; older males may initiate weight or shape change as means of dealing with workplace advancement, new sexual partners, or health concerns. Eating disorders have been diagnosed in males from 10 to 60 years of age, even though onset in the majority of cases is in the teens and early twenties.

About 18% of males with eating disorders have a gay orientation, approximately four or five times the average for the population as a whole, but still a minority (Fichter and Dasher, 1987). The reason for this higher percentage appears to be the increased valuation of thinness, especially thin muscularity, in the gay culture rather than any intrinsic consequence of sexual orientation. Males with gay orientation who have bulimia are at increased risk for HIV infection due to impulsive, unprotected sexual behavior. Many young males with anorexia are simply asexual.

Prevalence of Eating Disorders in Males

The widely quoted ratio of 10 females to 1 male for people with eating disorders is derived from presentations at clinics and hospitals, and is a serious underestimation of eating disorders among males (Sweeting et al., 2015). Population-based surveys are more accurate and typically find a ratio of 3.6:1 (Akgul et al., 2015), and an almost equal prevalence when the female-based diagnostic criteria and assumptions are taken into account. Most recent community-based studies support a ratio of 1:2–3 of males to females with some form of eating disorder (Hudson et al., 2007; Woodside et al., 2001). DSM-5 has eliminated references to amenorrhea in eating disorder diagnoses and now requires a gender-neutral finding of significant restriction of energy intake.

Diagnosis

There are multiple contributions to the underdiagnosis of eating disorders in men and boys. Males, and society in general, stigmatize males with eating disorders more than females (Griffiths, Mond, Li, et al, 2015; Griffiths, Mond, Murray, et al., 2014; MacLean et al., 2015). In one study, health care providers perceived eating disorders and anabolic-androgenic steroid use less favorably than cocaine use (Yu, Hildebrandt, and Lanzieri, 2015). Diagnostic criteria and standardized testing are normed for females, with some recent improvement. Clinicians share unvoiced social assumptions that eating disorders are female disorders. Thus, the first concern in assessing male patients is simply to think of eating disorders as a diagnostic possibility rather than to overlook abnormal eating and preoccupation with body image as "guy behavior." For some time, physicians dismissed the possibility of eating disorders in males because boys and men did not fit within archaic psychoanalytic formulations or because they could not manifest amenorrhea. Yet the first report of anorexia in the English language, in the late 1500s, as well as the first modern studies in England by Sir William Gull in 1873, included males.

Diagnosis of an eating disorder in males is made by criteria similar to those used for females, with some differences. Diagnosis is made simply and accurately by a brief set of questions and responses in the patient's history and interview, and *not by ruling out all conceivable medical possibilities*. Anorexia nervosa requires the presence of (1) medically significant reduction of energy intake (with or without binge-purge features); (2) a morbid fear of becoming fat and/or a relentless drive for thinness, leading to substantial and sustained weight loss over at least 3 months; (3) general medical signs of starvation; and (4), for many patients, a distorted perception of body image, not recognizing their thinness (ego-syntonic symptom). Abnormality of reproductive hormones (low testosterone, LH, FSH), like amenorrhea, is a secondary consequence of weight loss rather than an intrinsic part of the disorder.

Males with bulimia nervosa who are in the normal or mildly overweight range experience binge eating followed in 80% of cases by purging and in 20% by other forms of compensation such as overexercise or additional food restriction. Increasingly recognized is the presence of binge-eating disorder in male patients—binge eating with no purging or any other compensation (Pope et al., 2006). Binge-eating disorder occurs primarily in adult males, usually in their thirties to fifties, and is more common than anorexia nervosa or bulimia nervosa. Most studies find an equal prevalence of binge-eating disorder in males and females. It is often intermixed with mild to severe medical obesity. Male patients with bulimia are more likely than females to have the companion disorders of substance abuse and antisocial personality features. In contrast, most males who have anorexia with restricting subtype have self-critical, anxious, persevering, perfectionist, or obsessive-compulsive personality features.

The issue is not settled as to whether there are somewhat fewer males than females with eating disorders because males are less exposed than females to social pressures promoting thinness or because they have intrinsic biological protection against eating disorders. Media are increasingly promoting male drive for slim muscularity.

Risk Factors

Males who participate in sports, hobbies, or vocations requiring thinness for appearance or performance, or both, develop eating disordered behaviors more commonly than do other males (Thiel, Gottfried, and Hesse, 1993). About 18% of male high school students who wrestle show some form of eating disordered behavior and thinking during the wrestling season (Oppliger et al., 1993), although most of them improve spontaneously when the season is over. A high percentage of males in wrestling, gymnastics, swimming, track, horse racing, and football are vulnerable to eating disorders, with the desired direction of weight change determined by the nature of the sport. Football defensive players have been increasing in weight year by year. Before stricter regulations were recently put in place in some states, many wrestlers attempted to wrestle in artificially low weight categories by dieting and dehydration through fluid restriction or diuretics. The deaths of three wrestlers, reported in the media, have highlighted the dangers of rapid and excessive weight loss. Other sports in which primarily males participate, such as bodybuilding and football, may require artificial gains in weight, resulting in the use of anabolic-androgenic steroids. The jury is out on whether the common use of creatinine supplements to increase muscle mass is unhealthy. Male weightlifters are especially subject to muscle dysmorphia (Olivardia, Pope, and Hudson, 2000) and eating disorders (Ruffolo et al., 2006). Adolescent males with gynecomastia are very sensitive about chest shape and may initiate dieting to get rid of their breasts (Fisher and Fornari, 1990). Surgical reduction can be successful.

"Reverse" Anorexia Nervosa, Muscle Dysmorphia, and Body Dysmorphic Disorder

One form of eating disorder occurs almost exclusively in men and boys. Males who think of themselves as never big enough, never muscular enough, even though large and "cut," may suffer from "reverse" anorexia nervosa, considered by some to be a form of body dysmorphic disorder— more specifically, muscle dysmorphia. The literature has blossomed with studies on "reverse" anorexia nervosa compared with and contrasted with muscle dysmorphia and body dysmorphic disorder (Dingemans et al., 2012). *DSM-5* includes Body Dysmorphic Disorder under the category of Obsessive-Compulsive and Related Disorders; Body Dysmorphic Disorder is a general diagnosis requiring preoccupation with a perceived defect or flaw in physical appearance that is not observable to others or is considered insignificant by others. Males with hugely defined muscularity and very low body fat are not adequately included in the Body Dysmorphic Disorder category. *DSM-5* includes Muscle Dysmorphia as a specifier within Body Dysmorphic Disorder, describing it as a syndrome characterized by a person's preoccupation with the idea that "his or her physique" is too small or not sufficiently muscular (predominantly males). There is reason to consider "reverse" anorexia nervosa as overlapping with but different from muscle dysmorphia. Muscle dysmorphic disorder within the body dysmorphic disorder category focuses on the perception of smallness rather than on the abnormal eating and athletic behaviors of "reverse" anorexia nervosa, which is characterized by the relentless desire and drive for bigness, usually along with the objective reality of great muscularity. I suggest *macromusculophilia* (desire for huge muscles) and *microsomatophobia* (fear of being too small) as more precise terms for the condition—the first term recognizing the strong desire for large muscles in association with, in the second term, a morbid fear of having a small body. The term *"reverse" anorexia nervosa* is awkward linguistically but has the advantage of implying that the condition is a mirror image of the common perceptual distortion found in anorexia nervosa of being too large despite being, in reality, medically starved.

The following is a brief summary based on a progress note for an incarcerated male with "reverse" anorexia nervosa (macromusculophilia with microsomatophobia), who gave permission to share his story anonymously (nonspecific features are modified). The patient was a 30-year-old man serving out a prison sentence for burglary. He was in treatment for anxiety and depression, treated with sertraline, when I was asked to evaluate him for a second opinion. It soon became clear that he was also suffering from "reverse" anorexia nervosa in the context of defending himself in the prison environment. The patient viewed his body as too small and his muscles as not big enough. He was teased as a child for being small. In prison he embarked on a program of muscle development and increased weight. He worked out 3–4 hours every other day. He did not engage in cardiovascular activities such as running because of fear of losing weight. His stated goal was "to look huge." "I'm eating crazy." "I just want to be muscular. I don't want to be fat. I want to be huge." Despite his enormous biceps, he said that "my biceps don't look large enough from my viewpoint." His ideal was "all muscle, no fat, built like a bull or ox or horse." He was preoccupied for much of the day thinking about how to build up his body. He discounted comments that he was very muscular and huge. "I've been asking people how big I look—thinking about my body almost all day—once someone starts being a smart ass and saying I can't get any bigger, then I start thinking I need to do more workout." He lifted up to 700 pounds of weights.

"I'm doing 700 pounds half way; 435 all the way down." "I want to be so big that I'll look intimidating." He continued on sertraline and a few cognitive behavioral therapy (CBT) sessions until he was moved to probation status.

Comparison of Diagnosis and Body Dissatisfaction in Males and Females

Very starved male and female patients are similar medically with the exception that the male starts with a lower reserve percentage of body fat and a higher lean muscle mass, allowing him less weight loss before the onset of ketosis from protein breakdown. Males appear to be less attentive to taking vitamins while dieting and may suffer more vitamin deficiency syndromes. In contrast to the occurrence of amenorrhea in females, males have no comparable "signal" that alerts a family and others to the medical consequences of weight loss. In addition, boys and men who suspect they may have an eating disorder often perceive, accurately, stigma from society, from females with eating disorders, and from peers, and thus they may be hesitant to discuss this possibility with clinicians. Unfortunately, many professionals also fail to recognize eating disorders in male patients, through either theoretical bias or lack of diagnostic training. Not uncommonly, in our program we treat male patients whose eating disorders were recognized only belatedly because of denial of illness or stigma, or were refused treatment in other programs simply because they are male.

Men in general are more dissatisfied with their bodies from the waist up, while women are predominantly dissatisfied with their bodies from the waist down. Most men and boys with anorexia find that relentless self-starving does not produce the shape change they desire, despite drastic weight change; they become morbidly afraid of being fat, despite evident thinness, if some body part, especially the abdomen, has not been visibly reduced. There is a strong possibility that the cultural pattern of valuing thinness in women has not been followed by men because, in the early to mid-1980s, the thin, cachectic male became socially identified with possible AIDS.

Males, compared with females, develop within a different social learning experience regarding ideal body weight and shape, have a different hormonal milieu, value different goals in sports, diet for different and more personal reasons, may have different comorbid disorders, and will be

Table 13.1. Clinical features of males with eating disorders

- Feeling of increased stigma from self, from society, and from female peers with eating disorders.
- Less recognition from professionals of the possibility of an eating disorder. Increased probability of occurrence among participants in sports requiring weight loss for performance or appearance and among persons with vulnerable personality, childhood obesity, or gay orientation. Screening tests often underscore males.
- Increased probability of comorbid substance abuse as well as presence of OCD or depression.
- Anorexia nervosa usually associated with low plasma testosterone, low LH, and low FSH.
- Preoccupation with abdomen, chest, shoulders, arms, upper body.
- Binge-eating disorder as common as in females, often associated with obesity.

returning to a different gender role in society. For all these reasons, in diagnosis and treatment, it is of great importance for the clinician to recognize and treat males with eating disorders while respecting the male-specific components. Clinical features of males with eating disorders are summarized in table 13.1

Is an Eating Disorder a Form of Addiction?

The meaning of the term *addiction* has been broadened considerably in recent years. Previously, it referred to a condition of physical dependence with medically recognizable withdrawal features, as well as causing functional impairment including negative consequences to society. Eating disorders, especially "reverse" anorexia nervosa and muscle dysmorphia, do not result in physical dependence in the way opiate or alcohol use disorders can cause physical dependence. Males who are medically or otherwise interrupted in their quest for huge muscularity with low body fat can and do experience psychological withdrawal, sometimes accentuated by the physiologic withdrawal from anabolic-androgenic steroids. The question of what the term *addiction* covers is a semantic one, but the clinical condition is a reality. Interruption of any of the eating disorder subgroups, all of which are to some degree ego-syntonic, may well lead to psychological distress and a form of mourning before healthier thinking and behavior are established.

Medical Evaluation

In the history-taking part of the evaluation, unless the patient has been referred with a diagnosis of an eating disorder, the physician, physician's assistant, or advanced registered nurse practitioner can make the diagnosis in a straightforward manner by appropriate questions as described in chapter 1. It is helpful to have a short set of diagnostic screening questions for each common behavioral disorder and age group, comparable to the CAGE questionnaire for alcohol abuse. A comparable set of screening questions regarding eating disorders is the SCOFF questionnaire (Morgan, Reid, and Lacey, 1999).

A young male patient's participation in a higher-risk sport that emphasizes thinness for appearance or performance goals should alert the physician to pose diagnostic questions even in a routine physical, as should unexplained low potassium, weight loss of more than 15 pounds, parotid gland swelling (from purging), or nonspecific gastrointestinal discomfort. The primary care physician should ask about changes in eating and exercise history and any changes in the results of the physical examination compared with previous visits. Once the diagnosis of an eating disorder is made, or if the patient has been referred to the primary care clinician with a diagnosis of an eating disorder, the circumstances around the onset of weight loss or binge-purge activities should be explored, especially the reason for weight or shape change and the methods of weight loss. Of interest is that with mixed-gender twins, the male twin may be at increased risk of anorexia nervosa resulting from the intrauterine hormonal milieu resulting from hormonal production by the female twin (Procopio and Marriott, 2007), suggesting that gender effects begin as early as in utero.

Eating disorders almost always come as "package deals," with one to several comorbid psychiatric diagnoses separate from the eating disorder. Depression is seen in 50%–70% of males with eating disorders, comparable to the number for females. Other diagnoses are more likely in males than in females. At times, the comorbid condition—such as substance abuse, OCD, or impulsive, antisocial personality traits—will determine the long-term prognosis more than the eating disorder itself. If street drugs have been used, their relationship to the eating disorder should be explored; for example, it is not uncommon for patients to snort a line of cocaine to inhibit an urge to binge or to promote further weight loss. The presence and medical consequences of compulsive exercising, including "march hemo-globinuria" (blood in the urine) and stress fractures, should be noted.

The history of the male patient with an eating disorder includes changes in sexual desire and functioning, usually a decrease in sexual drive, sexual fantasies, and masturbation frequency, in proportion to weight loss. Sexual orientation should be determined because of the health implications of un-protected sex, either heterosexual or homosexual. Physical examination notes the general degree of emaciation and decline in lean muscle mass, as well as general medical findings including vital signs. Bulimia nervosa is less obvious on physical examination; patients may be secretive about binge-purge behav-iors. With obese males, screening questions should be asked to determine whether binge-eating disorder is present.

Laboratory studies for male patients, in addition to the general evalu-ation noted above, include serum testosterone level (both total testoster-one and free testosterone) if weight loss is present. Normal absolute testosterone varies typically from 340 to 800 ng/dL, while free testoster-one is usually in the range of 1.8–6.8 ng/dL (for ages 20–49). Testosterone declines in proportion to weight loss (Andersen, Wirth, and Strahlman, 1982). LH and FSH are correspondingly diminished in anorexia nervosa because the changes in gonadotropins are due to central hypothalamic hy-pogonadism secondary to starvation, rather than increasing in level as would be expected with a failing gonad. Testicular examination often re-veals testes that are decreased in size in anorexia nervosa, comparable to the testicular volume of prepubertal males. If unprotected sex or intrave-nous drug use is disclosed in the history, then a request for HIV testing is appropriate (Ramsay, Catalan, and Gazzard, 1992).

For males with binge-eating disorder, the medical complications of the commonly associated obesity should be evaluated through lipid panel test-ing, with attention to the presence of type 2 diabetes mellitus and hyper-tension. Any male with anorexic levels of weight loss for more than 6 months should generally be referred for a DEXA scan to assess for loss of bone mineral density. Osteoporosis and osteopenia are common in chronic eating disorders (anorexia nervosa and bulimia nervosa). Males, somewhat surprisingly, have even worse deficiencies in bone mineral density than females with eating disorders (Mehler et al., 2008).

Treatment

The treatment of low-weight males with anorexia nervosa is similar to that of underweight females, while addressing a few additional, male-specific concerns (Andersen, 1990). The general goals of all eating disorder treatments are as follows:

1. To normalize weight, with a healthy goal weight range of about 4 pounds (e.g., 143–147 pounds for case 1 at the beginning of this chapter). A subset of patients with bulimia nervosa are mildly underweight, and this contributes to binge urges if not corrected.
2. To normalize eating behavior by teaching patients how to choose balanced, adequate meals anywhere, anytime, whether by oneself, in a school cafeteria, at a family meal, or at a celebration.
3. To challenge and change the patient's overvaluation of the benefits of weight loss or shape change, using CBT. This is the core of lasting treatment benefits and involves helping the individual learn to deal with fundamental issues in living, such as identity formation, mood regulation, and harassment, and to gain a sense of control.
4. To reach a decision about whether the comorbid medical and psychiatric diagnoses are secondary (in which case, these conditions—for example, hypothermia—improve on their own) or primary, perhaps predisposing the patient to the disorder (e.g., preexisting depressive disorder), and whether they are long-lasting, as in the case of osteoporosis caused by the eating disorder.
5. To provide treatment that prepares males for return to their gender-specific social roles as well as to work out issues in sexuality. Males especially need work to accurately identify and express feelings.

There is merit to the consideration of physiologic replacement of testosterone for adolescents and adults who have reached all or most of their axial height. In the case of males with anorexia who have documented low levels of testosterone, there are no definitive studies regarding the specific benefits of testosterone replacement versus allowing hormone levels to return naturally. If testosterone replacement is chosen during the weight restoration phase, the typical mode currently used is a topical gel, with a 5 mg per day dose. Once full weight restoration has been attained, supplemental testosterone is discontinued.

Testosterone level is reassessed one month later to determine whether an adequate weight has been reached for the patient's normal hormone production. Because virtually all late adolescent and adult males of normal weight should be producing normal amounts of testosterone, a continued low level usually indicates inadequate weight or persisting testicular disorder independent of weight. The therapeutic use of testosterone for males with anorexia is based on an extension of testosterone use for underweight patients with AIDS or for burn patients. Caution would be indicated for males who are not yet close to full height and maximal bone growth, because testosterone can cause premature closure of the bony growth plate. The eventual benefits versus risks of this short-term anabolic hormone need to be rigorously studied.

Males with eating disorders are most commonly treated for most of their inpatient / day hospital stay in our program in mixed-gender groups, with two important additional treatments. Our experience is that males benefit, first, from enhanced strength training, with an emphasis on strength not appearance, and second, from participation in groups for boys and young men with their fathers or siblings. Ideally, the strength training exercises are guided by a team member trained in exercise physiology, starting "low and slow," building up to moderate levels of resistance, and emphasizing good form to enhance lean muscle development and decrease the tendency for early weight restoration to be in the abdominal area. When restored weight is concentrated in the abdomen, it provokes fears of becoming fat and concerns about repeating the body weight distribution that may have prompted the dieting originally.

Monitoring of liver function, hemoglobin, and other laboratory tests typically continues during testosterone replacement. There is some concern about long-term testicular deficiency in male patients who have had an eating disorder, a result noted in a study showing that 2 of 11 males who returned to a healthy weight remained oligospermic or azoospermic. The physician should ask the patient about the return of normal sexual drive, fantasy, and sexual function during the weight restoration process. Often the male patient's social behavior and spontaneous discussion of sexually related topics will indicate a return to more normal hormone production. Flirting with staff members and signs of masturbatory activity are signals of improved weight and testosterone production. The addition of testosterone to the weight restoration of male patients with anorexia is not a settled issue and is not mandatory.

Groups for teen boys and young men with their fathers and brothers have, in our experience, proved very beneficial to improving the often frayed relationships within the family. Teen boys and young men generally suffer from alexithymia, not having words for their feelings. One patient, for example, would come home, fatigued from a day of work, walk past his father and go to his room. The father would angrily come after his son and demand to know why his son was ignoring him and would not stop to talk with him. The son would become angry in return, and a long-standing distressed relationship worsened. After several groups with patient and father, the patient learned to come home and say to his father, "Dad, I am tired and worn out from tough customers; I'll spend some time in my room and then we can talk." As a result of disclosing his feeling to his father, the son allowed the father to relate to his son's fatigue and wait till later for a chat. A simple illustrative story we use in father-son-brother groups is that boys stop learning colors beyond those in a small crayon pack they receive in grade school. Their range of colors learned is limited to blue, red, green, yellow, brown, and black. Seldom do they identify mauve, fuchsia, salmon, or teal. The same limitation goes for feelings—anger is quickly learned and all too often may be the only feeling employed. In groups using CBT, sons learn to say: "When I come home tired, I feel tired and a little depressed; I am not sad or ignoring you. I need some space and quiet." Fathers learn to say: "Thank you for sharing your feelings. That makes sense that you would feel that way. I know you are not ignoring me." Distressed father-son relationships improve regularly.

We often treat servicemen in their forties and fifties who have developed an eating disorder in response to being required to lose weight and increase fitness to pass annual physical performance and medical examinations. They have generally responded well to treatment because their jobs are on the line.

A group that may be overlooked is long-term prisoners who develop "reverse" anorexia nervosa (macromusculophilia) to protect themselves from other, predatory prisoners or gangs, as described for one patient earlier in the chapter. Another patient, a 40-year-old male prisoner, began each day with 900 sit-ups despite knee injuries. He also performed hundreds of push-ups each day to avoid becoming fat from his involuntary intramuscular antipsychotic medications. Some incarcerated men go on hunger strikes to achieve leniency from prison restrictions, attaining anorexic weights.

What Is a Healthy Weight for Recovering Males with Anorexia?

In determining a healthy weight, the rule of thumb is to ask the body for the answer rather than an insurance table, although "ideal body weights" from standard tables may be used for the short-term goal in acute treatment. If the patient was at a stable weight and height for some time prior to the eating disorder and this was not an obese weight, then the pre-illness weight may be a good target for fully grown men. When an individual has grown taller during an illness of several years, the goal weight may not be obvious. Here, the Metropolitan Life "Ideal Body Weight" scales or the mean matched population weight chart may be reasonable initial choices, but final weight range should be modified according to the body's messages that it is functioning in a stable range. Specific signs of a return to a healthy body weight are present when the following conditions are met:

- Full normalization of temperature control with no signs of hypothermia.
- Normal patterns of hunger before meals and satiety afterward.
- Restoration of normal LH, FSH, and testosterone levels.
- Normal TSH level, if low when the individual was ill.
- Return to normal cues for eating, in place of mental preoccupation with food due to the psychobiology of starvation.

Continued mental preoccupation with weight and shape is a different issue, not yielding to the simpler measures of weight restoration but usually requiring expert psychotherapy, most clearly accomplished with CBT. As with the return of normal estrogen levels, normal testosterone is a necessary but not sufficient guideline for determination of a normal weight range. It is important for patients to understand that body functioning may not be fully normal until healthy behaviors have continued and weight has been stable in a healthy range for 6–9 months or longer after acute weight restoration. A final weight appropriate for age, height, and individual physiology will be worked out during the year after initial treatment is concluded, a year of intensive relapse prevention. The patient needs to be reassured that the disproportionate concentration of some weight in the abdominal area during weight restoration is a natural occurrence; this weight will be redistributed during the year of relapse prevention and psychological growth after acute care.

The male patient with bulimia suffers medical consequences similar to those for females, with medical symptoms divided between the consequences of weight loss, if present, and the specific problems associated with the particular purging behaviors. Binges themselves are uncomfortable physically and psychologically, triggering urges to purge or otherwise compensate for the excessive calories ingested, but generally have fewer medical complications than the purges (except for the rare gastric rupture). Hypokalemia with resulting arrhythmias is the most common serious medical complication of purging. Tender, enlarged parotid glands may be the most obvious medical sign. If a male with bulimia is HIV positive (usually resulting from comorbid IV substance abuse or unprotected sex, often due to an impulsive personality or bipolar II mood disorder), then appropriate treatment should be offered according to the best recent studies.

When binge-eating disorder is diagnosed in an obese male, treatments are directed first toward improvement of the binge-eating disorder through a combination of nutritional guidance, CBT, and often an SSRI, typically fluoxetine, sertraline, or escitalopram. Once the binge eating behaviors are improved, the second phase of treatment involves directing attention to the overweight or frank obesity, deciding whether it should be treated because of medical complications or whether the patient should be encouraged to develop overall cardiovascular fitness and attain greater lean muscle mass while accepting a weight up to a BMI of 28 or so. Evidence is good that a BMI from 25 to 28, along with good cardiovascular fitness, low body fat, and no hypertension, may be compatible with excellent health and is best accepted, rather than being characterized by relentless and ineffective dieting. Interestingly, in one study, older males with a BMI of less than 22.7 had the highest mortality (Breeze et al., 2006). Simply telling a patient in a weight range with BMI of 26–30 to lose weight is easy for physicians to recommend but much harder to carry out, and sometimes is not necessary if fitness goals are defined.

If weight loss is sought, one runs into all the problems of trying to trick the body into attaining and, more importantly, maintaining a lower weight than the body weight during the active binge-eating disorder. It is sometimes possible to obtain moderate, long-lasting changes in the "set point" of an individual's weight through improved choices of healthy foods, with the emphasis on choosing balanced food groups rather than limiting calories; addition of moderate, regular exercise; and improvement of stress management. The role of alcohol use, either solitary drinking or in a social context, in disinhibiting eating behavior in males must be explored and discussed. The increased eating associated with alcohol binges (the latter present in 60%–70% of first-year college students) is often passed off as normal behavior but may be a substantial contributor to undesired weight increase.

Finally, males with eating disorders who have had any sustained underweight for 6 months or more should be tested for bone mineral density with a DEXA scan. There is less likelihood that the clinician will think of osteoporosis in association with a male patient. However, males with anorexia experience more osteoporosis than do females (Andersen, Watson, and Schlechte, 2000). The contributing factors to the pathogenesis of osteoporosis in men appear to include low testosterone and, as in females, diminished calcium intake, lowered body weight, elevated cortisol, and the like. The best current treatments for osteoporosis in male patients include moderate exercise through low-impact weight-bearing activities (avoiding high-impact sports, which increase fracture risk), prompt restoration to normal body weight, restoration of natural production of testosterone, and fully adequate calcium (1,500 mg/day) and vitamin D (800–1,000 IU/day) intake. (Use of bisphosphonates for osteoporosis in men is not yet validated but may be considered.) A return to normal weight, involvement in low-impact weight-bearing activities, and normal testosterone production are the major contributing factors to improved bone mineral density.

The prognosis for males with anorexia nervosa is the same as or better than that for females (Strober et al., 2006). Any beliefs that maleness is by itself an adverse risk factor for recovery from eating disorders need to be updated by evidence-based studies supporting the fact that males have an excellent prognosis if treated promptly and fully. Individuals with eating disorders can be better off after remission through successful treatment than if they had never had the disorder (although it's a tough way to go) because they will have learned to deal more effectively with the sociocultural forces that overvalue weight and shape changes. A book accessible to the general public, *Making Weight: Men's Conflicts with Food, Weight, Shape, and Appearance* (Andersen, Cohn, and Holbrook, 2000), offers more details about men's issues with food, weight, shape, and appearance.

Some "pearls" and tips about the diagnosis and treatment of eating disorders in male patients are listed in table 13.2.

Summary

Men and boys develop eating disorders more frequently than was previously believed, in a ratio of approximately one male to two or three females. Many fewer seek medical care, however, indicating multiple roadblocks for males—especially shame, clinicians' failure to recognize this disorder in male patients, non-acceptance in treatment facilities, assumptions on the part of caregivers of sexual orientation, and fear of being treated like females. Males with eating disorders have a plurality of body image choices compared with females: very thin, mesomorphic, or overdeveloped. The common desire of almost all males with eating disordered behaviors is to achieve lean muscularity, with minimal body fat and favoring upper body development. If lean muscularity is not possible, then huge muscularity or extreme thinness are the next most commonly sought-after goals. The media have increasingly presented body image ideals for men that are as impossible to achieve as the starved images are for women. The socially and commercially mandated ideal physique for men has become more intensely promoted since about 1990. Males are more likely to develop eating disorders for specific personal reasons rather than a sociocultural endorsement of slimness for all men. Some of the more common reasons are to avoid being teased for childhood obesity, to improve sports performance, to avoid medical illnesses, and to improve a gay relationship. Males are often more concerned with shape than weight.

Screening tests used to identify males with eating disorders often under-score or omit male symptoms. A brief informed clinical evaluation is usually sufficient. Diagnosis is similar for male and female patients with anorexia nervosa or bulimia nervosa, but generally only males develop "reverse" anorexia, a condition in which fear of smallness dominates despite huge muscular development, predisposing these patients to use of anabolic-androgenic steroids. More precise terms to describe the psychopathology of males attempting to achieve overly defined muscularity with low body fat, despite perceptions of being still too small and underdeveloped, are

Table 13.2. Clinical "pearls" for the diagnosis and treatment of eating disorders in males

- Boys and men tend to feel fat only at weights above population norms, whereas women generally feel fat even when objectively thin.
- Males tend to be more concerned with shape than with weight and predominantly want to change the body waist-up rather than waist-down. The most frequently desired body image is lean muscularity; the alternatives are huge muscularity or extreme thinness.
- Males more often diet for very specific, personal reasons rather than because of a general cultural endorsement of thinness.
- Males with eating disorders are less well recognized by clinicians, who may not think of the diagnosis for male patients. They also are under-recognized because of the perception of stigma on their part and a resulting reluctance to seek either diagnosis or treatment.
- While not a proven therapy, there is merit to considering short-term replacement of testosterone during the weight restoration phase for males with anorexia, especially for those at or close to maximal height.
- Although being gay increases the risk for an eating disorder because of stringent sociocultural body image ideals, the majority of males with eating disorders are not gay or bisexual. Many young males with anorexia are asexual.
- Males with eating disorders develop osteoporosis as frequently as and with even more severity than females, most likely tied to the gender-specific contributing factor of low testosterone as well as the gender-shared contribution of low calcium intake, low body weight, elevated cortisol, and probably excessive consumption of diet sodas.
- Males especially benefit from resistance exercises during weight restoration; these exercises improve morale, provide a sense that the individual is making a personal contribution toward a desired body shape, resulting in an increased percentage of lean muscle mass, helping to decrease relapse, and providing a setting in which to work out with other males.
- Males, rarely females, may have "reverse" anorexia, in which they exercise relentlessly and attempt to increase their body weight because of the perception that they are never large enough, even though they may objectively be very muscular with extreme muscle definition. In contrast to the more common "drive for thinness," these males experience a "drive for bigness."
- Males with "reverse" anorexia nervosa are liable to use anabolic-androgenic s teroids to attain the "bigness" they desire: extreme muscularity with little body fat. This syndrome overlaps with muscle dysmorphia.

Table 13.2. (*continued*)

- Males with diminished bone density should avoid high-impact sports activities until there is an improvement in bone strength. After a healthy weight, freedom from binge-purge behaviors, and a healthy attitude toward food, weight, and shape are attained and maintained for several months, they can return to their chosen sports activities. Some males need to stay away from wrestling, figure skating, modeling, or other activities that promote weight loss if they continue to have a high drive for thinness.
- Wherever possible, it is beneficial to have some male-specific components in the eating disorder program. These components include "guys-only" groups (comparable to women-only rape survivor groups), consideration of testosterone replacement, strength training programs, and individual therapy that addresses issues of gender orientation, decisions about sports and vocational goals, and, especially, improved relationships with fathers and peers, as well as return to a chosen gender lifestyle.

macromusculophilia and microsomatophobia: a strong desire for huge muscles associated with a fear of having a small body. Treatment needs to appreciate male concerns, including establishing support groups for male patients, striving for improved relationships with fathers, implementing strength training, and occasionally using testosterone supplementation. Gay males are about five times more likely to develop an eating disorder than the general population, but still constitute a minority of cases. Male patients have a prognosis as good as or better than that for females. Increased concern for prevention of eating disorders in males is essential but neglected (Cohn et al., 2016).

REFERENCES

Akgul S, Akdemir D, Kara M, et al. 2015. The understanding of risk factors for eating disorders in male adolescents. *International Journal of Adolescent Medicine and Health* 28:91–96.

Andersen A E (ed.). 1990. *Males with Eating Disorders*. New York: Brunner/Mazel.

Andersen A, Cohn L, and Holbrook T. 2000. *Making Weight: Men's Conflicts with Food, Weight, Shape, and Appearance*. Carlsbad, CA: Gurze Books.

Andersen A E, Watson T, and Schlechte J. 2000. Osteoporosis and osteopenia in men with eating disorders. *Lancet* 355:1967–68.

Breeze E, Clarke R, Shipley M, et al. 2006. Cause-specific mortality in old age in relation to body mass index in middle age and in old age: Follow-up of the Whitehall cohort of male civil servants. *International Journal of Epidemiology* 35:169–78.

Chi K R. 2015. Masculinity: Men's makeover. *Nature* 526:S12–13.

Cohn L, Murrary SB, Walen A, et al. 2016. Including the excluded: Males and gender minorities in eating disorders prevention. *Eating Disorders* 24:114–20

Dingemans AE, van Rood YR, de Groot I, and Van Furth EF. 2012. Body dysmorphic disorder in patients with an eating disorder: Prevalence and characteristics. *International Journal of Eating Disorders* 45:562–69.

Fichter MM and Dasher C. 1987. Symptomatology, psychosexual development, and gender identity in 42 anorexic males. *Psychological Medicine* 17:409–18.

Fisher M and Fornari V. 1990. Gynecomastia as a precipitant of eating disorders in adolescent males. *International Journal of Eating Disorders* 9:115–19.

Griffiths S, Mond JM, Li A, et al. 2015. Self-stigma of seeking treatment and being male predict an increased likelihood of having an undiagnosed eating disorder. *International Journal of Eating Disorders* 48:775–78.

Griffiths S, Mond JM, Murray SB, et al. 2014. Young peoples' stigmatizing attitudes and beliefs about anorexia nervosa and muscle dysmorphia. *International Journal of Eating Disorders* 47:189–95.

Gull WW. 1873. Anorexia nervosa (apepsia hysterica). *British Medical Journal* 2:527–28.

Hobza CL, Walker KE, Yakushko O, and Peugh JL. 2007. What about men? Social comparison and the effects of media images on body and self-esteem. *Psychology of Men and Masculinity* 8:161–72.

Hudson JI, Hiripi E, Pope HG Jr., and Kessler RC. 2007. The prevalence and correlates of eating disorders in the National Comorbidity Survey Replication. *Biological Psychiatry* 61:348–58.

MacLean A, Sweeting H, Walker L, et al. 2015. "It's not healthy and it's decidedly not masculine": A media analysis of UK newspaper representations of eating disorders in males. *BMJ* dx.doi.org/10.1136/bmjopen-2014-007468.

Mehler PS, Sabel AL, Watson T, and Andersen AE. 2008. High risk of osteoporosis in male eating disordered patients. *International Journal of Eating Disorders* 41:666–72.

Morgan JF, Reid F, and Lacey JH. 1999. The SCOFF Questionnaire: Assessment of a new screening tool for eating disorders. *BMJ* 319:1467–68.

Olivardia R, Pope HG, and Hudson JI. 2000. Muscle dysmorphia in male weight-lifters: A case-control study. *American Journal of Psychiatry* 157:1291–96.

Oppliger RA, Landry GL, Foster SW, and Lambrecht AC. 1993. Bulimic behaviors among interscholastic wrestlers: A statewide survey. *Pediatrics* 91:826–31.

Pope HG, Lalonde JK, Pindyck LJ, et al. 2006. Binge eating disorder: A stable syndrome. *American Journal of Psychiatry* 163:2181–83.

Pritchard M and Cramblitt B. 2014. Media influence on drive for thinness and drive for muscularity. *Sex Roles* 71:208–18.

Procopio M and Marriott P. 2007. Intrauterine hormonal environment and risk of developing anorexia nervosa. *Archives of General Psychiatry* 64:1402–8.

Ramsay N, Catalan J, and Gazzard B. 1992. Eating disorders in men with HIV infection. *British Journal of Psychiatry* 160:404–7.

Reas KL and Stedal K. 2015. Eating disorders in men aged midlife and beyond. *Maturitas* 81:248–55.

Ruffolo JS, Phillips KA, Menard W, Fay C, and Weisberg RB. 2006. Comorbidity of body dysmorphic disorder and eating disorders: Severity of psychopathology and body image disturbance. *International Journal of Eating Disorders* 39:11–19.

Schreiber GB, Robins M, Striegel-Moore R, Obarzanek RD, Morrison JH, and Wright DJ. 1996. Weight modification efforts reported by black and white preadolescent girls. *Pediatrics* 98:63–70.

Soto Ruiz MN, Marin Fernández B, Aquinaga Ontoso A, et al. 2015. Analysis of body image perception of university students in Navarra. *Nutricion Hospitalaria* 31:2269–75.

Strober M, Freeman R, Lampert C, Diamond J, Teplinsky C, and DeAntonio M. 2006. Are there gender differences in core symptoms, temperament, and short-term prospective outcome in anorexia nervosa? *International Journal of Eating Disorders* 39:570–75.

Sweeting H, Walker L, MacLean A, et al. 2015. Prevalence of eating disorders in males: A review of rates reported in academic research and UK mass media. *International Journal of Men's Health* doi: 10.3149/jmh.1402.86.

Thiel A, Gottfried H, and Hesse FW. 1993. Subclinical eating disorders in male athletes: A study of the low weight category in rowers and wrestlers. *Acta Psychologica Scandinavica* 88:259–65.

Welch E, Ghaderi A, and Swenne I. 2015. A comparison of clinical characteristics between adolescent males and females with eating disorders. *BMC Psychiatry* 15:45.

Woodside BD, Garfinkel PE, Lin E, Goering P, Kaplan AS, Goldbloom DS, and Kennedy SH. 2001. Comparison of men with full or partial eating disorders, men without eating disorders, and women with eating disorders in the community. *American Journal of Psychiatry* 158:570–74.

Yu J, Hildebrandt T, and Lanzieri N. 2015. Healthcare professionals' stigmatization of men with anabolic androgenic steroid use and eating disorders. *Body Image* 15:49–53.

Zhang C. 2014. What can we learn from the history of male anorexia nervosa? *Journal of Eating Disorders* 2:138.

14

Using Medical Information
Psychotherapeutically

Arnold E. Andersen, MD

Common Questions

What is psychoeducation?

How can clinicians use medical information psychotherapeutically for patients who have eating disorders?

Can you scare patients into healthy behavior?

Will medical information, if accurately presented, demoralize patients who have eating disorders?

Which medical tests offer the best possibility for psychotherapeutic use?

When is medical information not appropriate for psychotherapeutic feedback?

What information is helpful to families?

How can new genetic information help families understand eating disorders and decrease guilt?

Case 1

C.Y. was a 47-year-old surgeon whose wife persuaded him to come for evaluation for an eating disorder because of compulsive exercising and weight loss. The patient had insisted that he was overweight at 185 pounds and 5 feet 10 inches tall. Three years before evaluation, he began a strenuous exercise program of long-distance running, swimming, and bicycling. His father's death at about that time had caused him to fear that he might, like his father, be at risk of death from cardiac disease. Also, his older daughter was preparing to leave for college. His weight decreased to 130 pounds. He counted calories and limited fat grams to 10 grams a day, including monosaturated lipids. Despite feeling cold, becoming irritable at suggestions to decrease his several hours a day of exercise, and suffering two ankle sprains and knee pain, he continued his program.

At evaluation, C.Y. insisted he was only practicing healthy behaviors. He met criteria for anorexia nervosa in a male but would not accept the diagnosis until his DEXA scan and testosterone blood levels were shared with him. He met the criteria for osteoporosis, with a femoral neck bone mineral density of $T = -2.7$ standard deviations below normal and an L1–5 finding of $T = -2.3$ standard deviations. His testosterone was 180 ng/dL (normal 340–800). Gentle confrontation with these data allowed him to accept treatment, which included vigorous exercise but at a much more reasonable level, a gradual increase in weight to 165 pounds, coming to terms with his fears of mortality, and establishing a more adult-to-adult relationship with his daughter, including acceptance of her transition to becoming a college student. His marriage improved. Providing him with reading material about bone density loss in males (Andersen, Watson, and Schlechte, 2000) was helpful, as he was a clinical researcher as well as a surgeon.

Case 2

S.J. was a 20-year-old engineering student at the top of her class. In the course of her eating disorder, in addition to restricting her food intake, she began to abuse laxatives. She developed significant electrolyte problems, which were corrected in treatment. She was presented with information in a published study that 80% of calories ingested are absorbed despite laxative use excessive enough to lose 6 L of diarrhea fluid a day (Bo-Linn et al., 1983). When she read this information, she said, "It doesn't make sense to do things that don't work," and stopped using laxatives. S.J. went on to recover her weight and cease all purging behavior, as well as to change her core beliefs that thinness was essential to her sense of control and effectiveness. Medical information produced a helpful psychotherapeutic response.

Background

Eating disorders are characterized, according to Hilde Bruch (1979), by denial of thinness, denial of illness, and denial of sexuality. Patients with eating disorders, especially anorexia nervosa, often live an intellectualized life, from the neck up, with little attention to the reality of what is happening to their bodies. They often appear to produce "insightful" responses in psychotherapy but then show no change in illness behaviors or illness-based abnormal thinking.

Clinicians can use medical tests that document significant changes in body function in a number of different ways while interacting with patients who have eating disorders. First, medical information may simply be screened from the patient and never presented (the paternalistic style). Second, information may be presented in a neutral manner with neither psychotherapeutic discussion nor blame (the *Dragnet* style: "Just the facts, ma'am"). Third, information may, unfortunately, be used to blame or scare patients (club the victim). Scaring patients does not last for long, though, and certainly not long enough for motivation and engagement in successful treatment. Last, and preferably, information can be used psychotherapeutically (the ideal use). *Psychoeducation* means the use of information about the nature of the disorder and medical test results in a manner that respects the patient, empowers her or him to become a partner in decision making, and helps draw out the implications of accepting versus refusing treatment. Accurate and therapeutically presented information is vital for family members to become co-therapists and to relieve their apprehension and guilt or self-blame.

Psychotherapeutic Use of Medical Tests

The goal of using medical information psychotherapeutically is to form a therapeutic alliance with the healthy side of the patient to overcome her or his denial of the illness or denial of the seriousness of the illness. It is an attempt to form a working partnership with patients to help them interrupt the belief that they do not have an illness or that it has no significant consequences. Blaming patients for medical consequences is inappropriate because they often already have significant self-blame. Scaring patients doesn't work; at best, it produces a short-term alteration in behavior.

The following suggestions for possible therapeutic use of medical information are based on experience (Yager and Andersen, 2005), but not on any established studies with statistical confirmation. Good background reading for the clinician is a chapter on psychoeducation by Garner et al. (1985), which has stood the test of time. Presenting accurate medical information, both from current medical test results and on expected symptoms during the course of recovery, will reassure the anxious, fearful patient. It will also increase respect for the staff through the patient's awareness that this illness is understandable and predictable to the staff, as well as treatable.

Vital Signs and Acute Medical Instability

When a patient is seen for a diagnostic evaluation or first admitted and has electrolyte disturbances with associated EKG changes, information about these test results may help the patient either accept the diagnosis and the need to begin treatment or, if already admitted, to accept the need for staff-directed treatment instead of self-directed efforts. This information generally is best presented by using the laboratory reports themselves, which show normal levels as well as the patient's results. Along with presentation of the medical information, an explanation of the significance and cause of the results is helpful so that the prescribed treatment will make sense. Unfortunately, many patients with restricting anorexia nervosa have normal laboratory values despite marked cachexia. Fairburn (1995) reviewed the physiology of anorexia nervosa.

Bone Mineral Density by DEXA Scan

A dual-energy X-ray absorptiometry scan often provides graphic visual evidence that the patient has a serious medical problem. This information is usually first received by the clinician in the form of a graph that compares the patient's results with those of healthy, same-gender individuals at different ages (fig. 14.1). When the DEXA results for a patient with anorexia are traced across the graph, it is easy to show the patient that she or he has the same bone density as 70-year-old individuals. A typical response is, "Oh, my goodness. I never realized that this was happening," or, "I didn't know it was this serious." The patient can be reassured that the problem, while it may not be completely ameliorated, can be treated with increasingly effective methods. Here, too, facts are presented: because the lifetime maximum bone density is usually reached, at the latest, by the twenties (some recent studies suggest by age 17 or 18), with the maximum rate of accumulation in the mid-teens, there is an urgency in attempting to build a healthy "bone bank for retirement." Active research is now taking place to address the problem, and most patients with deficient bone

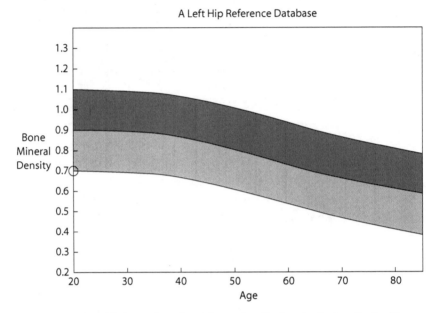

Figure 14.1. Visual information about bone density in a typical patient with anorexia nervosa can be used psychotherapeuetically. The figure shows that the patient's bone density is equal to that of a 70-year-old woman. The middle line is the average bone density for age.

mineral density have a number of years to correct the deficiency, which responds slowly to treatment. Incidentally, studies have demonstrated that estrogens are relatively ineffective in restoring bone density for the starved patient with anorexia (Mehler and MacKenzie, 2009)—another reason for restoration of full body weight. The DEXA scan is widely available, moderate in cost, accurate (Winston, Alwazeer, and Bankhart, 2008), and low in radiation (a tenth that of a chest X-ray).

Magnetic Resonance Imaging

While a brain MRI scan is not indicated for all patients, individuals with atypical features or a history of seizure or brain injury require an MRI for differential diagnosis and to assess the contribution of structural brain change to mental functioning. When an MRI is obtained for a patient with anorexia, it often shows enlarged ventricles and decreased brain volume. Patients may be astounded to see that their MRI is similar to that of a patient who has Alzheimer's disease, which also shows enlarged ventricles and decreased brain substance. Assurance can be given that most recent studies demonstrate recovery of brain size in anorexia nervosa with effective treatment and weight restoration, but it is not certain that all brain abnormalities are eventually improved (Swayze et al., 2003).

Gastrointestinal Changes

Patients can be shown published studies reporting that for most patients with anorexia nervosa, abdominal distress is improved with renutrition and supportive medical care without the need for medication or GI studies (e.g., Waldholtz and Andersen, 1990). It is hard for the patient to concentrate during therapy when she or he has significant abdominal distress. Published information about the return to normal gastric emptying, decreased bloating, and normalization of the speed of GI transit time helps the patient tolerate the temporary refeeding symptomatology affecting the GI tract, knowing that it is temporary, will improve, and is a consequence of the illness. Anorexia nervosa doubles the transit time of the GI tract.

Signs of Medical Starvation

Discussion of the signs and symptoms of medical starvation may help the patient accept that he or she is medically starved and not simply healthy in a way that causes others to be envious. Low T3 and increased reverse T3 levels, signs of acrocyanosis, and small, shrunken ovaries on a sonogram are all evidence that the body is truly starved. It may help to refer to the studies of Keys, Brozek, and Hemscheo in *The Biology of Human Starvation* (1950) showing that many of the psychological changes and much of the social isolation and altered eating behavior come from starvation, not the core anorexia nervosa psychopathology. "Marcie, that slowness of thinking and the difficulty in finishing the personal journaling assignment come from the effects of starvation on the brain. They will improve soon." Most of the medical symptoms in anorexia nervosa are understandable as the biology of starvation.

Status of Reproductive Hormones

Presenting patients with information documenting low estrogen in females or low testosterone in males and comparing these results with normal values may help individuals accept that they have an illness. Even though patients with anorexia nervosa often avoid discussions about sexuality, some want to have families in the future. Information about their low reproductive hormone levels may help them accept necessary weight restoration. The subsequent demonstration that these values usually become normal with return to a healthy weight will often reassure patients and especially their parents that no permanent damage has occurred. "There is nothing broken. Your reproductive hormones have gone back to a prepubertal state, and they will almost always return to normal when your weight is fully normal, your eating pattern is normal, your stress levels are lower. The body has mechanisms for dealing with famine from humankind's long experience with shortages of food. The body thinks it is in a famine. When you let it know that the 'famine' is over, the hormones will return to normal over several months." It is important for women who expect to be sexually active to know that they may become pregnant before their first period because the ovum is shed before that time, and they therefore should take appropriate precautions.

Allergies and Complaints of Lactose Intolerance

Nutritional rehabilitation is substantially hindered if patients have significant food allergies and/or lactose intolerance. Some patients complain that virtually all foods they eat cause allergic responses. Other individuals complain of GI symptoms after eating dairy products, denying themselves the beneficial protein and calcium content of these foods. Refeeding is often greatly assisted by requesting a formal consultation, early in treatment, for breath hydrogen testing to confirm or rule out lactose intolerance and allergies to specific foods. About 80% of patients complaining of lactose intolerance do not have confirmation of this on objective testing. Similarly, many fears of a generalized allergic response to foods or additives are not sustained on medical testing. Normal responses on these tests will allow nutritional rehabilitation to proceed with as few limitations as possible and will generally decrease the phobic quality of these foods in the patient's mind.

Abuse of Laxatives

Information about the ineffectiveness of laxatives may help patients undergo a program of cessation or tapering of laxative use after recognizing its ineffectiveness in producing the desired goal (see Bo-Linn et al., 1983). Case 2 at the start of this chapter describes one such patient response.

Night Sweats

The first patient in whom night sweats were noted in our eating disorder service was a pathologist whose occupation brought her in contact with a variety of microorganisms, some of which were lethal. An extensive evaluation was undertaken for the TB mycobacterium and other microorganisms, and all results were negative. There was no evidence of any medical disorder besides the medical starvation of anorexia nervosa. When we inquired about this pattern in subsequent patients with anorexia nervosa who were undergoing weight restoration, they all acknowledged night sweats as a phenomenon.

Night sweats should be discussed with patients because when their normality is not recognized, they can worry patients or families, can cause unnecessary tests to be ordered, or can be considered psychosomatic. Patients can be alerted in advance to expect, usually within a week or two of being hospitalized for treatment of anorexia nervosa, that their feelings of coldness and objective hypothermia will probably improve in a sequence: first, a week or two into treatment, they will experience night sweats, sometimes drenching and requiring a change of night clothing; then there is a gradual leveling off of the sweating over the next two weeks; and, finally, there is a return to a state of normal temperature control without subjective coldness. Patients sometimes give increased respect to staff, rather than skepticism, when the prediction of night sweats is confirmed by experience. Interestingly, this phenomenon is observed in male patients as well as females, so estrogen return may not be involved but, rather, some aspect of hypothalamic regulation in the setting of increased nutrition, including changes in thyroid hormones or receptors.

When Is It Not Helpful to Give Medical Information to a Person with an Eating Disorder?

Clinical experience suggests that in several situations, sharing of medical information is not appropriate. Very young patients may simply not be able to understand the nature of medical data. If patients are too young or too starved, or if they have substantial deficits in intellect—making it difficult to form a working therapeutic relationship, especially for cognitive behavioral work—then medical information may produce only fear and no therapeutic response or may create a negative preoccupation. Some patients with vulnerable personality traits may internalize medical information to increase self-blame, but this can be anticipated and prevented by the manner of sharing information. Patients who are self-critical or depressed at the time the medical information is available may need to wait until the depression is improved and/or a psychotherapeutic relationship has been under way for a while. The goal of sharing medical information is not to frighten patients or increase their self-blame but to form an alliance with the patient against the illness.

One form of medical information, in our experience, is not helpful to most patients with anorexia nervosa: daily information about the patient's weight during intensive inpatient programs; and sometimes even in full-day (partial hospital) or outpatient programs. A preoccupation with daily weight, or learning to "eat your way out of hospital" by complying with the behavioral goals but not changing core beliefs, is not therapy. Not everyone agrees with this advice, but in our experience, daily sharing of the patient's body weight, which is more like a daily confrontation, has more drawbacks than benefits. A focus on weight obscures the fact that eating disorders have essentially nothing to do with food, weight, or shape, but are instead strategies to deal with issues in living, mood regulation, relationships, an adequate sense of control in life, and self-esteem.

Obviously, a time comes when patients need to know their weight. We usually tell them their weight and their goal weight range when they are in a healthy target range or have transitioned from inpatient treatment to partial hospital at 85%–90% of healthy weight. At that time, they are taught the rationale for a 4- to 5-pound range, rather than a single number—for example, 120–125 pounds for a 25-year-old woman who is 5 feet 3½ inches tall. They are told that it is normal to experience fluctuation within that 4- to 5-pound range. They are asked to concentrate, before that time, on understanding themselves and changing the thinking and behaviors that form the core of their eating disorders, while trusting us to prescribe nutrition as medication. We promise them, based on more than 20 years of experience, that we will not let them become overweight. At times, a patient with a personal and family history of obesity may need to have a target weight 10–15 pounds above the ideal weight. Weight, like height, follows a bell-shaped curve, and someone has to hold down the upper standard deviation from the average—although few women accept this fact. It is an important therapeutic goal to persuade the patient that the true goal weight will be determined in the year after intensive treatment, when both patient and therapist will ask the body where it functions well, using information from laboratory test results, absence of hypothermia, and the return of normal hunger and satiety, regular menses, and sexual drive and function.

The Role of Parents

Appropriate medical information may also reassure parents that the physical symptoms of the eating disorder are being addressed and that their daughter or son will not die. Parents often fear the worst. If the situation is desperate medically, certainly the possibility of a fatal outcome should not be withheld, but often parents' fears are greater than the situation warrants. Parents appreciate learning the difference between starvation-induced, reversible symptoms and serious short-term or long-term complications that need to be separately addressed with specific medical treatments. They may need to be given the medical information if they, too, are doubtful of the need for treatment and have their own form of denial of the illness. Parents are often reassured to know that few, if any, medical consequences are permanent. They usually welcome learning about the increasing evidence on the genetic contributions to the predisposition to eating disorders. This information allows them to consider the eating disorder as a true illness and not the fault of the family or the patient. At times, parents may disclose that they or another family member have struggled with an eating disorder or with other illnesses in the spectrum of eating disorders vulnerability, such as depression, anxiety disorders, or OCD.

The Method of Presenting Medical Information

Medical information is psychotherapeutic when it is presented as part of a planned approach aimed at forming a therapeutic alliance to defeat the denial of illness that is characteristic of eating disorders. Information is most convincing when shown in a formal report in which the patient herself or himself can see the results and, especially, can compare her or his results with normal values. Appreciation of the information through visual means tends to break down the intellectual denial of illness.

It may also help patients understand why they have difficulties with mental concentration and abdominal discomfort, or why the treatment team or clinician has prescribed limitations on high-impact activities, and so on. Information on the reversibility of reproductive hormone abnormalities may reassure patients who wish to have a family later. Medical information presented therapeutically rather than in a critical or even neutral manner may allow patients to give themselves permission to accept the refeeding process rather than being fearful or hostile recipients of the nutritional rehabilitation.

Accurate medical information also increases respect for the staff's knowledge when the patient is told about symptoms that probably will occur during the course of treatment, how these symptoms will be treated, and their transient nature. This includes information about possible night sweats during the refeeding process, gastrointestinal discomfort, refeeding edema, changes in mental concentration, and progressive increases in energy, to name but a few.

Summary

Conveying medical information about the physical consequences of an eating disorder to the patient is important so that the treatment team can give good care. In certain situations, or if the information is not presented with due care, some vulnerable patients may perceive the information critically, with negative effects on the clinician-patient relationship. But if the information is presented as we recommend, psychotherapeutically, it can be used to form an alliance with the patient, to establish the reality of the illness, and to diminish denial of the illness or its seriousness.

REFERENCES

Andersen AE, Watson T, and Schlechte J. 2000. Osteoporosis and osteopenia in men with eating disorders. *Lancet* 355:1967–68.

Bo-Linn GW, Santana CA, Morawski SG, and Fordtran JS. 1983. Purging and caloric absorption in bulimic patients and normal women. *Annals of Internal Medicine* 99:14.

Bruch H. 1979. *The Golden Cage*. New York: Vintage Press.

Fairburn CG. 1995. Physiology of anorexia nervosa. In: Brownell KD and Fairburn CG, eds. *Eating Disorders and Obesity*. New York: Guilford Press, pp. 251–54.

Garner D, Rockert W, Olmsted M, Johnson C, and Coscina D. 1985. Psychoeducational principles in the treatment of bulimia and anorexia nervosa. In: Garner D and Garfinkel P, eds. *Handbook of Psychotherapy for Anorexia Nervosa and Bulimia*. New York: Guilford Press, pp. 513–72.

Keys A, Brozek J, and Henscheo A. 1950. *The Biology of Human Starvation.* Minneapolis: University of Minnesota Press.

Mehler PS and MacKenzie TD. 2009. Treatment of osteopenia and osteoporosis in anorexia nervosa: A systematic review of the literature. *International Journal of Eating Disorders* 42:195–201.

Swayze VW, Andersen AE, Andreasen NC, Arndt S, Sato Y, and Ziebell S. 2003. Brain tissue volume segmentation in patients with anorexia nervosa before and after weight normalization. *International Journal of Eating Disorders* 33:33–44.

Waldholtz BD and Andersen AE. 1990. Gastrointestinal symptoms in anorexia nervosa: A prospective study. *Gastroenterology* 98:1415–14.

Winston AP, Alwazeer AEF, and Bankhart MJG. 2008. Screening for osteoporosis in anorexia nervosa: Prevalence and predictors of reduced bone mineral density. *International Journal of Eating Disorders* 41:284–87.

Yager J and Andersen AE. 2005. Clinical practice: Anorexia nervosa. *New England Journal of Medicine* 353:1481–82.

15

Ethical and Medicolegal Considerations in Treating Patients with Eating Disorders

Patricia Westmoreland, MD, and Philip S. Mehler, MD

Common Questions

What are the bioethical principles guiding the care of patients
with eating disorders?

What is meant by "coercion" in medical care?

What is the difference between certification and guardianship?

Why is it harder to certify patients with anorexia nervosa than
patients with other psychiatric illnesses?

Are there specific criteria that can be used to certify a patient with
anorexia nervosa?

Do patients with anorexia nervosa who are treated involuntarily
do as well as patients treated voluntarily?

What is meant by "harm reduction"?

What is the difference between palliative care and hospice care?

Does a patient with a severe eating disorder have to be competent
to make the decision to reject treatment and begin hospice
care?

ETHICAL PRINCIPLES

Case 1

M.A. was a 35-year-old female diagnosed with anorexia nervosa,
binge-purge subtype. She was first diagnosed with an eating disorder in
her early teens. She was treated on seven occasions and was eventually
able to live and function, albeit at a low weight. She maintained this weight

for 8 years. She then began having abdominal pain and was diagnosed with gallstone pancreatitis. She underwent multiple abdominal procedures and surgeries, as a result of which she began to use pain medications excessively. She also suffered from depression and anxiety, but she had a supportive family who set strong boundaries regarding the need for treatment. In addition, her family controlled her finances. M.A. was admitted to an inpatient level of care. At the time of admission, she weighed approximately 65 pounds (height 5 feet 3 inches; 52% of ideal body weight [IBW]). She refused to eat and would not accept nasogastric (NG) feeding. Her treating psychiatrist petitioned for inpatient certification and also requested court-ordered medications and involuntary tube feeding. M.A. was subsequently certified, and the court approved the petition for court-ordered medication and tube feeds. M.A. required a physical hold to insert tube and initiate feeding on several occasions. The certification was renewed at 3 months, uncontested by the patient. She was restored to her goal weight. During the weight restoration process, she was transitioned to 100% oral nutrition. She was discharged to outpatient treatment. Four months later, M.A. returned for a short hospital stay as a voluntary patient after having lost 10 pounds. She was again readmitted approximately a year thereafter. She was once again severely ill. Following a prolonged hospital stay that included certification, she was discharged to outpatient care, maintained her goal weight, and was engaged in gainful employment.

Comment: Although this patient had a long history of eating disorder and several protracted hospitalizations, she was eventually able to achieve and maintain a reasonable level of recovery. Certification was helpful in that it kept her in treatment when her body weight was so low that her cognitive distortions did not allow her to restore weight. In addition, having family who were able to maintain strong boundaries with her and support the treatment team was important in helping her through treatment. Even if she had eloped from treatment to escape the certification, her family would not have continued to support her financially, and she would have had few options other than to return to treatment.

Case 2

Y.D. was an 18-year-old female diagnosed with anorexia nervosa, restricting subtype. She was transferred to an inpatient eating disorder treatment program following treatment at a medical unit, where she had been admitted at a weight of 74 pounds. During her stay on the medical unit, she was fed via NG tube under guardianship laws. Y.D. had been treated on 11 prior occasions since age 11. She had required forced tube feeding in the past and had eloped from prior treatment facilities. Y.D. was diagnosed with comorbid posttraumatic stress disorder, depression, and conduct disorder. She was transferred from the medical unit to the inpatient eating disorder treatment unit on a mental health hold. The treating psychiatrist petitioned for certification. Y.D. was certified, and the petitions for involuntary medications and NG tube feeds were granted.

During her course of inpatient treatment she removed her NG tube on multiple occasions; she also purged via the tube and had several episodes of syncope. She refused to transition to an oral diet, despite the promise of more privileges on the unit, with a chance to transition to a lower level of care and go on outings off the unit. Y.D. "cheeked" the olanzapine and lorazepam she was prescribed and saved these medications, which she then took all at once. She told emergency room staff that her motivation for the overdose was that she was hoping to be discharged from eating disorder treatment. Emergency room staff opined that the patient was too ill from an eating disorder to be admitted to an acute psychiatric unit, a procedure that would normally be considered after a deliberate drug overdose.

Following her return to the inpatient eating disorder unit, Y.D. continued to repeatedly remove the NG tube (to such a point that her nostrils became inflamed and further NG tube insertion was considered harmful). In terms of her willingness to engage in recovery, Y.D. remained amotivated. As her weight was no longer critical (she had gained more than 20 pounds through NG tube feeding), the team agreed that she had reached maximum benefit under certification and petitioned the court to drop the certification. Y.D. agreed to minimal oral intake (just enough to ensure her weight and vital signs remained stable while disposition was arranged). She was discharged home at 85% IBW (106 lb) and has not returned for further treatment to the facility that certified her.

Comment: Although this patient certainly had the potential to recover, her comorbid diagnosis of conduct disorder led to her flouting rules on every occasion she could, increasing her resistance to treatment and decreasing her compliance with the treatment team. In addition, her parents differed on how best to proceed with treatment, and differences of opinion between the parents (and between parents and treatment team) greatly affected the patient's care. Her care was terminated when treatment reached the point that she was medically stable enough to leave and the treatment team believed it would be more harmful than helpful to continue NG feeding against her will.

The Principles of Modern Biomedical Ethics

Four guiding principles form the basis of modern biomedical ethics:

1. Respect for autonomy: The patient's informed choices take priority.
2. Beneficence: Doing what is best for patients, not always with their consent.
3. Nonmaleficence: First, do no harm—*primum non nocere*.
4. Justice: Balancing individual and social costs, benefits, risks.

These ethical principles take precedence over the treating physician's self-interest. Nonmaleficence and beneficence have historically been honored. In recent decades, respect for autonomy has become of increasing importance in medical practice. Social justice is the concept of fair, equitable, and appropriate treatment in the light of what is expected or owed to members of society.

These four guiding principles are applicable in most situations involving patient care. There are conflicts within and between these principles, however, that are relatively specific to anorexia nervosa, given the unique features of this psychiatric illness:

1. The interrelationship between the effects of medical starvation on cognition and the behavioral consequences of overvalued beliefs underlying the disorder.
2. The perception that anorexia nervosa is a voluntary disorder responsive to self-determination in both the development of the illness and the process of regaining health.
3. The moralizing that disorders of eating behavior and weight are disorders of personal failure.
4. The common stereotype of anorexia nervosa that limits the perception of illness to teenage Caucasian females.

5. The relatively robust appearance and behavior of many patients even with serious anorexia nervosa.
6. The multifactorial concept of etiology that generates competing approaches to treatment.
7. The reality of living in a society with increasing health care costs and the need to use health care resources wisely.

The following sections weigh these guiding principles against the reality of treating eating disorders.

Respect for Autonomy versus Beneficence

To respect autonomy one must acknowledge that patients have a right to hold views, make choices, and take actions based on their values and beliefs. Two concepts are essential for autonomy: liberty (independence from controlling influence) and agency (capacity for intentional action). Some distinguish capacity (a clinical decision) from competence (a legal decision), but this distinction is less important in practice because diminished capacity usually leads to a court finding of incompetence (Beauchamp and Childress, 2012). Capacity may change over the course of a patient's lifetime or illness. Patients' wishes to receive information and make decisions are not uniform across cultures; they are influenced by culture and community. It should not be assumed that all patients want the same amount of information about their condition or the same amount of autonomous choice. Respect for autonomy does not extend to persons who cannot act in an autonomous manner, such as those who are immature, incapacitated, or suicidal.

Individuals who have severe anorexia nervosa often appear more competent than they are (they talk the talk but do not walk the walk). They are intelligent and articulate and are often able to convince relatives as well as treatment providers that they are doing quite well, when, in fact, they are not. Patients with severe anorexia nervosa give the illusion of sanity even when they are driven by deadly irrationality, failing to appreciate that anorexia nervosa has the highest death rate of all psychiatric illnesses.

The principle of beneficence is the moral obligation to act for the benefit of others. Beneficence entails protecting and defending the rights of others, preventing harm from occurring to others, and removing conditions that will lead to harm. These rules present positive requirements for action. The idea that beneficence is the primary obligation in health care dates back to the time of Hippocrates, and physicians have historically relied mostly on their own judgments about what is in the best interests of the patient. In many cases, physicians override the wishes of the patient and justify this action by citing the goal of benefiting or reducing harm to the patient. This is termed paternalism. However, as modern medicine has led to an emphasis on a patient's rights to receive information and make independent judgments, paternalism is being challenged to a greater extent.

Carefully delineated respect for autonomy combined with experienced assessment of mental and behavioral functioning in anorexia nervosa will determine when beneficence trumps autonomy. Collecting accurate data on the patient's medical health (weight, blood pressure and pulse, EKG, laboratory test results), looking at the treatment history in its entirety, and taking into account the patient's wishes are essential when making a decision as to whether an individual with anorexia nervosa should, for example, be certified or allowed to refuse treatment.

Authentic Beneficence versus Authoritarian or Pseudo-Beneficence

True beneficence does not imply a patronizing or authoritarian approach. On the one hand, an out-of-date form of beneficence fails to discuss with the patient the diagnosis, treatment options, prognosis, and benefits and risks of having treatment or not. The "doctor knows best" attitude falls into this category, as does limiting the treatment options to an overly narrow category consisting only of the skill set of the clinician— even when this is not best suited to the needs of the patient. On the other hand, a false view of updated beneficence presents treatment options through a "cafeteria approach," with no guidance or specific recommendations. "Whatever the patient wants" is pseudo-beneficence and not in the best interests of the patient. The ethical clinician gives the patient a clear understanding of the diagnosis, treatment, and prognosis of anorexia nervosa and offers tailored recommendations based on his or her experience and on evidence from sound studies. The clinician should also acknowledge limitations in his or her training and accede to a request for a second opinion or a referral when appropriate. Not every clinician who can competently diagnose eating disorders can also treat all forms of eating disorder at every level of severity. Recognizing one's limitations is essential, and referring to a higher level of care when needed is in the patient's best interests.

Authentic beneficence grows out of empathy and appreciates the patient's struggles with giving up the perceived benefits of illness (anorexia is often ego-syntonic) for what seems to be perceived as a loss of control resulting from becoming healthy. Beneficence will acknowledge that although the patient's physical concerns (hair falling out, dry skin) may seem to be clinically less important than the threat of death or chronic illness, these concerns need to be incorporated into a treatment plan. Authentic beneficence always includes a biopsychosocial formulation that integrates palpable concern for a patient's suffering with the best available interventions to treat the medical, intrapsychic, and interpersonal aspects of the disorder.

Nonmaleficence versus (Unintended) Maleficence

The principle of nonmaleficence obligates us to abstain from causing harm to others. In addition to the obligation of beneficence, the Hippocratic Oath incorporates the obligation of *primum non nocere*—first, do no harm. The rules of nonmaleficence are negative prohibitions of action (they tell us what *not* to do) and provide a moral basis for legal prohibitions of certain forms of conduct. As medical care has become more sophisticated, so has our thinking about when it is appropriate to override the prima facie obligation to treat. Examples of when we override the obligation to treat are when treatment is futile or when the costs or burdens of treatment clearly outweigh the benefits. Much controversy still exists in this domain, however, and determinations of what is considered active killing (vs. letting die) continue to evolve. Active and passive forms of harm may occur in a number of other ways. An example of active harm is inappropriate refeeding (too-rapid refeeding, albeit well-intentioned). Another example may be deciding to certify and force-feed a patient with severe and enduring anorexia nervosa without fully considering the patient's treatment history, the wishes of the patient and family, and whether pursuing the goal of full weight restoration has a reasonable probability of achieving remission. An example of passive harm is not pursuing insurance authorization for treatment of a patient with anorexia nervosa.

Social Justice versus Business as Usual

Social justice views the patient's disorder as a tapestry in which individual and societal costs, needs, and benefits are interwoven. The term *distributive justice* refers to fair, equitable, and appropriate distribution of benefits as determined by the norms of that society. The patient is a de facto part of a broad social network of family members, caregivers, communities, governmental regulators, third-party payers, legislators, and judges. While each component of this social network, in theory, has the patient's welfare at its center, in practice each has its own self-serving goals, which may be in conflict with what is in the patient's best interests.

Legislatures have previously given lip service to parity, but seldom has this resulted in an impartial approach to all illnesses as worthy of comparable levels of care based on intensity of the illness. Psychiatric disorders have more limited health care insurance benefits than "medical disorders," and eating disorders, specifically, have seen the most stringent limitations in coverage. In contrast, "medical disorders" may have almost unlimited benefits. The result has been shorter inpatient treatments for anorexia nervosa despite evidence-based studies documenting that inpatient treatment short of full weight restoration leads to the propensity for a patient to suffer relapse and to be readmitted to inpatient care (Steinhausen et al., 2008). Repeat hospitalizations are considered "business as usual," while adequate length of stay is considered a money-losing proposition, although over the course of illness it may end up costing less.

True social justice does not tolerate disparities in service based on race, gender, or sexual orientation. Failure to reach out to diverse ethnic and racial communities—which, as data increasingly demonstrate, have a high and increasing prevalence of eating disorders—represents an injustice.

Advocacy for social justice includes a call for comprehensive treatment programs and adequate reimbursement of care, as well as a call for funding of both clinical and translational research studies. Increased knowledge of anorexia nervosa will lead to clinical advances, community education programs, screening for early diagnosis, and preventive intervention in demonstrated areas of effectiveness. Social justice advocacy also calls for an end to stigma regarding eating disorders in particular, interaction with legislative bodies for further actualization of parity, and a willingness to appear before administrative justices and other personnel within the justice system to plead the patient's case for funding. States that currently do not support involuntary treatments for patients with severe anorexia nervosa, even when clearly necessary in life-threatening cases, need to remediate this deficit, in view of the evidence that selective involuntary admission and treatment can be beneficial as well as life-saving (Elzakkers et al., 2014).

INVOLUNTARY TREATMENT

Coercion

Coercion, in medical care, is the practice of persuasion by using force or threats. It may exist on an informal basis (e.g., treatment contracts, achievement of certain privileges if patients demonstrate compliance with treatment) or be achieved through legal measures (involuntary treatment). Although patients might not refuse outright to enter treatment, many patients with anorexia nervosa feel they are coerced (albeit not involving legal measures) to enter treatment, either by family or by outpatient treatment providers who will no longer provide care for them as an outpatient unless they agree to complete treatment at a higher level of care. Coercive pressure to enter treatment does not necessarily undermine clinical progress or the formation of a therapeutic alliance (Schreyer et al., 2016). In addition, within weeks of entering treatment, patients are often able to acknowledge that, in retrospect, they needed treatment, even though they felt coerced at the time of admission (Guarda et al., 2007).

Despite studies that suggest coercion may produce a favorable outcome, Kendall (2014) comments that the use of coercive strategies for patients with anorexia nervosa indicates that "persons with anorexia nervosa are paradoxically understood as possessing the competence to make decisions to comply with treatment but not to refuse it." Accordingly, when patients enter treatment either voluntarily or as a result of coercion, their decisional capacity is not assessed. When they refuse certain aspects of their treatment, however, their decisional capacity becomes an issue. Thus, when clinicians consider involuntary treatment on the basis of a patient's refusal of a particular treatment goal, it appears that this decision is being made just because the patient is not complying with the plan of the treatment team, rather than on the basis of the patient's incompetence.

Coercive approaches also engender concern as to whether a patient's autonomy or liberty interests are being protected. If patients are compliant only to avoid involuntary treatment, their decision to comply with treatment may not be truly autonomous, and they are in effect involuntary patients without the protections of the law that are afforded to patients who are being certified.

Guardianship and Certification

Guardianship and certification are legal measures that are, in essence, formal means of coercion. They have come into play because patients with anorexia nervosa are often very reluctant to seek the life-saving treatment of weight gain. Weight gain, however, is critical to the success of treatment and is a significant predictor of a reduction in eating disorder pathology (Accurso et al., 2014). Weight gain is also paralleled by improvements in emotional and psychological well-being, as well as body in image perception and coping skills, and is imperative for patients' recovery (Long, Fitzgerald, and Hollin, 2012). Early response to treatment, as measured by early weight gain during the first 6 weeks of hospitalization, is especially important in terms of symptom improvement (Accurso et al., 2014; Wales et al., 2016). Younger age when beginning treatment and shorter duration of illness are also predictors of better outcome (Le Grange et al., 2014), whereas lower body mass index (BMI) on admission and older age (midlife adults) carry a poorer prognosis (Ackard et al., 2014; Nakamura et al., 2013). Thus, hospitalization and treatment, even if involuntary, should be considered *before* patients reach a severe and/or chronic stage of the illness. In practice, however, it is often the case that patients for whom involuntary treatment is considered are precisely the patients with the most serious forms of illness and who are least likely to benefit from further treatment.

Conversely, misplaced respect for patients' autonomy, thereby allowing patients to continue to lose weight and either refuse care or be admitted only at a critically low BMI, may lead to a fatal outcome (Holm et al., 2012; Nakamura et al., 2013). This concern is particularly relevant because the patients more likely to default from treatment are those who have the lowest BMIs and the highest impulsivity (as evidenced by suicidality and substance use) and are more psychologically ill (Huas et al., 2011).

Despite the increased risk of the illness becoming chronic (or the patient dying from the eating disorder), there is often reluctance on the part of family and the treatment team to initiate involuntary treatment.

Families, though relieved that their critically ill family member is being compelled to receive care, often bear the brunt of the patient's anger and indignation at being forced into treatment. Treatment providers worry that a push for involuntary treatment will disrupt the already fragile alliance between patient and treatment team and make further progress all but impossible. These concerns may be well founded in that therapeutic alliance is an important predictor of achieving a target weight and remaining in treatment (Bourion-Bedes et al., 2013; Sly et al., 2013). In addition, involuntary treatment at a time when a patient is beginning to contemplate the need for change and recovery may prove harmful for the patient's engagement in treatment (Douzenis and Michopoulos, 2015) These concerns, however, must be weighed against concerns about future morbidity and mortality if a patient with severe anorexia nervosa continues to refuse life-saving care (Arcelus et al., 2011). Furthermore, patients with anorexia nervosa have been found to ultimately agree with the need for compulsory treatment once their weight is restored (Tan et al., 2010).

Guardianship versus Certification

Guardianship and certification differ in terms of the type of treatment that may be meted out under each statute (medical care vs. psychiatric care) and the venue for that treatment. Treatment under guardianship laws may occur as an inpatient on a medical unit or, to ensure medical treatment, on a psychiatric unit or as an outpatient, and the guardian has latitude as to where the patient (who, under guardianship law, is defined as the "ward") resides while receiving care. In contrast, treatment under certification can take place only on an inpatient psychiatric unit. The certification may be transferred to an outpatient status only after the patient no longer meets criteria for inpatient psychiatric treatment.

Significantly more has been written on certification than guardianship for patients who have eating disorders, but guardianship has been successfully used to treat patients with eating disorders who are severely medically ill (Born et al., 2015; Griffiths et al., 1997). Nonetheless, the appointment of a guardian may be problematic for patients with anorexia nervosa. Not only is treatment under guardianship laws limited in nature, but the guardian is called upon to make decisions that are often opposite to those desired by the ward. The guardian may find it extremely difficult to deal with a ward who actively opposes treatment and blames the guardian for taking away his or her freedom.

Guardianship is useful in assisting with medical treatment decisions for patients with anorexia nervosa who are critically medically ill and refusing basic medical treatment such as replacement of electrolytes and IV fluids or nutrition (through NG or nasojejunal tube). However, once these medical interventions have been successful and the patient is no longer in immediate medical danger, such interventions cannot be continued under guardianship laws. Guardianship also does not cover involuntary admission to an inpatient psychiatric unit, even if that unit is an eating disorder treatment unit. Therefore, guardianship is not an adequate intervention with respect to compelling psychiatric treatment for patients with severe anorexia nervosa once they become medically stable, are no longer at imminent risk, and are able to transfer from a medical unit to a psychiatric unit. The initiation of certification to a psychiatric unit must be made in accordance with the state's procedure for certification and use of emergency and involuntary psychiatric medications.

To psychiatrically hospitalize an individual involuntarily, a psychiatrist or other mental health practitioner must establish that the individual is a danger to himself or herself, a danger to others, or gravely disabled. The family of a patient with a severe eating disorder may contact either emergency services (such as police) or a mental health provider and request that their family member be evaluated for placement on a mental health hold. If there are grounds for the mental health hold (danger to self or other or, in some states, the presence of grave disability), the patient is placed on a hold and transferred to an emergency room.

If emergency room staff agree that continuing the mental health hold is warranted, the patient may then be admitted to a psychiatric unit for a short period of observation (usually several days, but variable from state to state). During this time-limited observation period, the treating psychiatrist may file for certification. The psychiatrist may also allow the patient to sign into treatment voluntarily or to leave; in both of these instances, the mental health hold is terminated. If the treating psychiatrist files for certification, the patient may either agree to the certification (i.e., stipulate) or contest the certification in court. If the patient is certified, the certification may not exceed a defined period (e.g., in Colorado, short-term certification is 3 months) (Colorado Revised Statute 27-65). Thereafter, further petitions must be filed to prolong involuntary treatment. While procedures and criteria vary across jurisdictions, providing involuntary medications to mentally ill patients is, in many jurisdictions, an additional step beyond certification. Moreover, involuntary tube feeding is achieved only through an additional petition. In Colorado, involuntary tube feeding is designated as a special procedure, much like electroconvulsive therapy (ECT), and requires a separate legal hearing.

Case Law and Certification

Courts in several states have applied certification statutes to the treatment of patients with eating disorders. Considering some of the decisions made by these courts is useful for analyzing the results of certifying patients with eating disorders. The courts have considered several important aspects of certification of patients with anorexia nervosa. These include the scope of the certifying court in involving itself in treatment decisions: whether it is in the court's purview to agree that a patient is best served by receiving treatment in another state, that accurate criteria are used when presenting an argument for certification, that the definition of grave disability does not necessitate that the patient be close to death, and that medications may be warranted in treating patients with eating disorders.

In the Matter of Joanne Kolodrubetz (1987). Ms. Kolodrubetz presented to a facility in Minnesota where she was certified because of severe anorexia nervosa. She was so ill that her life was repeatedly endangered by her behaviors when she was not in treatment. Following certification, she did not agree with the treatment modality at the facility and pursued the administrative complaint process. After that administrative process had run its course and the findings and recommendations were unsatisfactory to her, she petitioned the certifying court for relief. Under the Minnesota statute, the certifying court only makes the initial legal determination as to whether the patient meets statutory criteria for certification. Patients challenging the specific form of treatment at a facility must follow the Minnesota administrative review process. Indeed, the appellate court noted that the certifying court may not involve itself in treatment decisions and that the remedy for a patient who disagreed with the findings and recommendations generated by the administrative process was for the patient to file a lawsuit seeking damages. The legal standard in such a lawsuit was whether the treatment pursued by the facility was within accepted professional standards. There was no indication that the facility's treatment of Ms. Kolodrubetz fell outside that standard.

In the Matter of Molly Kellor (1994). The People appealed a Minnesota District Court case authorizing Ms. Kellor to receive treatment in an out-of-state facility. As noted above (*In the Matter of Joanne Kolodrubetz*), once the Minnesota certifying court makes a judicial determination, the court will not review specific treatment modalities.

Ms. Kellor was initially committed to a hospital for a period of 6 months, and then for a subsequent period of 12 months, to be transferred to a psychiatric facility once she was medically stable. Following her transfer to the psychiatric facility, Ms. Kellor continued to restore weight through tube feeding but gained little if any insight into her eating disorder and had a conflictual relationship with treatment staff. She sought transfer to an out-of-state facility specializing in the treatment of eating disorders, located in Tulsa, Oklahoma. The district court granted her request, finding that no in-state facility offered eating disorder–specific treatment in Minnesota and that under the Minnesota statute, the patient was entitled to receive appropriate treatment in the least restrictive setting. The People appealed the trial court's decision, claiming that the trial court improperly interfered with treatment decisions, and also contended that the trial court had no authority to commit Ms. Kellor to an out-of-state facility. The appellate court determined that while the trial court should not interfere with or monitor treatment decisions, there was evidence in the record supporting the trial court's determination that there was no facility in Minnesota that at the time could adequately treat Ms. Kellor's eating disorder. The appellate court held that the trial court has wide discretion in determining the least restrictive setting and agreed with transferring Ms. Kellor to an out-of-state facility.

In re S.A.M. (2005). S.A.M. appealed an Iowa District Court case that determined that she met the definition of a person with a serious mental impairment and as a result was likely to inflict physical injury upon self or others if allowed to remain at liberty. When filing the appeal, S.A.M. admitted that she suffered from a mental illness, anorexia nervosa, and therefore did not challenge the trial court's findings that she suffered from a serious mental impairment. However, S.A.M. challenged the trial court's finding that there was clear and convincing evidence that she was likely to inflict physical harm to self if she were allowed to remain at liberty. Given that S.A.M. had been able to maintain a stable body weight while in outpatient treatment just prior to being rehospitalized and had never suffered from metabolic abnormalities even at a lower body weight, the reviewing court determined that there was *not* clear and convincing evidence that it was "probable or reasonably expected" that S.A.M. was likely to inflict physical injury upon herself if she was allowed to remain at liberty. Therefore, the trial court's ruling was reversed.

People of the State of Colorado in the interest of P.A. (2012, 2013). Under the Colorado statutory scheme, the professional person associated with a facility designated for mental health treatment initiates the involuntary treatment process by filing a Notice of Certification for Short-Term Treatment with the district court in the appropriate venue. In Denver, the Denver Probate Court is a district court of limited jurisdiction, handling involuntary mental health treatment requests. Hearings involving the certification aspect only may be before a jury of six or before the court. In 12CA1024 and 13CA1350, P.A. requested court trials. In both instances, the trial court upheld the short-term certification for the statutory 3-month period, determining that P.A. was a danger to herself and was gravely disabled. The trial court also granted both involuntary medication administration authority to the designated facility regarding the respondent and authority to involuntarily place a feeding tube for the purposes of NG or nasojejunal feeding. P.A. appealed the court's decisions, alleging that because she had partially restored weight in the facility, she was no longer gravely disabled or a danger to self as she was no longer near death. The appellate court found that the definition of gravely disabled does not require that the respondent be imminently near death. Instead, the definition requires only that the respondent be in danger of serious physical harm because of an inability or failure to provide oneself with the essential human needs of food and medical care.

P.A. also appealed the order of the probate court that granted involuntary administration of medications. She asserted that the standard for involuntary medication set forth had not been met by clear and convincing evidence. The court of appeals ruled that P.A.'s mental illness had so impaired her judgment that she was incapable of participating in decisions affecting her health and that medication was needed to prevent the likelihood of her causing serious harm to herself, albeit indirectly. If she did not take medication, she would decompensate psychiatrically and (as a result) put herself in life-threatening danger by not taking in adequate nutrition. There were no viable alternatives to adequately treat her mental illness, and (to that end) her psychiatrist testified that she would not be able to successfully treat P.A.'s anorexia without medication.

When P.A. appealed her certification again in 2013, this was the second appeal in a period of just over one year involving a short-term commitment based on substantially similar circumstances. The court concluded that, based on these substantially similar circumstances—that is, P.A.'s lack of sustained recovery—the issues raised in the case were moot. Under the "mootness doctrine," an issue is moot when any judgment concerning the issue cannot have a practical effect on an existing controversy, and appellate courts will not render opinions on the merits of an appeal when the issues presented are moot because of subsequent events. Thus, the court declined to reconsider the issues presented by P.A.

Certifying Patients with Eating Disorders

The frequency with which patients with anorexia nervosa are certified ranges from 8% to as high as 44% (Clausen and Jones, 2014; Elzakkers et al., 2014). The differences in percentage of patients treated involuntarily may be explained both by differences in patient populations and by differences in local regulations or procedures as well as across hospitals.

For several reasons, certification of a patient with anorexia nervosa differs from that of a patient with any other major psychiatric illness, such as bipolar disorder or schizophrenia. Patients with anorexia nervosa have been described as presenting with a "pocket of irrationality operating within a sea of personal rationality regarding all other matters" (Carney, 2014). A review on the topic of assessing subtle forms of incompetence is pertinent in this regard (Gutheil and Bursztajn, 1986). First, with anorexia nervosa, the patient's competence is usually suspect only in the narrow area of self-nutrition / body image, and patients with anorexia nervosa do not appear disorganized or illogical in general conversation. Second, patients with anorexia nervosa are usually intelligent and articulate and have a good grasp of the legal issues at hand, even when their cognition is compromised by malnutrition; they are usually well groomed and dress in a manner designed to conceal their extreme emaciation. Third, because the illness has been of several months or years duration by the time it comes to medical or psychiatric attention, the medical danger typically associated with anorexia nervosa is often perceived not to be imminent. Fourth, patients with eating disorders usually provide the court with a rational explanation for their behavior, and they do not usually express an intent to die; on the contrary, they usually express an intent to continue living but with a continued reduction in weight (Appelbaum and Rumpf, 1998). Finally, judges or magistrates may find it difficult to distinguish an eating disorder from culturally normative weight concerns, given media and social emphasis on thinness.

Certification of patients with anorexia nervosa is most likely to be triggered by a patient having a longer duration of illness, a greater number of prior admissions, more comorbidities, a higher incidence of self-harm, and a greater severity of medical illness (e.g., having a very low BMI or a high risk of refeeding syndrome) (Ayton, Keen, and Las, 2009; Carney et al., 2008; Clausen and Jones, 2014; Douzenis and Michopoulos, 2015). Duration of illness may also be a significant predictor of involuntary treatment. The characteristics of patients who are treated involuntarily, noted in the cases above, speak not only to the severity of their illness but also to the complexity of their situation as a whole.

There are no definitive criteria regarding when to certify versus not certify a patient with a severe eating disorder. Criteria that have been suggested as favoring certification include medical comorbidities such as seizures, syncopal episodes, hypoglycemia, organic brain syndromes, cardiac arrhythmias, severe bradycardia, renal compromise, volume depletion, tetany, and rapidly diminished exercise tolerance (Holm et al., 2012). Psychiatric comorbidities such as suicidal ideation or self-harming behavior are also likely to bring about involuntary treatment.

Outcome of Certification

Patients who are treated involuntarily take a longer time to restore weight, are more often hospitalized on a locked psychiatric unit, are more likely to be tube-fed, and may also be more prone to refeeding syndrome (Clausen and Jones, 2014). Despite beginning their course of treatment with more severe symptoms and comorbidities and having a longer and potentially more complicated inpatient stay, patients who undergo involuntary treatment have BMIs at discharge similar to those of patients treated voluntarily (Clausen and Jones, 2014; Elzakkers et al., 2014). However, mortality in the 5 years following a compulsory admission is higher than that of patients treated voluntarily (Ward et al., 2015). Despite this statistic, approximately 20 years following admission, this difference was found to be attenuated and, although the standardized mortality in the compulsory treatment group remained higher, the difference between the two groups declined over time. Thus there was no significant difference between certified patients and those who were treated voluntarily when differences were measured two decades later. This reflects a prior finding that the risk of premature death among patients with anorexia peaks within the first 10 years of follow-up (Franko et al., 2013). It has also been suggested that poor outcome for certified patients is probably not the result of certification in itself but rather because these patients have other validated poor prognostic factors such as comorbid psychiatric illnesses and older age at admission (Ayton, Keen, and Las, 2009; Ramsey et al., 1999).

Involuntary tube feeding, while beneficial in the short term, may also lack benefit in the long term, as it generally cannot continue indefinitely. In addition, patients who require involuntary tube feeding for a prolonged time are those who are most recalcitrant in their attitudes toward and motivation for recovery. Another reason that certification may not be helpful is repeated elopements from treatment. It may also prove futile to treat patients who are chronically ill, have required multiple prior treatments, have never had a sustained period of wellness despite extensive interventions, and steadfastly communicate that their life is not worth living.

TREATMENT OF SEVERE AND ENDURING EATING DISORDERS

Patients with severe and enduring eating disorders (SEED) are a subgroup of patients whose illness is long-standing and life-threatening. While the likelihood of recovery has been reported to plateau after 6–12 years of illness (Robinson 2009, 2014), others suggest that the chances of recovery plateau later in the illness. Regardless, patients with SEED have a very low likelihood of recovery, poor adaptive function, high levels of symptoms, and comorbid physical and psychological ills, and they require the regular attention of a multidisciplinary team (Hay and Touyz, 2015; Robinson, 2009, 2014). Patients with SEED present with signs and symptoms of a severe eating disorder (such as BMI below 13) and physical sequelae of long-standing illness (e.g., osteoporosis, renal failure, bowel disease due to laxative abuse). The symptoms of their eating disorders profoundly interfere with their quality of life. Patients with SEED may be as impaired by symptoms of their disorder as are individuals who suffer from other serious chronic mental illnesses such as schizophrenia. The burden on caregivers is noted to be substantially higher than that of caring for a relative with schizophrenia or bipolar disorder (Schmidt et al., 2016). Patients with SEED often suffer from depression as well as social isolation and stigmatization. If involuntary treatment has been unsuccessful, then managing these cases may require trying a novel treatment modality or a shift in the goal of treatment from cure to harm reduction or, ultimately, to palliative or hospice care.

Fluoxetine has proved useful for patients with bulimia (Yager et al., 2010), and lisdexamfetamine has been used to successfully treat binge-eating disorders (Citrome, 2015). However, there is a lack of credible scientific evidence for the use of psychiatric medications in treating eating disorders per se. Several novel treatment modalities have been considered for patients with SEED. Deep brain stimulation, transcranial direct current stimulation, transcranial magnetic stimulation, and ECT have all been used to treat patients with eating disorders, especially those with a severe and enduring form of the illness (Andrews et al., 2014; Coman et al., 2014; Ferguson, 1993; McClelland et al., 2013; Oudijn et al., 2013; Sauvaget et al., 2015; Zhang et al., 2013). (Further discussion of these is beyond the scope of this chapter.) Most of these treatments are in the early stages of use for patients with eating disorders, and there is no guarantee that these treatments will lead to cure or remission. Patients with chronic and severe anorexia nervosa may then look for a compromise between cure, harm reduction, palliative care, and an inevitable death. However, a recent study offers optimism even for the most chronically ill patients with anorexia nervosa and bulimia. It gives reason for pause before summarily labelling a patient as SEEDs.

Harm reduction means treatment directed toward enabling an individual to continue living and being in less danger of immediate death, while conceding that the treatment is less than a full course of care and is directed only toward maintaining a minimal (albeit acceptable) level of care for the individual involved. Harm reduction involves deemphasizing weight gain and placing increased emphasis on quality of life and function, even though the latter may be somewhat limited (Hay and Touyz, 2015).

Palliation means preventing or relieving suffering in addition to supporting the best possible quality of life for patients who are facing a severe or life-threatening illness. Palliative care involves managing pain, shortness of breath, nausea, fatigue, and cognitive symptoms (sadness, grief, depression, anxiety and delirium).

A futile act is one that is considered pointless or useless. Very little has been written regarding futility and psychiatric illness, and those who have given consideration to the topic have asked whether there is really a psychiatric illness for which every treatment has been tried and no hope remains. Given that anorexia nervosa has a poor prognosis in only a subset of patients and that their psychiatric condition leads directly to their death (i.e., not eating, because of anorexia nervosa, leads to malnutrition and subsequent death), the question arises as to when to continue pursuing active treatment versus either engaging in a harm reduction type of care or conceding that continuing care (except that directed toward a less painful death) is futile.

Harm Reduction

The goal of the harm reduction model is to help patients attain (and then maintain) a reasonable level of functioning at a lower than optimal weight, rather than subjecting them to a full course of treatment (i.e., a prolonged hospital stay to achieve and maintain ideal body weight). Finding meaning and purpose in life is emphasized, and symptom remission (beyond that required to keep these patients from needing hospitalization) is deemphasized. Candidates for harm reduction are those patients who have endured multiple prior eating disorder treatments with minimal success and those for whom full weight restoration has not been sustainable or for whom quality of life close to their goal weight has been unacceptable to them. Patients who undergo harm reduction treatment are cared for as outpatients once they have attained an agreed upon (though less than ideal) body weight at an inpatient or residential level of care and once they are out of immediate medical danger. They are then allowed to remain at a weight that is sufficient to enable them to have a reasonable quality of life, even if they cannot work or be fully independent.

In this model, patients with a BMI below 13 are at highest risk of death, whereas those with a BMI above 15 are at the lower end of the risk spectrum. However, no matter what the patient's BMI, the individual's level of risk may be increased if he or she experiences rapid weight loss or other medical problems (such as electrolyte abnormalities secondary to purging). Patients undergoing a harm reduction model of care are also at great risk of further morbidity and early mortality if they develop medical problems such as a viral illness, pneumonia, or a fracture (Robinson, 2009, 2014). These comorbidities may lead to rapid decompensation and death.

Patients who receive treatment according to the harm reduction model must be closely monitored. They must have regular visits with their outpatient team, consisting of a psychiatrist or primary care physician, dietician, and therapist. If their weight drops below the agreed upon weight or laboratory test results become significantly abnormal (e.g., rising transaminase levels; hypoglycemia; drop in white blood cell count; abnormalities in potassium, bicarbonate, magnesium, or sodium; changes in EKG), they must be hospitalized so as to restore the amount of weight they have lost or to normalize laboratory test results. Patients undergoing harm reduction should also be monitored for depression, hopelessness, and suicidal ideation. It is well known that suicide attempts, with a high risk of being fatal, are made by people who are habituated to pain because of their experience with physical pain (Joiner, 2006). Patients with severe and chronic eating disorders often attempt suicide using highly lethal means because they are well accustomed to pain, given their experience of starvation, binge eating, purging, and the medical complications of their eating disorder, as well as habituation to other forms of self-injurious behavior (e.g., cutting and substance use).

Palliative Care

The goal of palliation is to reduce suffering through comfort care, including but not limited to management of pain. Patients who undergo palliative care are those for whom any further treatment (whether active treatment, with the goal of normalizing weight, or harm reduction) is unlikely to resolve or decrease their illness and suffering and whose goal is to be comfortable during the remainder of their life, albeit likely to be an abbreviated one. Continuing to treat these patients is more harmful than beneficial, and they are unable to accede to the terms necessary for a harm reduction model to work in their favor. Patients who elect to undergo palliative care often have untreatable comorbidities such as severe major depressive disorder that does not respond to treatment. Candidates for palliative care have usually had multiple prior treatments and no remission in symptoms or ability to sustain any weight gain. They see no reason to strive for a continued existence. Although the term *palliative care* (symptomatic relief from pain or physical or mental stress) is not synonymous with *hospice care*, these terms are frequently conflated. Symptomatic relief includes (but is not limited to) analgesics for pain associated with osteoporosis and stress fractures, wound care for decubitus ulcers, and medications to reduce anxiety symptoms, depression and perseverative, obsessive thinking and to improve sleep. Palliative care may take place in the patient's home, in a hospital, in a skilled nursing unit, or ultimately, but not necessarily, in a hospice care unit.

FUTILITY

Case 3

M.M. was 56 years old when she was admitted to an inpatient eating disorder treatment unit. She had suffered from anorexia nervosa, restricting subtype, since her teens and had had multiple prior treatments. She had managed to function relatively well for 8 years, but had suffered relapses several times over the preceding 5 years. She became progressively more ill at each admission. M.M.'s eating disorder was complicated by major depressive disorder, recurrent, with poor response to medications. She underwent ECT and developed delirium, leading to the discontinuation of ECT. She had two adult children with eating disorders, with whom she had a contentious relationship. M.M. wanted to leave treatment. An ethics consultation was requested to assess decisional capacity. The consultant opined that M.M. lacked capacity, but raised questions about her ability to recover, given the chronicity of her illness. A mental health hold was placed but was dropped when M.M. contracted for weight restoration to a certain point (i.e., harm reduction). However, she was unable to overcome her entrenched behavior of caloric restriction and struggled to gain weight, especially after her transition to a partial hospital program (PHP).

Insurance labeled M.M. as "chronic" and unlikely to benefit from continued care. Her insurance company refused to fund further PHP care as she was "too sick" for PHP, but then refused to fund inpatient care as she was "too chronic." Insurance terminated, and M.M. left treatment. She relapsed immediately following discharge. She became severely depressed. She came close to committing suicide on two occasions and was readmitted to an inpatient eating disorder treatment unit, but was so ill she required treatment on a medical unit. A capacity evaluation was performed, and M.M. was deemed to have decisional capacity. In addition, her brother had durable power of attorney and agreed with her decision to return home to hospice care. The remainder of her family struggled with this decision but eventually came to terms with M.M.'s decision. The patient died several weeks after arriving home.

Comment: The patient's lifelong battle with her eating disorder as well as her depression, which was not responsive to treatment, led to her feeling that she did not have a reasonable quality of life. While she had previously had a period during which she was in remission from eating disorder symptoms, during the latter part of her life she was unable to return to that state. The treatment team assessed that a very reasonable effort had been made to assist this patient in returning to health, but noted more and more distress with each admission as she struggled to cope with immense depression and very severe body image concerns; the team concluded that further active treatment would do more harm than good. At the time she decided to begin hospice care she was deemed to have capacity to make this decision, and treatment team members (and, in time, her family) were able to see that allowing her to die on her terms was ultimately better than continuing to try to force treatment or have her complete suicide in a violent manner.

Decisional Capacity

Patients who are subjected to involuntary treatment are often those who are the most severely and chronically ill and who therefore have the highest risk of death. Despite the truism of this statement, it does not necessarily mean that these patients *should* be certified merely because the symptoms and signs of their clinical condition meet the burden of proof for certification—which in most jurisdiction is clear and convincing evidence. Patients who have been ill for a long time may be least likely to benefit from certification. Although they may be more likely to be deemed incompetent regarding decisional capacity, they have a wealth of experience with their illness and may be the most capable of judging the quality of their lives and whether that quality justifies continued attempts at active treatment, harm reduction, or palliative or hospice care.

The concept of futility has sparked a contentious debate as it pertains to anorexia nervosa. There are several arguments against futility in this disease. First, there is a lack of clarity as to what is meant by the term *end stage* as it applies to an eating disorder, even if the eating disorder becomes severe or chronic. Unlike terminal cancer, in which there may be little or no hope of cure, most medical complications of anorexia nervosa are treatable, even in their most severe form (Westmoreland et al., 2016). What makes anorexia nervosa untreatable is not the lack of a known or available cure but rather the patient's inability or refusal to accept that his or her critically low weight is life-threatening. Patients with severe anorexia nervosa often say they want to live but then eschew the very treatment (eating and weight restoration) required to save their lives. A severely ill patient stating that he or she wishes to live who then rejects life-saving care raises the question as to whether this patient has the decisional capacity required to refuse treatment.

Decisional capacity is an individual's ability to understand information about his or her condition, reason through the information needed to make a decision about care, appreciate the consequences of the decision that he or she makes, and communicate his or her choice. It is questionable whether patients with severe eating disorders have the capacity to decide that further treatment is futile, when the core symptom of their illness is a cognitive distortion about nutrition and weight gain and when they do not believe that starving themselves is life-threatening. A recent study of decision-making capacity in patients with anorexia nervosa found poorer decision-making capacity in these patients, whose intolerance of uncertainty and myopia regarding the future underlie their deficits in decision making (Adoue et al., 2015). Because cognitive distortions often normalize with weight gain, it has been asked whether treatment providers are not obligated to treat patients so that their cognitive distortions resolve and their decision making is no longer impaired (Geppert, 2015).

In two cases in which patients with SEED were allowed to refuse treatment, leading to their death, both patients appear to have embarked on the path toward death despite having questionable decision-making capacity. In one of the first published cases discussing end-of-life care for a patient with anorexia nervosa, O'Neill, Crowther, and Sampson (1994) reported that a 24-year-old who had suffered from anorexia nervosa for at least 7 years and had been hospitalized on 11 occasions over 5 years was admitted to a hospice unit. Prior treatment had included NG feeding and psychotropic medications. At the time of her hospice admission, the patient was severely underweight and suffering from pressure sores, urinary incontinence, and multiple fractures. She continued to exercise despite her treating physician's concern that doing so in the setting of lumbar spine fractures could lead to paraplegia. A week after admission to the hospice unit, she developed delirium and died. While the decision to admit this patient to hospice care was apparently a joint decision between the psychiatric consultant, hospice medical director, the patient's family, and the patient herself, her decision-making capacity does not appear to have been evaluated before the decision to admit her to hospice.

The second case dealt with a 30-year-old patient with a history of chronic anorexia nervosa (Lopez, Yager, and Feinstein, 2010). According to her treatment providers, she had reached a point in her treatment where either forcing her into involuntary treatment or waiting for her to voluntarily engage in treatment was unlikely to cure her eating disorder or even afford her a decent quality of life. Active treatment was terminated and hospice care was instituted. However, she was reluctant to discuss end-of-life issues and insisted that she would not die, nor did she want to die. Her health continued to decline, and she died 3 weeks after admission to a hospice care unit. Despite questions about her capacity, her treatment providers remarked that even if she had been declared legally incompetent regarding her ability to make treatment decisions, "Then what?"—indicating that capacity may not be the final arbiter in deciding futility. Rather, they noted, patients with a poor prognosis who continue to decline physiologically and psychologically and appear to be facing a terminal course should be given the more humane choice of hospice care, rather than being forced into a treatment stay with an undoubtedly questionable prognosis.

In a more recent review on the topic, patients who chose to succumb to their illness were noted to be competent in their decision making when they elected to pursue end-of-life care (Campbell and Aulisio, 2012). These patients were older than those described by McNeil et al. (1994) and Lopez et al. (2010) and had had longer periods of failed treatments, and their refusals of life-sustaining care had been consistent over a longer period.

Case Law and Futility

Two recent cases from the United Kingdom argue opposing sides of the futility debate.

Local Authority vs. E (2012). A patient with a severe and chronic eating disorder had previously executed two advance directives refusing compulsory feeding. Her parents and physicians argued that she was comparatively well when she executed the directives, and they asked that she be allowed to die with dignity. However, the judge ruled that Ms. E suffered from the same cognitive distortions at the time of the court case as she did at the time she executed the directives. The judge noted that the value of life trumps the presumption that further treatment will fail and ordered that involuntary treatment be tried in this case. Critics of this decision have suggested that supporting the will of the patient to the best possible extent, with the additional support of the family, might have been a better course of action than the formulation of "best interests" (with the objective of saving the life of a patient who did not want to live and whose family supported her decision to die) (Ryan and Callaghan, 2014).

NHS Foundation Trust vs. Ms. X (2014). In this case, the court declined to subject Ms. X, who had had anorexia nervosa for 14 years, to forced feeding, even though she had been deemed to lack capacity with regard to her eating disorder. The judge characterized forced feeding against her wishes as amounting to inhumane treatment interfering with her autonomy. The judge also attempted to distinguish between feeding and weight gain and psychosocial treatment that focuses on quality of life (McKenzie, 2015). However, this approach fails to take into consideration that weight gain during inpatient treatment is a significant predictor of clinical outcome following discharge, even though it is unclear whether weight gain exerts a causal effect or is, instead, a marker for readiness to tolerate weight restoration and to engage in life beyond the eating disorder (Lund et al., 2014; Steinhausen et al., 2009). In addition, it has been argued that treatments seeking only to improve quality of life may be unlikely to produce lasting change unless accompanied by a reduction in eating disorder symptoms and an improvement in weight (Bamford et al., 2015).

Framework for End-of-Life Decisions

Eating disorder professionals are trying to strike a balance between opposing futility outright and succumbing to a "slippery slope" argument that would make all patients with SEED inherently eligible for end-of-life care. The need for compassion, perhaps above capacity, has been noted, so that patients are not forced into an intolerable living situation merely because they are deemed to lack capacity. On the other hand, when the illness itself compromises a patient's ability to make a fully competent decision, overriding a patient's autonomy may be justified under the doctrine of paternalism in an effort to save that patient's life and return him or her to a state where he or she can make an informed and competent decision.

A framework that balances patients' wishes with legitimate concerns about allowing someone with impaired decision-making capacity to refuse further treatment has been proposed. In a recent editorial on this topic, McKinney (2015) suggested that treatment-refusal decisions about further episodes of care should be made under the following conditions: (1) decisions must be made at a time when the patient is competent (i.e., between episodes), (2) the patient must have a realistic expectation about outcome (must know that refusing nutrition will lead to death), (3) the patient's decision to die must be based on a realistic assessment of current quality of life and the low probability that current or future treatment will succeed, and (4) the patient must be consistent in communicating his or her desires. Each case must be considered in a nuanced and thoughtful manner. There is a justifiable reluctance on the part of eating disorder professionals to undertake any treatment that bears little hope of advancing a patient's quality of life, directly opposes the wishes of the patient and family, and simply extends a life of suffering, even if the patient has diminished capacity. As has been suggested, surely even a patient who does not have decision-making capacity is still likely to be capable of appraising his or her suffering (Kendall, 2014; Yager, 2015). Futility should therefore be considered on a case-by-case basis and applied when considering a particular treatment intervention, at a particular time, for a particular patient.

Summary

Ethical principles assist us in determining the best course of action for patients with anorexia nervosa. Certification and guardianship may be helpful in treating these patients, especially those who are in the earlier stages of the illness. Given the poor prognosis for patients with chronic and life-threatening anorexia nervosa, the high recidivism rate of these patients, and the chronic suffering endured by patients with severe and enduring eating disorders, it is important to realistically assess each patient's capacity for recovery or ability to engage in a harm reduction model. At the same time, one must remain in touch with the wishes of the patient, family, and treatment team. The burden on caregivers and stewardship in the expenditure of health care resources should also be considered when deciding whether involuntary treatment, novel treatments, harm reduction, palliative care, or end-of-life care be recommended for a particular patient.

End-of-life care is controversial, but it may be of expanding relevance for a narrowly defined set of patients with anorexia nervosa whose illness is severe and enduring. Failure to consider end-of-life care as an option for patients with a chronic and severe psychiatric illness such as anorexia nervosa may perpetuate the stigma of mental illness as separate from physical illness in terms of the compassion we afford its sufferers. Thus, while it is important to adjust the usual treatment paradigm of anorexia nervosa to include involuntary treatment, novel treatments, and harm reduction and palliative care, there is also a need to educate ourselves about the possibility of futility as it pertains to patients with eating disorders, especially those with severe and enduring forms of the illness (Westmoreland and Mehler, in press).

REFERENCES

Accurso E, Ciao A, Fitzsimmons-Craft E, et al. 2014. Is weight gain really a catalyst for broader recovery? The impact of weight gain on psychological symptoms in treatment of adolescent anorexia nervosa. *Behavioral Research and Therapy* 56:1–6.

Ackard D, Richter S, Egan A, and Cronemeyer C. 2014. Poor outcome and death among youth, young adults, and midlife adults with eating disorders: An investigation of risk factors by age of assessment. *International Journal of Eating Disorders* 47:825–35.

Adoue C, Jaussent I, Olié E, et al. 2015. A further assessment of decision-making in anorexia nervosa. *European Psychiatry* 30:121–27.

Andrews JT, Seide M, Guarda AS, and Redgrave GW. 2014. Electroconvulsive therapy in an adolescent with severe major depression and anorexia nervosa. *Journal of Child and Adolescent Psychopharmacology* 24(2):94–98.

Appelbaum PS and Rumpf T. 1998. Civil commitment of the anorexic patient. *General Hospital Psychiatry* 20:225–30.

Arcelus J, Mitchell AJ, Wales J, and Nielsen S. 2011. Mortality rates in patients with anorexia nervosa and other eating disorders: A meta-analysis of 36 studies. *Archives of General Psychiatry* 68:724–31.

Ayton A, Keen C, and Las B. 2009. Pros and cons of using the mental health act for severe eating disorder in adolescents. *European Eating Disorders Review* 17:14–23.

Bamford B, Barras C, Sly R, et al. 2015. Eating disorder symptoms and quality of life: Where should clinicians place their focus in severe and enduring anorexia nervosa? *International Journal of Eating Disorders* 48:19–25.

Beauchamp TL and Childress JF. 2012. *Principles of Biomedical Ethics*, 7th ed. Oxford: Oxford University Press.

Born C, de la Fontaine L, Winter B, et al. 2015. First results of a refeeding program in a psychiatric intensive care unit for patients with extreme anorexia nervosa. *BMC Psychiatry* 15:57.

Bourion-Bedes S, Baumann C, Kermarrec S, et al. 2013. Prognostic value of early therapeutic alliance in weight recovery: A prospective cohort of 108 adolescents with anorexia nervosa. *Journal of Adolescent Health* 52:344–50.

Campbell AT and Aulisio MP. 2012. The stigma of "mental illness": End stage anorexia and treatment refusal. *International Journal of Eating Disorders* 45:627–34.

Carney T. 2014. The incredible complexity of being? Degrees of influence, coercion, and control of the "autonomy" of severe and enduring anorexia nervosa patients. *Bioethical Inquiry* 11:41–42.

Carney T, Tait D, Richardson A, and Touyz S. 2008. Why (and when) clinicians compel treatment of anorexia nervosa patients. *European Eating Disorders Review* 16:199–206.

Citrome L. 2015. Lisdexamfetamine for binge eating disorder in adults: A systematic review of the efficacy and safety profile for this newly approved indication—what is the number needed to treat, number needed to harm and the likelihood of being helped or harmed. *International Journal of Clinical Practice* 69(4):410–21.

Clausen L and Jones J. 2014. A systematic review of the frequency, duration, type and effect of involuntary treatment for people with anorexia nervosa, and an analysis of patient characteristics. *Journal of Eating Disorders* 2(29):1–10.

Coman A, Skårderud F, Reas DL, and Hoffman BM. 2014. The ethics of neuromodulation for anorexia nervosa: A focus on TMS. *Journal of Eating Disorders* 2(10):1–7.

Douzenis A and Michopoulos L. 2015. Involuntary admission: The case of anorexia nervosa. *International Journal of Law and Psychiatry* 39:31–35.

Eddy KT, Tabri N, Thomas JJ, et al. 2017. Recovery from anorexia nervosa and bulimia nervosa at 22-year follow-up. *Journal of Clinical Psychiatry*, 78(2): 184–89.

Elzakkers I, Danner UN, Hoek HW, et al. 2014. Compulsory treatment in anorexia nervosa: A review. *International Journal of Eating Disorders* 47:845–52.

Ferguson JM. 1993. The use of electroconvulsive therapy in patients with intractable anorexia nervosa. *International Journal of Eating Disorders* 13(2):195–201.

Franko DL, Keshaviah A, Eddy KT, et al. 2013. A longitudinal investigation of mortality in anorexia nervosa and bulimia nervosa. *American Journal of Psychiatry* 170:917–25.

Geppert CMA. 2015. Futility in chronic anorexia nervosa: A concept whose time has not yet come. *American Journal of Bioethics* 15(7):34–43.

Griffiths R A, Beaumont P J V, Russell J, et al. 1997. The use of guardianship legislation for anorexia nervosa: A report of 15 cases. *Australian and New Zealand Journal of Psychiatry* 31:525–31.

Guarda A S, Pinto A M, Coughlin J W, et al. 2007. Perceived coercion and change in perceived need for admission in patients hospitalized for eating disorders. *American Journal of Psychiatry* 164:108–14.

Gutheil T G and Bursztajn H. 1986. Clinicians' guidelines for assessing and presenting subtle forms of patient incompetence in legal settings. *American Journal of Psychiatry* 143:1020–23.

Hay P and Touyz S. 2015. Treatment of patients with severe and enduring eating disorders. *Current Opinion in Psychiatry* 28:473–77.

Holm J S, Brixen K, Andries A, et al. 2012. Reflections on involuntary treatment in the prevention of fatal anorexia nervosa: A review of five cases. *International Journal of Eating Disorders* 45:93–100.

Huas C, Godart N, Foulon C, et al. 2011. Predictors of dropout from inpatient treatment for anorexia nervosa: Data from a large French sample. *Psychiatry Research* 185:421–26.

In the Matter of Joanne Kolodrubetz, 411 N.W. 2d 528 (Minn. App. 1987).

In the Matter of Molly Kellor, 520 N.W. 2d 9 (Minn. Ct. App. 1994).

In re S.A.M., 695 N.W. 2d 506 (Iowa App. 2005).

Joiner T. 2006. *Why People Die by Suicide*. Cambridge MA: Harvard University Press.

Kendall S. 2014. Anorexia nervosa: The diagnosis. *Bioethical Inquiry* 11:31–40.

Le Grange D, Fitzsimmons-Craft E, Crosby R, et al. 2014. Predictors and moderators of outcome for severe and enduring anorexia nervosa. *Behavioral Research and Therapy* 56:91–98.

Local Authority v. E., E W H C 1639, 2012.

Long C, Fitzgerald K A, and Hollin C. 2012. Treatment of chronic anorexia nervosa: A 4-year follow-up of adult patients treated in an acute inpatient setting. *Clinical Psychiatry and Psychotherapy* 19:1–13.

Lopez A, Yager J, and Feinstein R E. 2010. Medical futility and psychiatry: Palliative care and hospice care as a last resort in the treatment of refractory anorexia nervosa. *International Journal of Eating Disorders* 43:372–77.

Lund B C, Hernandez E R, Yates W R, and Mitchell J R. 2014. Rate of inpatient weight restoration predicts outcome in anorexia nervosa. *International Journal of Eating Disorders* 42:301–5.

McClelland J, Bozhilova N, Nestler S, et al. 2013. Improvements in symptoms following neuronavigated repetitive transcranial magnetic stimulation (r-TMS) in severe and enduring anorexia nervosa: Findings from two case studies. *European Eating Disorders Review* 21:500–506.

McKenzie R. 2015. Ms. X: A promising new view of anorexia nervosa, futility, and end-of-life decisions in a very recent English case. *American Journal of Bioethics* 15(7):57–58.

McKinney C. 2015. Is resistance (n)ever futile? A response to "Futility in Chronic Anorexia Nervosa: A Concept Whose Time Has Not Yet Come" by Cynthia Geppert. *American Journal of Bioethics* 15(7):53–54.

Nakamura M, Yasunaga H, Shimada T, et al. 2013. Body mass index and in-hospital mortality in anorexia nervosa: Data from the Japanese Diagnosis Procedure Combination Database. *Eating and Weight Disorders* 18:437–39.

NHS Foundation Trust v. Ms. X, EWCOP 35, 2014.

O'Neill J, Crowther T, and Sampson G. 1994. Anorexia nervosa: Palliative care of terminal psychiatric disease. *American Journal of Hospice and Palliative Care* 11(6):36–38.

Oudijn MS, Storosum JG, Nelis E, and Denys D. 2013. Is deep brain stimulation a treatment option for anorexia nervosa? *BMC Psychiatry* 13(277):1–9.

People of the State of Colorado in the interest of P.A. 12CA1024, (Col. App. 2012), unpublished.

People of the State of Colorado in the interest of P.A. 13CA1350, (Col. App. 2013), unpublished.

Ramsey R, Ward A, Treasure J, et al. 1999. Compulsory treatment in anorexia nervosa: Short-term benefits and long-term mortality. *British Journal of Psychiatry* 175:147–53.

Robinson P. 2009. *Severe and Enduring Eating Disorder (SEED). Management of Complex Presentations of Anorexia and Bulimia Nervosa*. Chichester, UK: John Wiley and Sons.

———.2014. Severe and enduring eating disorders: Recognition and management. *Advances in Psychiatric Treatment* 20:392–401.

Ryan CJ and Callaghan S. 2014. Treatment refusal in anorexia nervosa: The hardest cases. *Bioethical Inquiry* 11:43–45.

Sauvaget A, Trojak B, Bulteau S, et al. 2015. Transcranial direct current stimulation (t-DCS) in behavioral and food addiction: A systematic review of efficacy, technical and methodological issues. *Frontiers in Neuroscience* 9(349):1–14.

Schmidt U, Adan R, Böhm I, et al. 2016. Eating disorders: The big issue. *Lancet* 3(4):313–15.

Schreyer C, Coughlin J, Makhzoumi S, and Redgrave G. 2016. Perceived coercion in inpatients with anorexia nervosa: Associations with illness severity and hospital course. *International Journal of Eating Disorders* 49(4):407–12.

Sly R, Morgan JF, Mountford VA, and Lacey JH. 2013. Predicting premature termination of hospitalised treatment for anorexia nervosa: The roles of therapeutic alliance, motivation, and behaviour change. *Eating Behaviors* 14:119–23

Steinhausen HC, Grigoroiu-Serbanescu M, Boyadjieva S, Jürgen K, and Neumärker K-J. 2008. Course and predictors of rehospitalization in adolescent anorexia nervosa in a multisite study. *International Journal of Eating Disorders* 41(1):29–36.

Steinhausen HC, Grigoroiu-Serbanescu M, Boyadjieva S, et al. 2009. The relevance of body weight in medium-term to long-term course of adolescent anorexia nervosa: Findings from a multi-site study. *International Journal of Eating Disorders* 42:19–25.

Tan J, Stewart A, Fitzpatrick R, and Hope T. 2010. Attitudes of patients with anorexia nervosa to compulsory treatment and coercion. *International Journal of Law and Psychiatry* 33:13–19.

Wales J, Brewin N, Cashmore R, et al. 2016. Predictors of positive treatment outcome in people with anorexia nervosa treated in a specialized inpatient unit: The role of early response to treatment. *European Eating Disorders Review* 24:417–24.

Ward A, Ramsay R, Russell, and Treasure J. 2015. Follow-up mortality study of compulsorily treated patients with anorexia nervosa. *International Journal of Eating Disorders* 48:860–65.

Westmoreland P, Krantz MJ, and Mehler PS. 2016. Medical complications of anorexia nervosa and bulimia nervosa. *American Journal of Medicine* 129(1):30–37.

Westmoreland P and Mehler PS. In press. Law and psychiatry: Caring for patients with severe and enduring eating disorders (SEED): Certification, harm reduction, palliative care, and the question of futility. *Journal of Psychiatric Practice* 22(4).

Yager J. 2015. The futility of arguing about medical futility in anorexia nervosa: The question is how you would handle highly specific circumstances. *American Journal of Bioethics* 15(7):47–50.

Yager J, Devlin MJ, Halmi K, et al. 2010. *Practice Guidelines for the Treatment of Patients with Eating Disorders*, 3rd ed. Arlington, VA: American Psychiatric Association.

Zhang HW, Li D-Y, Zhao J, et al. 2013. Metabolic imaging of deep brain stimulation in anorexia nervosa: A ^{18}F-FDG PET/CT study. *Clinical Nuclear Medicine* 38(12):943–48.

16

Medical Information for Nonmedical Clinicians and Educators

Arnold E. Andersen, MD

Common Questions

What background medical knowledge is needed by nonmedical health and education professionals (psychotherapists, experiential therapists, social workers, nutritionists, educators, coaches) who play a role in identifying, treating, or preventing eating disorders?

How do you approach a student, athlete, or friend whom you think may have an eating disorder?

When do you refer a person with a possible eating disorder to a physician?

What medical components of care may non–medically trained health professionals or educators carry out?

What are some safeguards against legal consequences for an adverse medical outcome while treating or advising a client/patient or student with an eating disorder?

What ethical concerns are present for nonmedical clinicians and educators when interacting with clients/patients or students with eating disorders?

What role does the educator play in the course of eating disorders?

What published resources are available to families?

Case 1

Mr. B was a coach for a university cheerleading club that performed at major sports events. Chad, a third-year cheerleader, was 5 feet 10 inches tall and weighed 160 pounds. He complained that he could not lift Jill, who was 5 feet 5 inches and 125 pounds, over his head in a complicated, show-stopping half-time program for the basketball season. Chad asked Mr. B to suggest to Jill that she lose 10–15 pounds. After listening to Chad's concerns, Mr. B suggested that Chad would benefit from a trainer-guided program to increase lean muscle mass, especially increasing strength in his shoulders, back, and quadriceps, so that he could lift Jill in the routines required. The coach explained that Jill ate normally and was in a healthy, thin-normal range of body fat at 18%, and he expressed concern that he might provoke eating-disordered behavior in an otherwise healthy young woman by suggesting weight loss. Mr. B recognized the ethical aspects of the gender disparity in completing cheerleader routines, and rather than suggesting the usual change of asking the young woman to lose weight, suggested that the young man gain more strength in a fitness program; both students could benefit from this "win-win" philosophy. As for many male gymnasts of his height, Chad's frame would carry extra muscle mass well.

Case 2

L.M., a 12-year-old female, had developed pubertal changes slightly earlier than her peers. In a health class in the fifth grade, she, like every other student in the class, was weighed in front of the class, with the teacher commenting on the weight status of each student. L.M. was told that she was about 10 pounds overweight and should lose some weight. She felt ashamed and criticized. She started a program of severe dietary restriction, cutting out sweets and fats, adding exercise, and becoming preoccupied with the calorie and fat content of foods. Within 6 months she met the criteria for anorexia nervosa, including loss of menstrual periods.

For the next 6 years L.M. required continued regular care for her low weight, her morbid fear of fatness, the development of binge-purge behaviors, and overexercising. She avoided social events involving food. When she went to Europe on a student exchange program, she was referred to an experienced clinician who helped to stabilize her weight, change her core psychological overvalued beliefs in the necessity of extreme thinness, and begin a pattern of healthier weight and eating. She remains preoccupied with weight but has had return of her menstrual periods and continues in psychotherapy.

What Non-Medically Trained Clinicians and Educators Need to Know about Eating Disorders

Effects of Out-of-Control Dieting and Excessive Weight Loss

The most common abnormal eating pattern in high school and college students is to skip breakfast, eat a light lunch, and then have to fight hunger later in the day. Sometimes this restrained eating or chronic dieting pattern, through perseverance, results in the desired thinness, but many times it leads to binge eating behavior later in the day. Most people self-regulate body weight in a narrow 4- to 5-pound range called the "set point." This range of weight is not fixed in stone but tends to be fairly consistent for each individual. Significant lowering of weight below this point often leads to involuntary preoccupation with thoughts of food, decreased mental attention, becoming more isolative or irritable, feeling colder than peers, and changing eating behavior toward either eating slowly and in small bites or gulping food ravenously. In studies by Keys and others in the 1940s on volunteers who underwent experimental starvation to help prepare the United States to take care of returning prisoners of war, these changes were documented as being effects of starvation (Keys, Brozek, and Henscheo, 1950). Many of the signs and symptoms of what is called anorexia nervosa are in fact the mental and physical changes of starvation. The component that is truly at the core of the eating disordered illness is an internalized overvaluation of the benefits of slimness or shape change and the driven behaviors employed to achieve these ends.

Effects of Binge and Purge Behavior

Binge eating behavior is driven by three factors: hunger, distressed moods, and habit patterns related to time of day or place. Initially, binges simply start as a response to food restriction, weight loss, and hunger. Gradually, binges become triggered by distressed moods such as anxiety about a test, a low mood resulting from a relationship upset, anger at perceived unfairness, or feelings of boredom and emptiness. Binge behavior is not an ineffective or "dumb" behavior; it helps in the triggering situations, temporarily, somewhat like a drug fix—but then creates more problems than it solves.

Most binge eating behavior initially represents an attempt at an anorexic weight that did not work because the body has refused to accept this degree of deprivation, allowing hunger to break through despite willpower.

Anorexia nervosa of the restricting type is possible only in individuals with the genetic endowment of strong perseverance. The diagnosis of bulimia nervosa requires binge episodes, even though people often mislabel purging behavior as bulimia. The term *bulimia* comes from the words for "ox-hunger." However, purging behavior takes place in 80% of individuals who experience regular binge behavior; it is initiated because of the fear of fatness due to the unwanted binge calories, as well as gastric medical distress from the binge. The 20% of individuals who binge but do not purge compensate in other ways: through heroic exercise or through even more severe restriction of food intake. While binges are uncomfortable, the purging usually produces the more dangerous medical symptoms, including a low serum potassium level that can cause heart irregularity, dehydration due to loss of fluids, bleeding from the esophagus, chest pain, loss of dental enamel, and enlarged parotid glands (the glands that swell in front of the ears during mumps), to name but a few.

Healthy Nutrition

Educators, coaches, nutritionists, psychotherapists, and experiential therapists are often asked to describe good nutritional patterns. There are so many fads and fallacies in the area of nutrition that informal though sincere psychoeducation or guidance in nutritional selection is commonly loaded with bias, personal misinformation, and economically driven misinformation about food choices. Registered dieticians are the most qualified to give accurate advice. In some states, it is illegal for anyone but a physician or a registered dietician to prescribe nutrition.

Many students and athletes count fat grams as much as calories. The preoccupation with fat grams, without distinguishing healthy lipids (monounsaturates such as olive oil, fish, nuts) from unhealthy lipids (trans fats, saturated fats), is a completely unscientific holdover from recent decades when all fats were considered bad. From the 1970s through the 1990s, the average weight of US citizens increased while fat consumption dropped. The average student who is counting fat grams tries to live on 0–10 grams of fat a day. A truly prudent program of nutrition would allow 25%–30% of daily energy intake as healthy fats. Attempts at 0, 5, or 10 grams of fat are unnecessary, unpalatable, and usually unsuccessful.

For male students and athletes who are wanting to bulk up with lean muscle, carbohydrates have become the recent phobia. Magazines touting muscle development hype low-carb diets as the secret to success. Here again, there is a vast difference between unrefined carbohydrates (grains, fruits, vegetables) and highly refined carbohydrates (white bread, sugar). Avoiding highly refined carbohydrates is reasonable, whereas avoiding unrefined carbohydrates is unhealthy. There is increasing evidence that, in males, the brain connections between the prefrontal cortex, where executive judgment is centered, and the amygdala, where emotions and impulses are primarily experienced, are not fully formed until about age 25. While this is an oversimplification of a profound neurodevelopmental process, the basic finding is supported by research. The implication is that many strongly desired but unwise activities during adolescence and early adulthood (driving drunk with a sense of immunity from crashes, going to war, engaging in extreme nutritional programs to bulk up) are pursued with no recognition of their dangers.

Multiple studies support the finding that dieting rarely works. The usual use of the word *diet* refers to an attempt to reduce weight quickly by a program that is overly low in calories and poor in nutritional balance. The only weight change plan that works in the long run is a lifetime nutritional plan: eating every day to stay in a healthy range, or, if some weight change is medically indicated or is a reasonable personal goal, eating for the desired set point so that the program does not need to be changed when the goal weight range is reached. For example, a young woman who is 5 feet 4 inches tall and weighs 140 pounds, with visible excess abdominal obesity, and wants to weigh 125 pounds should eat the number of calories (with a balance in nutrition) that would maintain a young woman at 125 pounds, so that when she has achieved that weight, she does not have to change her eating habits. Most diet programs that advertise, say, "40 pounds lost in 10 weeks" never give follow-up at 1, 2, or 5 years to state how many dieters have maintained their weight loss. The behind-the-scenes answer is almost none.

Educators, nonmedical health professionals, nutritionists, and coaches should encourage students to think of *diet* as a bad four-letter word. They should instead advocate a small cluster of healthy behaviors: good balanced nutrition, regular exercise, and good stress management, along with adequate sleep. Inadequate sleep has been shown to increase snacking and overeating, only recently recognized as an important contributor to abnormal eating patterns.

Evidence is accumulating that there is no benefit from taking vitamins if one is eating a balanced nutritional diet (evidence disputed by economic interests). A major factor in helping students to eat nutritionally is to have available attractive, tasty, healthy snacks and meals and to remove all soft drink machines from schools and sports facilities. An occasional soda pop will not hurt most people, but it is too easy to become accustomed to the taste and mouth texture of concentrated sweets and trans fats (in the form of doughnuts, for example). The best defense nutritionally is a good offense. Studies in Norway have shown that simply having bowls of fruit in a classroom will increase students' likelihood of choosing fruits for part of their daily food intake (Bere et al., 2015).

Healthy Weight

Normal body weight, like height, is distributed in the human population in a bell-shaped curve. Most media promote an unhealthy thinness or impossibly lean muscularity (McCabe and Ricciardelli, 2005). The narrow ranges suggested by insurance company tables or other charts for individual weights are often used inaccurately. These weights are averages, not norms. The real measures of health include a percentage of body fat that is appropriate for age and gender, the location of fat distribution (pear shape vs. apple shape), the resting heart rate, absence of signs of starvation, normal patterns of hunger and satiety, and abandonment of the idea that there are any bad foods or foods that should be phobically avoided. Too many physicians tell patients what to weigh within a too-narrow range, basing their recommendations on average insurance table numbers for longest lifespan—for example, stating that a 5 foot 4 inch woman should weigh 120 pounds. Instead, the appropriate approach is to take a full personal and family history, use multiple measures of fitness, and identify a range of healthy weight for the individual. Studies have shown that patients with anorexia nervosa, in general, will pursue low weight more strongly than profound religious goals. For example, Roman Catholic girls may skip going to mass because of the calories in the wafer (Graham, Spencer, and Andersen, 1991).

Exercise

The United States is as much an underfit as an overfat nation, as well as a nation that has irrationally invested moral and emotional meaning in artificially thin or muscular ideals. With only a few exceptions, the body self-regulates weight in a narrow range when eating is driven by normal cycles of hunger and satiety (rather than in response to emotional needs) and when daily life includes moderate energy output in any form of exercise or physical activity. In general, we encourage "couch potatoes" to get moving and engage in three to five moderate-exercise periods of 30–40 minutes each per week, such as walking. At the same time, we guide compulsive exercisers to choose moderate, prudent exercise rather than driven, inappropriate exercise. (See chapter 12 on athletes and eating disorders.)

Diagnostic Approaches

There is nothing sacred about asking screening questions to sort out whether a person may have an eating disorder, nor is the asking confined to health professionals. Educators, therapists, coaches, and others can use the same SCOFF questionnaire that primary care physicians use (see chapter 1 and table 1.6) and can add their own questions. These questions should cover the following general areas: Are you extremely concerned about your weight? Does attaining a different weight or shape dominate your life? Are you dieting? Have you lost significant weight? Do you experience binge eating or other out-of-control eating? Do you purge after meals? Do you exercise compulsively? Does an overvaluation of the benefits of slimness or shape change override normal concerns? Some school systems have used the EAT-26 (Eating Attitudes Test) for screening for eating disorders (D'Souza, Forman, and Austin, 2005).

Risk Factors

Eating disorders usually occur in individuals with known risk factors (see chapter 1). The more numerous the risk factors and the more severe they are, the higher is the probability of a person's developing an eating disorder. Risk factors include participation in sports or interest groups that encourage weight loss; a family history of obesity, anxiety, eating disorder, or depression; sensitive, self-critical, persevering personality traits; excess weight gain during childhood or during early puberty; gay orientation in males; and comments from influential individuals (teachers, coaches, and educators) promoting weight loss. Teachers may influence students in unhealthy or healthy habits (see the section "Information for Educators" below for more on this topic).

When to Refer an Individual to a Physician

It is good practice, at the beginning of psychotherapy, for any patient (including student) with an eating disorder to have a medical evaluation (table 16.1). This procedure may disclose hidden medical complications
resulting from the eating disorder, but at a minimum it offers a baseline
against which to measure future medical symptoms. It is helpful for the
therapist to have an established relationship with a primary care physician with expertise in treating people with eating disorders. This elimi-
nates the possibility of an inexperienced medical approach to patients
whom the therapist may refer for evaluation and avoids unnecessary, excessive testing. Subjective complaints that should lead to prompt referral
to a primary care physician include constant coldness, faintness or light-
headedness, heart palpitations or chest pain, shortness of breath, abdominal pain, or frequent purging behavior as evidenced by the individual's
saying that she or he uses many diuretics or laxatives a day—and certainly
if ipecac, an over-the-counter medicine to induce vomiting in children
who have eaten poison, is used. (Ipecac is no longer recommended for poison response.) Common sense and professional judgment will also guide
therapists and educators to refer patients or students when they note
significant weight loss, a thin, bony appearance, bluish hands, a cold hand-
shake, or an overall appearance of bad health. Information from parents

**Table 16.1. When to refer a client or student with a suspected eating disorder
to a primary care physician**

- At the beginning of psychotherapy treatment, for evaluation and to establish a
  liaison relationship
- When the client or student has any of the following symptoms:
  - Severe or rapid weight loss
  - Dizziness, lightheadedness, fainting (hypotension)
  - Uncontrolled binge-purge behavior (electrolytes often abnormal; EKG may be
    abnormal)
  - Constant coldness
  - Medical distress such as chest pain (often from purging behavior) or
    abdominal pain
- For psychopharmacologic augmentation (preferably by a psychiatrist) to
  psychotherapy
- For periodic check-ups or weighing (weighing often may be performed by
  physician's assistant or nurse)

or friends about excessive purging behavior should also generally lead to referral.

At times, medical referral is deferred because an individual is developing insight. It is important to realize that while "insight" is critical, there is a huge difference between intellectual insight and behavior-changing insight. Insight is useless unless it leads to sustained behavioral change. Valuing intellectual insight in the presence of continued severe weight loss, a failure to restore weight, or lack of change in significant binge-purge behavior is an illusion. The patient has not made progress when she or he gains and then loses weight, with multiple excuses and promises to do better next session. Behavior is behavior is behavior.

When to Accept an Individual for Therapy on Referral from a Physician

Accepting a client/patient from a physician should, ideally, involve sufficient assurance from the physician that the individual is well enough to come for nonmedical treatment, primarily psychotherapy and experiential therapy (table 16.2). It is important to record agreements regarding when the patient should be referred back to the physician and to set up both regular and as-needed communication between therapist (or coach, for student athletes) and physician. Also important is to establish who performs what roles in shared medical functions, such as weighing the patient. It is inappropriate to refer an individual for treatment without specifying who will monitor weight or binge-purge behavior. Agreements should be in writing, and contacts should be recorded in the medical record. Table 16.3 summarizes the components of effective collaboration.

Table 16.2. When to accept a client/patient for psychotherapy or experiential therapy from a referring physician

- After medical evaluation is under way
- After establishing a frequency-of-contact schedule and conditions for the client/patient's return to see the physician
- After decisions are made on frequency of checking body weight and who will weigh the client/patient
- After deciding who will instruct the client/patient on healthy nutrition and prescribe a nutritional program (physician or registered dietician)

Table 16.3. How team members should collaborate effectively in the care of a patient with an eating disorder

- Establish a regular, agreed-on communication schedule.
- Set up clear, specific conditions for referrals (e.g., to dietician, social worker).
- Clearly define the roles of the various team members.
- Share techniques guiding the overall treatment.
- Set goals for client/patient care within each discipline that are specific, time-limited, achievable, and ratable.
- Decide who is "captain of the ship."
- Decide on a single, consistent guiding psychotherapeutic strategy, such as CBT.

Medical Responsibilities That Can Be Carried Out by Non–Medically Trained Health Professionals

A medical degree or other specific training is not required to weigh an individual or to encourage healthy behaviors such as good nutrition. These are commonsense practices that can be carried out by nonmedical professionals and certainly are performed frequently by coaches and educators, as well as by formally trained nutritionists and physicians. Coaches often monitor athletes' resting heart rate. The key here is to be clear on who does what, and under what conditions the patient or student needs to be referred back to the physician. Some psychologically trained therapists do not like the idea of weighing a patient, or they carry outmoded ideas that weighing would somehow interfere with psychotherapy. Sometimes it is simply not practical or is too expensive for an individual to return to a doctor's office for weekly weighing when it can be done in a therapist's or nutritionist's office. Agreements need to be recorded about a weight minimum or a lack of progress in weight restoration that will prompt referral to more intensive medical treatments. A psychotherapist can ask a patient to keep a nutritional record so as to assess compliance with the nutritional prescription, emotionally based alterations in eating, or the presence of binge-purge behaviors. The patient can use a simple 3×5 index card or a laptop or iPad to record each day, in columns, the time of day, food eaten, emotions experienced, and events taking place. This record can form the basis for beginning a psychotherapy session.

How to Avoid Legal Problems

The key to avoiding legal problems in comprehensive care includes good recordkeeping, decisions about when to refer an individual to a physician (erring on the side of more rather than fewer referrals), documentation of regular communication with the primary care physician and other team members (see table 16.3), and acting with knowledge and common sense. Letting a person lose weight in front of your eyes because she or he is developing "insight," failing to refer someone who looks very ill, perpetuating irrelevant or out-of-date details about calories or fat grams in place of sound nutrition, failing to document communications with a primary care physician—all would open one to being included in litigation if adverse medical consequences arise. This does not mean that referral is necessary for mild but improving starvation, occasional binge-purge behavior, and so on. It takes time, knowledge, and development of professional judgment to balance the intrusiveness of medical referrals versus their necessity after the initial evaluation. Working within your limits of qualified training is essential, as is having a team-oriented approach (see chapter 2). Litigation is rarely a concern when treatment is sound, adequate records are kept, and good patient-clinician relationships are maintained. When these guidelines are followed, the treatment and education of clients/patients, students, or athletes with eating disorders will be satisfying and effective.

Information for Educators

The most common question asked by educators is how they should approach a student who may have an eating disorder. We provide some guidelines (for educators and others) in table 16.4. Seeing that a student is losing significant weight, seeing a student consistently exiting after meals or snacks to use the restroom, or becoming aware of significant mental preoccupation with weight and shape should all alert the educator to the possibility of an eating disorder. Educators are often approached by a student's friends who tell them about behaviors that an educator might not see directly. The best tactic is simply to approach the student and say that you are concerned that an eating disorder may be present and that it is essential for her or him to see a trained individual or eating disorder clinic for an evaluation. Depending on the age of the student, the parents may be informed and their help solicited.

Table 16.4. How to approach a person you suspect may have an eating disorder

- Educate yourself about eating disorders from accurate sources.
- Be caring but firm in approaching the person.
- Share your concern about the possibility of an eating disorder being present. Share what you have observed, in a kindly way, as evidence for the presence of a problem.
- Gently but firmly tell the person to schedule an appointment with a qualified health professional or eating disorder clinic for assessment, and then "I'll be off your case."
- Don't oversimplify the issue or assume that time will improve the disorder.
- Don't imply that bulimia nervosa is less serious because there is no obvious emaciation.
- Express your concern privately.
- Don't diagnose.
- Don't become the therapist or savior or offer short-term, oversimplified solutions.
- Do act in an emergency, such as the presence of chest pain, suicidal thinking, or passing out, and get help immediately.
- Assure the person that you will maintain friendship through the process of becoming well.
- Encourage the continuation of spiritual growth without "spiritualizing" or "moralizing" the problem.
- Be direct and nonpunitive.
- Avoid arguing.
- If there is no response, consider sharing your concern with an authority figure, such as a teacher, coach, or parent.

Educators have multiple important roles. One role is preventive intervention, an ideal that is seldom achieved but is increasingly possible (Piran, 2004; Russell-Mayhew, Arthur, and Ewashen, 2007). Educators may attempt to prevent eating disorders by talking with students about symptoms, but this approach has the contrary effect of probably increasing the tendency to develop eating disorders. Instead of more information about signs and symptoms, students need to know how to develop skills of healthy thinking and behavior in a media-saturated atmosphere that emphasizes thinness or shape change as the most important achievement in life. As Runi Gresko (1993), Norway's leading educational expert on prevention of eating disorders in schools, advised, "Eating disorders are not prevented by talking about eating disorders."

Almost certainly, if primary prevention is possible, it will happen by insulating vulnerable individuals from our culture's relentless demands for thinness. That eating disorders can be prevented is only partially and selectively proven, but there are hints that the keys to successful prevention include teaching increased assertiveness, especially to young girls; helping individuals to become critical of media claims promoting the value of thinness; increasing body self-esteem; and teaching valuation of the normal diversity of weights, while strongly encouraging fitness at every set point. Girls benefit by moving from an observational, judgmental, and objectified view of body to an operational, instrumental, and functional view, seeing the body in terms of what it allows one to do, not primarily how it looks. Setting minimum weights and BMIs below which a student is not allowed to participate in a sport or activity (wrestling, ballet) shows some promise of decreasing the behavioral incentive for further slimming.

Weighing young people in schools, even when the staff concern is overtly about health, certainly produces no result except to embarrass, distress, or humiliate the student; it leads to psychological distress, at a minimum, and promotes unhealthy and unnecessary dieting. Spotlighting an individual's weight as being excessive may be the starting point for an eating disorder (see case 2 in this chapter). Educators are role models who need to take seriously their responsibility to teach fitness behaviors in place of dieting and to stress the normality of a wide range of weights. Their personal examples of fitness behaviors and healthy weight ranges, as well as their openness to discussion, are essential.

There is increasing evidence that for mild cases of eating disorders, especially bulimia nervosa, self-help modules through Internet-assisted computer methods may be effective (Ljotsson et al., 2007). Educators are usually up to date on information available on the Internet, and this medium may offer young sufferers the most helpful program for their needs. Educators can sensitize students to the perils of "pro-anorexia" websites by exploring such sites with the students and teaching them to critique and deglamorize them.

Information for Coaches

There is increasing evidence that setting lowest acceptable weights and maximum rates for weight loss and body fat loss for participation in sports helps to decrease the onset or perpetuation of eating disorders, especially in wrestling, ballet, and long-distance running. When there is no advantage to further weight loss in ballet or wrestling ("You will have to leave the program if you lose more weight"), then there is less incentive to keep on losing. In Wisconsin, for example, a legislative action requires high school wrestlers to limit the amount of weight lost for qualification for a particular wrestling weight category and has set minimum body fat levels for eligibility to participate. These efforts, partially a response to the deaths of several young wrestlers associated with weight loss practices in the 1990s, appear to be effective.

In sports where weight for achievement of performance goals or appearance may be in conflict with an individual's health needs, ethical and health decisions must be integrated, with the athlete's best interests being the first concern. An individual whose performance in sports is maximized only when there are signs of abnormal eating behavior, or when there is distressed thinking about weight and eating patterns, needs to be counseled about the relative importance of health versus performance. Unfortunately, many young men and women live in a bubble of illusory invulnerability, failing to appreciate that some performance goals are simply not worth the health costs. Elite athletes are often driven internally as well as externally through a narrow focus of interest, relentless perseverance, and self-critique. Reports have documented the presence of the "elite athlete triad" of abnormal eating, weight loss, and osteoporosis in young female athletes (Sundgot-Borgen, 1994). Mild to moderate eating disorder syndromes are missed or overlooked when these athletes are performing with excellence. Case 1 in this chapter suggests that women often carry a disproportionate burden to lose weight in couples' sports such as cheerleading and pairs skating. The male partner could just as well be advised to get strength training. It is this author's opinion that the lower and lower weights and younger ages characteristic of female gymnasts in recent Olympics present ethical concerns. Bonci et al. (2008) describe how athletic trainers can help to prevent, detect, and manage eating disorders in athletes. Support for a healthier body habitus for female gymnasts may have been evident at the 2016 Olympics in Brazil.

Information for Parents

Parents play major roles in shaping the course of eating disorders in their children. Although too often blamed when they are in fact doing their best, parents do sometimes exert excess pressure for girls to be thin and boys to be muscular (McCabe et al., 2007). Only recently appreciated are the stresses experienced by parents living with a child with anorexia nervosa (Kyriacou, Treasure, and Schmidt, 2008) and the needs of the siblings of adolescent girls with anorexia (Honey and Halse, 2007). Treasure (1997) has written a survival guide for families, friends, and sufferers. (Additional books for both families and professionals are listed under "Suggested Readings" below.)

The role of the parents varies with the age of the child with the eating disorder: the younger the child, the more involved the family must be. Families need support, information, and a sense of realistic optimism about the outcome of treatment for eating disorders. Parents also have a role in monitoring computer usage by their children, allowing appropriate changes as children reach their later teen years. Pro-anorexia sites are abysmally silly and unattractive from the viewpoint of an adult without an eating disorder and with good self-esteem, but they may have a strange fascination for a subgroup of teens. Talking about these issues openly from a neutral viewpoint may be helpful. Research provides robust findings that having regular family meals most days of the week decreases the probability of a teen developing an eating disorder or drug abuse problem (Ackard and Neumark-Sztainer, 2001; Fulkerson et al., 2006). Parents benefit from knowing about the increasingly well-documented contributions to eating disorders, helping them understand that these are true illnesses, not simply a lack of effort or a result of following social fads.

Summary

A combination of medical knowledge, common sense, and a good working relationship with medical professionals allows the shared treatment of clients/patients and students who have eating disorders, as well as the possibility of prevention and, certainly, the early identification of eating disorders. Good recordkeeping, documenting regular communication with a medical professional, having a low threshold for referral when appropriate, and recognizing the ethical aspect of weight and shape change versus performance goals—all will enhance the significant role of nonmedical mental health professionals, educators, coaches, and nutritionists in the care of young people. The recognition, treatment, and prevention of eating disorders involves a "village" or community of caring, concerned individuals who are knowledgeable, thoughtful, and proactive.

SUGGESTED READINGS

Hill, Laura, David Dagg, Michael Levine, Linda Smolak, Sara Johnson, Sonja A. Stotz, and Nancy Little. *Family Eating Disorders Manual: Guiding Families through the Maze of Eating Disorders*. Columbus, OH: Center for Balanced Living, 2012.

Kortink, Joanna, and Greta Noordenbos (trans. Valerie Thompson). *Ending Emotional Eating: A New Solution for Eating and Weight Problems*. Kindle Version, 2014 [a European perspective].

Lock, James, and Daniel Le Grange. *Help Your Teenager Beat an Eating Disorder*. New York: Guilford Press, 2015.

Noordenbos, Greta. *Recovery from Eating Disorders: A Guide for Clinicians and Their Clients*. Hoboken, NJ: Wiley-Blackwell, 2013.

Treasure, Janet. *Anorexia Nervosa: A Survival Guide for Families, Friends, and Sufferers*. East Sussex, UK: Psychology Press, 1997.

Treasure, Janet, Gráinne Smith, and Anna Crane A. *Skills-Based Caring for a Loved One with an Eating Disorder*. New York: Taylor and Francis, 2017.

REFERENCES

Ackard DM and Neumark-Sztainer D. 2001. Family mealtime while growing up: Associations with symptoms of bulimia nervosa. *Eating Disorders* 9:239–49.

Bere E, te Velde SJ, Småstuen MC, et al. 2015. One year of free school fruit in Norway—7 years of follow-up. *International Journal of Behavioral Nutrition and Physical Activity* 12:139.

Bonci CM, Bonci LJ, Granger LR, et al. 2008. National Athletic Trainers' Association position statement: Preventing, detecting, and managing disordered eating in athletes. *Journal of Athletic Training* 43:80–108.

D'Souza CM, Forman SF, and Austin SB. 2005. Follow-up evaluation of a high school eating disorders screening program: Knowledge, awareness and self-referral. *Journal of Adolescent Health* 36:208–13.

Fulkerson JA, Story M, Mellin A, Leffert N, Neumark-Sztainer D, and French SA. 2006. Family dinner meal frequency and adolescent development: Relationships with developmental assets and high-risk behaviors. *Journal of Adolescent Health* 39:337–45.

Graham MA, Spencer W, and Andersen AE. 1991. Altered religious practice in patients with eating disorders. *International Journal of Eating Disorders* 10:239–43.

Gresko, R. 1993. Personal communication.

Honey A and Halse C. 2007. Looking after well siblings of adolescent girls with anorexia: An important parental role. *Child: Care, Health, and Development* 33:5–58.

Keys A, Brozek J, and Henscheo A. 1950. *The Biology of Human Starvation*. Minneapolis: University of Minnesota Press.

Kyriacou O, Treasure J, and Schmidt U. 2008. Understanding how parents cope with living with someone with anorexia nervosa: Modeling the factors that are associated with carer distress. *International Journal of Eating Disorders* 41:233–42.

Ljotsson B, Lundin C, Mitsell K, Carlbring P, Ramklint M, and Ghaderi A. 2007. Remote treatment of bulimia nervosa and binge eating disorder: A randomized trial of Internet-assisted cognitive behavioral therapy. *Behaviour Research and Therapy* 45:649–61.

McCabe MP and Ricciardelli LA. 2005. A prospective study of pressures from parents, peers, and the media on extreme weight change behaviors among adolescent boys and girls. *Behaviour Research and Therapy* 43:653–68.

McCabe MP, Ricciardelli LA, Stanford J, Holt K, Keegan S, and Miller L. 2007. Where is all the pressure coming from? Messages from mothers and teachers about preschool children's appearance, diet and exercise. *European Eating Disorders Review* 15:221–30.

Piran J. 2004. Teachers: On "being" (rather than "doing") prevention. *Eating Disorders* 12:1–9.

Russell-Mayhew S, Arthur N, and Ewashen C. 2007. Targeting students, teachers and parents in a wellness-based prevention program in schools. *Eating Disorders* 15:159–81.

Sundgot-Borgen J. 1994. Risk and trigger factors for the development of eating disorders in female elite athletes. *Medicine and Science in Sports and Exercise* 26:414–19.

Treasure J. 1997. *Anorexia Nervosa: A Survival Guide for Families, Friends, and Sufferers.* East Sussex, UK: Psychology Press.

17

Innovative Psychological Treatments of Eating Disorders

Arnold E. Andersen, MD

Common Questions

How can asking patients to write a letter to their illness ("You are my friend because . . ."; "You are my enemy because . . .") increase their engagement in treatment and in becoming coinvestigators with the clinician?

How can clinicians use the power of narrative stories to convey important psychoeducational information about eating disorders?

How can clinicians use a sequence of psychotherapeutic methods to comprehensively treat patients with eating disorders?

Letters I Write to My Illness*

Most patients have, at a minimum, ambivalence about treatment and often are in frank denial about the seriousness of their disorder. Entry into a treatment program means only that a patient is physically present. The real challenge is persuading patients to find motivation and engage in treatment. The core of treatment of eating disorders is psychotherapy. Eating one's way out of treatment results in a revolving door to readmission. Based on two seminal and heuristic publications by the London group led by Janet Treasure and Lucy Serpell and their colleagues (Serpell et al., 1999;

*Pages 327–32 are based on L. Serpell, J. Treasure, J. Teasdale, and V. Sullivan, "Anorexia Nervosa: Friend or Foe?" *International Journal of Eating Disorders* 25:177–86, 1999; and L. Serpell and J. Treasure, "Bulimia Nervosa: Friend or Foe? The Pros and Cons of Bulimia Nervosa," *International Journal of Eating Disorders* 32:164–70, 2002.

Serpell and Treasure, 2002), we have found that writing "A Letter to My Illness" results in a patient's enhanced engagement and increased motivation. In addition, patients become partners in the journey to wellness.

What does not work? Scaring patients does not work. While they need psychoeducation about the medical, social, and developmental risks of their eating disorders, this information alone is not sufficient. Speaking in psychobabble or in other overly technical terms may result in nods, but little internal understanding. Authoritarian approaches may work in some surgical specialties, but not with eating disorders. Authoritative, yes; authoritarian, no.

Why are engagement and motivation challenging issues for patients with eating disorders? Anorexia nervosa is almost always ego-syntonic. Patients with anorexia nervosa do not see themselves as ill, or if they grudgingly acknowledge their illness, they have enormous fear of becoming fat and losing control. Patients with bulimia nervosa most often have a strong sense of shame and are filled with guilt. In contrast to other psychiatric illnesses such as schizophrenia or major depressive disorders, eating disorders are functional and adaptive, giving patients rules and routines, rituals and methods of dealing with a variety of issues, including existential fears of maturation, self-treatment for dysphoria, strategies for controlling families, and multiple other age- and gender-specific issues.

How do patients with eating disorders present to the therapist? They often present with arms folded, prepared to resist, feeling cornered and threatened. They generally suffer from alexithymia, finding it hard or impossible to identify feelings except for the "feeling" (really a thought) that "I feel fat." Insight into the seriousness of the disorder is lacking. They are most commonly entangled in their illness, believing "I AM my eating disorder," rather than "I HAVE an eating disorder," as one would say about having influenza.

The publications of Serpell and Treasure et al. have been too much overlooked, for a number of reasons: they present results free of statistics, have no control group, prescribe no medications, involve no laboratory studies, include no genetic studies or brain imaging. These publications are simply enormously useful. Writing "A Letter to My Illness" is a useful and widely applicable approach to enhancing the engagement of patients in treatment and to increasing motivation.

Background of the Benefits of Writing

In *Fasting Girls*, Joan Brumberg of Cornell University examined the diaries of girls of the nineteenth century. She found that girls of more than a century ago experienced menarche much later than girls today; as a result, they were able to navigate the shoals of puberty later, within a more structured social context (Brumberg, 2000). The Nun Study of Aging and Alzheimer's Disease, which began in 1986, analyzed the autobiographies of women entering a religious order at an average age of 22. The investigators correlated the linguistic density of these early autobiographies with the onset of cognitive impairment and Alzheimer's disease: the more linguistically dense the autobiographies at this early age, the later the onset of cognitive impairment (Iacono et al., 2009). Powerful!

The practical side of the process: Ask patients 2–4 days after admission to write on one sheet of paper "A Letter to My Illness: You Are My Friend Because . . . ," responding in paragraphs or bullet points or in any manner comfortable for them. Then ask them to write on a second sheet of paper "A Letter to My Illness: You Are My Enemy Because . . ." The patient then reads her or his letters aloud to the team (or to the therapist) the next day. It is often astounding how a seemingly tongue-tied, alexithymic patient responds fluently to this task.

Writing these letters accomplishes a number of goals. (1) The focus is changed from a spotlight on the patient, who may feel pushed into a corner, to a focus on the illness. The patient is okay; the Illness is not. (2) The patient becomes a co-investigator with the therapy team/therapist: "We are on the same side." (3) The writing process respects the intelligence of the patient. (4) It engages more of the patient's hidden brain-based skills than question and answers. (5) It individualizes the patient's history and psychodynamic themes. (6) It utilizes a patient's most recent functioning activity: school (for the younger patient) and work (for the older patient) are usually continued despite the presence of severe illness. Starved, cachectic patients and patients who binge or binge-purge tend to go to school or to work no matter what. (7) It uses the language of the patient, not the language of the therapist—it is a stealth entry into the patient's experiences.

There are multiple benefits for the therapist/therapy team. (1) This process integrates well with cognitive behavioral therapy (CBT). Meaningful therapy almost always involves homework, both with these letters and with CBT. (2) These letters individualize the patient—each letter is unique; no longer is the patient simply another starved, cold, resistant patient in a long queue of similar-appearing patients. Looking forward to what these patients write increases the pleasure for the therapist/team and decreases the burn-out potential. (3) These letters bring the patient out from the wallpaper—patients stand out separate from their illness. (4) The therapist has the privilege of finding out what is going on "behind the curtain" of the illness. (5) It sets up a life-long pattern of self-investigation and insight that can contribute to continued effective treatment. (6) Letters written close to discharge are an effective measure of treatment progress and, as the example below illustrates, are a measure of long-term recovery.

Letters Written during Illness and after Sustained Recovery

This is how a 49-year-old married woman viewed her illness 30 years ago:

You Are My Friend:
- Because it makes me feel in control
- Because I am thinner than everyone else and I like that
- Because it makes me feel confident and strong
- Because I can read a cookbook and it makes my hunger go away
- Because I like my clothes loose
- Because people compliment me on how skinny I am

You Are My Enemy:
- Because I always think about food and I am tired of it
- Because I sometimes feel like I am going crazy
- Because I can't spend time with my sisters to go shopping because I haven't run yet and I have to do that first all the time
- Because I can't go out to eat with my family
- Because I don't want to socialize or talk to people anymore. I have no friends
- Because I am anxious and frightened all the time
- Because I am tired and don't feel good

This is what the patient writes now, in her sustained recovery:

You Are My Friend Today:

- Because when I am stressed it makes me not have to think about anything
- Because I still like to be skinnier than others

You Are My Enemy Today:

- Because it would not let me be a part of my friends and family's life
- Because it would not let me try new things
- Because it keeps me from dealing with my real emotions
- Because it makes my family worry about me
- Because I know it is behavior I do when I am not dealing with my real issues
- Because I am proud that I recovered and I don't want to fall back into old behaviors

[Note: Patients are told about "normative cultural distress," a shrewd concept, described by Rodin, Silberstein, and Striegel-Moore (1985), reassuring patients that having occasional thoughts about dieting and giving lip service with peers to the desire to be thinner (while having dessert) is quite normal, provided the behaviors are healthy and eating disordered thinking does not dominate their lives.]

Some patients write what is almost a romance or love story about their eating disorder: "You are my friend because you are always there for me; you rescued me when things were chaotic—my boyfriend left me; my family moved to a new area; no one liked me in the new school; everyone was thinner than I was. But I could depend on you to help me. Never go away. I need you." Details of their lives are revealed as they face their illness, rather than facing someone who, in their eyes, is going to take away their way of life.

Here's a letter by a young man with anorexia nervosa:

You are my friend because our relationship has lasted 18 years. We have been through many trials and challenges together, but we have always managed to get back together because our relationship has taken priority over everything else. School became a threat to us, but we stayed firm to preserve our relationship. I was tempted to make long-term commitments, but this would have forced me into adulthood before I was ready. You were exciting.

You are my enemy because you have stolen so much from me. Every time I turn my back and let my guard down you are there to pilfer more. I despise you. Where is my identity? It has been stolen. Where is the athlete? Gone! You have taken small pieces of my self-esteem consistently over time. You are crafty. I demand you return my life, my spirit, my core. You are slippery, illusory, and cunning.

This letter was written by a gay man with bulimia nervosa:

I grew up with a very abusive, neglectful mother. My father was an alcoholic. I was picked on constantly by other kids. I became very looks and body conscious and would try anything to be attractive. When I started lifting weights, I liked the reaction I got from people being intimidated. Nobody picked on me any more or bullied me. If you are not thin, muscular, and sexy, you are invisible. Being thin, muscular, and attractive is all I have to offer. Our culture wants everyone to be beautiful and young.

In summary, writing a letter to their eating disorder is an innovative method to increase patients' engagement and motivation in treatment. This method also benefits therapists/therapy teams by individualizing treatment and forming a therapeutic alliance.

Stories I Tell My Patients

Storytelling is an old and honored art. Great literature conveys its message to us in stories. In a way, the stories remain the same—they tell of life, love, death, birth, hope, loss, discovery, fear, quest, beauty, humor, truth, falsehood, despair, faith, and all the other issues of life. Some time ago I felt stuck in interacting with my patients in psychotherapy, and on rounds I realized we were trading words rather than making real progress. I began to tell short stories to find a way around the intellectualized defenses and to get to the issues. It seemed to get attention, sometimes sowing a seed, sometimes challenging a wall of resistance. No matter how old we get, we can relate to roses and bike trips, to shadows and catsup. Sometimes the challenge of treatment may be helped by stories.

Where Are You When You Are Eating?

A group of four high school students were having lunch at the new Southwestern Grill on a Saturday afternoon. It was a fun restaurant—with real cactus plants, warm colors, and authentic food. After the food arrived,

John immediately thought back to how his wrestling coach had warned him about getting too fat in the off-season. With mechanical action he ate, but his mind was on that interaction and on his determination that he would never again be criticized for his weight. "Hey, get off my case, Coach," he wished he could say, but John couldn't get off his own case. Gun to the head, he couldn't say after the meal what he had eaten.

Sue got nervous as soon as she took one look at the tortilla chips and mango salsa the waiter put on the table before they even ordered, and once her Santa Fe chicken salad arrived, Sue feared that she would never fit into her prom dress in a few weeks. While her jaws worked, she saw herself trying to squeeze into her beautiful gown, its seams tearing on the dance floor. The image felt so real that she could sense her rising anger and disgust about her hips. Food? What food? The plate was clean, but so was any memory of the food.

Joan ordered a plank steak with hot peppers, but you would never know it if you asked her afterward. That food, that smell, that plate radiated anxiety and brought her back to when her boyfriend had patted her on the hips and said she was getting a little heavy. Her stomach churned and she could barely swallow. She relived the rage that had boiled inside, but she stuffed down the anger so she wouldn't lose the boyfriend. She thought of all the things she could have said, but never did.

Brad decided on the house special, which sounded good when the waiter described it to him. While he was eating, he had no idea what the food tasted like. It was like a silent movie. He said some things to the others but couldn't remember what. It was a script. His mind was on those years in junior high school when he was teased mercilessly as a "fat slob." The humiliation was still there, tingling in his bones, even 3 or 4 years later, and it was certainly more real than the flavors of the house special. His body was drenched in sweat, and even with these close friends he was afraid that they were judging him.

When they got together on campus on Monday afternoon, it was funny, sad, and puzzling. None of them could remember what they had had for lunch on Saturday. In fact, none of them could remember their morning showers or even what they'd studied in their classes moments earlier. Their minds were everywhere else. One look at their abdomens and hips for Sue and Joan sent them into old tapes of how much they disliked their bodies.

One look at their chests and shoulders sent John and Brad into a panic about the past and the future. They were there, but they weren't there.

Comment: Jon Kabat-Zinn (1990), a pioneer of the powerful therapeutic method of mindfulness, which has shown utility across many diagnoses, asked a question of the audience during a lecture: "When you took a shower this morning, where were you?" Almost everyone in the audience smiled. Almost no one had been really in the shower, feeling the water, letting it play over the hair and run down the body in warm rivulets of pleasing sensation. Some were into their schedule for the day. Some worried about yesterday's sessions. Others rehearsed the anger they had swallowed when talking to their supervisors the day before. Almost no one was where they were, as far as their minds were concerned.

We can help our patients deal with meals by having them practice here-and-now mindfulness about the process of eating—being present with all their feelings, especially the pleasant sensations the body is set up to perceive when hunger is satisfied, and with a social interaction that is real not mechanical. When clinicians and therapists first practice being where they are at that moment, with full awareness, without judgment, with openness to what thoughts and feelings are going on, they are on their way to helping patients be mindful. Let's help our patients, when they are taking meals, to be really present, to experience taste and scent and social interaction, letting the past stay in the past, and the future in the future. Being healthy means being aware of and enjoying the sensations of eating in a social context. Be mindful. Help our patients be mindful. Let's give that "monkey mind" some rest.

Follow Your Star

Sam: "Our Day Program for Eating Disorders is close to completion for this group. You've all worked very hard. I'd like to hear what your plans are after the group is over."

Brittany: "I'm excited by all the expectations I have. I expect to be free of all the preoccupation with weight I used to have. I expect to get a perfect job, and to do it perfectly. My expectation for relationships is to have lots of friends, to never argue again with my family, and to make every day a sunny one for myself and everyone around me. That's the star I'm following."

Ted: "I'm excited too, but my expectations are way different. I expect my life will be all positive thinking, no more negatives. Those urges to binge and purge will all be gone. I expect to exercise with perfect form and moderation; no more of the out-of-control exercise. My star is sending me strong rays letting me know that I can't fail."

Brynn: "There are going to be a lot of stars in the sky for me, too. My boyfriend tells me that he expects me never to compare myself with others like I used to do. That was the pits—always seeing myself as fat and stupid. Never again. I expect I'll be a perfect French major with my improved concentration. In fact, I'm calling my star 'ma belle etoile,' French for 'my beautiful star.'"

Sam: "I can tell you are all enthusiastic about being free from your eating disorders. You've all worked hard to put anorexia and bulimia behind you. Let me try out an idea and see what you think. I'm going to suggest you follow a different star, one I put in capitals: STAR. To my mind, expectations are demands in disguise. They are recipes for disappointment, not that you mean to do that. There's also some passivity to expectations—a kind of demand that things should happen a certain way, or that a certain event should happen. What do you think of substituting the STAR system of *goals* in place of *expectations*? Use the STAR memory trick.

"The S stands for Specific—not vague, like being a perfect student or being completely happy each day. How would you know what a perfect student is? Or what a perfect day is? In contrast, consider a specific goal like learning 30 phrases of conversational Spanish. That's clear and specific.

"The T stands for Time-Limited—for example, having a goal of learning 30 phrases of Spanish in 30 days. That gets you out of the having to do it yesterday, or never getting around to it.

"The A stands for Achievable—meaning your goal is very reasonable and can be accomplished by normal human beings. Almost anyone can learn 30 phrases of Spanish, as opposed to being a perfect Spanish student. Perfection isn't achievable, and the alternative is to set yourself up for the self-label of being a failure when you are not fulfilling your expectation of being a perfect student.

"The R stands for Ratable—the goal can be measured. Measured, not judged. For example, you can ask a Spanish-speaking friend to listen to your answers when she reads out the phrases in English and you answer in

Spanish. Compare that with the unratable expectation of being a perfect language student, or always being cheerful every day—everybody's going to be grumpy some days. By the way, if you expect to be cheerful every day and get out of bed grumpy, you can have a goal of going back to bed and getting out on the opposite side.

"So, now you can have a goal of 30 phrases of Spanish in 30 days, a specific, time-limited, achievable, and ratable goal that will be satisfying to accomplish. What do you guys think?"

Brittany: "That makes sense. I feel a lot of pressure off my shoulders. I didn't realize I had been painting myself into a corner with my expectations."

Ted: "I know I can plan on doing 30 minutes of moderate exercise a day, four days a week, in place of the expectation of a perfect moderate workout."

Brynn: "It feels like I'm getting away with something when I don't have to be perfect in fulfilling my expectations, but I like it. You're right. I wouldn't know when I had become a perfect French student."

Sam: "Well, guys, let's try following the STAR plan for goals after group is over, instead of impossible expectations. These two words, *impossible* and *expectation*, are sort of redundant, anyway. The neat thing about goals is that they can be changed when it's appropriate. They're flexible. They can be modified to more or fewer, to speed them up or slow them down. There's only a learning experience, not demands in disguise. See you for the final session next week."

Comment: So many of our patients have perfectionist traits and suffer from unreasonable expectations and then think of themselves as failures. Expectations are seldom achievable and usually reflect all-or-none reasoning. What a recipe for disappointment and failure! Saying "I expect never to argue with my parents again" is like expecting warm weather in January in Iowa. Sometimes it happens, but don't expect it. You'll be very disappointed. How much better are the STAR goals—patients usually feel relieved and freer with STAR goals instead of expectations. You can flex goals—they can be revised as experience shows that you can learn 30 Spanish phrases in 15 days, or maybe need 45 days. It works for our relationships with patients to have treatment goals, not expectations. We're vulnerable to our own impossible expectations and feeling worn out because these hidden expectations are not specific or achievable. Go for goals. Follow the STAR.

Halt Bad Dog

It kept lunging at her. Tamara felt as if she was being attacked by a bad dog. The attack continued relentlessly. She placed her hands on her throat for protection. "How did I get myself into this position? I swore it would never happen again. I said I'd never let myself get this vulnerable." All she could think of was running away. But she knew from past experience that it would follow her wherever she went. She couldn't outrun it. Running didn't help. She'd like to call a friend, but there wasn't time. The assault grew stronger. Her breath grew very rapid and shallow. She knew she couldn't avoid it any longer. So she opened the freezer, took out the quart of macadamia nut ice cream, and swallowed it in chunks as fast as she could. Then came the last of the brownies.

Her mother called out to her: "What's wrong Tamara?"

"Nothing, Mom. I had the crazy idea I was being attacked by a bad dog."

"That's silly, Tamara," her mother said. "Our miniature dachshund never attacks anyone. She would give her hot dog to a burglar."

"Yes, Mom, I know."

In her weekly session, Tamara explained to Kay, her therapist, how it felt. "The attack got stronger and stronger, and I wanted to say 'Stop,' but it didn't stop." Kay gently told Tamara that she had indeed suffered an attack, a binge attack, which Tamara had related in her own somewhat dramatic way. Kay decided to use the concept of a dog attack, and she shared an approach with Tamara.

"Tamara, let's think of your binge urges as attacks by a bad dog. And then let's stop them by saying, 'Halt Bad Dog.'"

"Kay, that's nuts. Even I, with my dramatic tendencies, know there's no real dog."

"Yes, Tamara, but that's a better analogy than you may realize. Here's what I mean. Most binge urges, like alcohol urges, occur when a person feels crummy. The alcohol rehabilitation counselors have taught many alcohol-abusing patients to say 'HALT" when they have an urge to drink. That's a shorthand way of saying, 'Are you Hungry, Angry, Lonely, or Tired?'—four of the biggest triggers for an alcohol binge. Asking yourself which specific crummy or dysphoric feeling you have as soon as the binge urge starts allows you to deal directly with the trigger, and that stops the attack. You've learned in therapy to practice specific, different, approaches when you are hungry, or angry, or lonely, or tired. I'm going to suggest you not only say 'HALT' to stop the dog in its tracks, but say 'HALT BAD DOG!'

"You know the HALT feeling words. Continue the mnemonic: BAD stands for Bored, Anxious, or Depressed. DOG stands for Demoralized, Overwhelmed, and Given up. The moment you feel that attack coming— and I do want you to continue to visualize it as a bad dog attacking—say out loud, if no one is close to you, or say to yourself, 'HALT BAD DOG.' Then deal directly with whichever feeling is asking for a pseudo-solution through a binge—the bad dog attack really is halted. Try it, Tamara."

Comment: The HALT mnemonic has been used with alcohol-abusing patients for some time. It applies just as well to binge urges. Frank, my cotherapist and an expert social worker, and I decided in our group to try out a more complete phrase: HALT BAD DOG. The key is getting a patient to inhibit the binge response for just a little while so that, while sitting on the urge, there is enough time to give the dysphoria a name. Our patients then use the different approaches they have learned for different types of emotional distress. Once an accurate name is given, by thinking HALT BAD DOG to remind themselves, they can use the appropriate action plan. Some people carry reminders on 3 × 5 index cards or a smart phone in their pocket, one for each letter of HALT BAD DOG. It gives power to the patient to know that these attacks can be slowed down, held off, and then avoided completely. Try it with your patients. Ruff. Ruff.

The 5:36 Express from Paddington Station

Paddington Station was as busy as usual, with end-of-day commuters rushing to their train compartments to head for home. London was grimy, soot filled the air . . . it would be oh so pleasant to return to the countryside for a long summer evening. As everyone knows from reading Agatha Christie and other British mystery writers, murders take place on the Paddington Express. Today, it was not to be murder, but something that seemed almost as awful—at least to Jane. You enter British trains, at least the older ones, directly from the train platform, stepping up into a carriage through the little swinging doors. Jane briskly entered her compartment and uttered a sigh of relief that she would be alone for the journey, alone with her thoughts, letting the work of the day slide from her mind with each passing mile. Just as the train was about to leave the platform, a burly man with a handlebar mustache jerked open the door and entered. Oh well, you can't always control those things. But things soon became worse than simply having to share a compartment. The burly man needed a shave and a bath. As soon as the train picked up speed, he pulled out an enormous salami that reeked of garlic. Then he opened a tin of sardines. Jane was not sure what the last straw was—taking off his shoes and socks to clip his toenails, or spreading out the dirty contents of his suitcase on the vacant seats.

Jane thought to herself: "Now what are my options? I can kill him and throw him from the train, but I wouldn't want to take someone's life. I could jump from the train myself and hope for the best. That would not be very helpful either. The train must be going 55 miles an hour. I could pitch a fit, jump up and down, cry, scream, and glare at him, but I know the other carriages in the train are full, so there is nowhere else for him to go. I suppose I can settle back, read my book, let the unpleasant man be as he is. Then I will breathe a sigh of relief when he gets off at his stop or when I get off at mine, whichever comes first.

And that is what Jane did on the 5:36 from Paddington Station. The unpleasant man, with his inconsiderate behavior, his salami, his sardines, his socks and nail clippings, his untidy suitcase into which he stuffed all the dirty clothes he had spread around him, that unpleasant person and all the unpleasantness that went with him, left the train about halfway to Jane's destination. After Jane had aired the compartment out, she pulled out her knitting, settled into a pleasant routine, and enjoyed the remainder of her trip. No murder today on the 5:36 from Paddington. No jumping out of the window of a speeding train. What she needed was patience and the knowledge that she would soon be without her unpleasant companion because either he would leave first or she would arrive at her station.

Comment: Spells of painful moods, depression, anxiety, boredom, loneliness, all are temporary states, much like the experience Jane had with the unpleasant man in her train compartment. We can help our patients during episodes of dysphoria by asking them to imagine they are on a train ride. Someone very unpleasant enters and creates an uncomfortable situation—

no joke, it's unpleasant to have this jerk on board. But you have to remind yourself that the unpleasant, almost unbearable, person will be getting off the train at his stop, or "Jane," our patient, will be getting off the train at her stop. It's a temporary situation. Knowing that this "person," a metaphor for a painful state of mind, is only temporary, and really believing that fact, will help a patient to practice "mindfully being with" that state of mood until it changes or goes away. The problem comes when a person tries to "murder" that mood state, to commit harm to self, becomes desperate about getting rid of the state of mind. These visitors to the compartments of our speeding lives enter without our consent from time to time. They are not pleasant. We validate the fact that they are unpleasant. But we teach our patients that we can tolerate them without taking desperate measures. In fact, we can go beyond "being with" these states of mind; we can become curious about them. "Now I wonder what caused that person to enter my compartment? What makes him so messy and unpleasant? Maybe he's got no place to go. And I did see that he was writing a poem. It could be he's not always totally unpleasant. Maybe he could teach me something if I stopped fuming and asked him a few questions, like: Who are you? What brings you here? How long do you plan to ride on my train?"

In the midst of our struggles to separate ourselves from unpleasant "visitors," we can do things that are much worse than putting up with these visitors. What is most important to remember is that these unpleasant visitors will be leaving the train.

Now, it's time to pull out one of the old Agatha Christie novels, or one of the films made from her novels, and enjoy a good murder mystery about the 5:36 from Paddington Station. Murders on the trains in mystery novels are okay. Having to murder temporary mood states in our lives is not okay.

Ask the Dry Cleaner

Meg wanted expert advice for anything important in her life. Her cosmetician always selected the perfect hair color for her. She wouldn't think of changing the arrangement of her living room without guidance from her trusted interior designer, Susie, who had designed the homes of some of the city's best families. Her bike came from a French firm that specialized in the titanium bicycles used in the Tour de France. Her yoga instructor guided each client with a personal fitness program.

But Meg had one area in which she was unsure of how to proceed—what should she weigh? Her gynecologist was working with her to figure out why her periods had stopped. Her physician, Dr. Ryan, thought she might be too thin. Meg thought, without saying so, that there was no way she was too thin. After her last visit with the doctor, Meg had a great idea—when she went to pick up her dry cleaning, she would ask Mrs. Lang if she was too thin. Mrs. Lang could remove any spot from any article of clothing. No stain was too tough.

The next day, Meg went to Mrs. Lang for her weekly laundry. "Mrs. Lang, I was wondering, do you think I am too thin?" she asked the lovely Mrs. Lang. Meg, as usual during cool weather, was wearing a mock turtleneck under an angora sweater, topped by her faux leather coat. "No, dear, I don't think you are too thin. You look beautiful to me," said the dry cleaner. "Thank you very much, Mrs. Lang. I appreciate your expert opinion."

Meg felt reassured. That doctor was an expert in hormones, of course, but she knew he couldn't be right about the weight. Not after hearing Mrs. Lang's opinion. It was so important to get advice from the right people.

Later that afternoon, Meg saw her dermatologist for evaluation of some sunspots on her cheek. She would need dermabrasion, but if that was necessary according to the specialist, Meg would not hesitate to make a follow-up appointment. After all, she valued expertise.

The comment from her gynecologist that Meg might be too thin still bothered her a bit. To confirm her own opinion about weight, Meg asked the UPS delivery woman about her weight. Ms. Lopez was a wonderful delivery person. Every new order from Amazon.com was placed neatly by Meg's front door. Ms. Lopez was 7 months pregnant but did not want to stop the job she loved until the ninth month. "No dear," said Ms. Lopez, "you don't look too thin to me. I wish I looked like you, but that's the way it goes with pregnancy. You'll know some day."

Dr. Ryan insisted Meg see a specialist at the hospital's eating disorder clinic. Meg did so in order not to displease Dr. Ryan, but knew it was a waste of time. At the clinic, after a thorough evaluation, they said to Meg: "We believe you meet criteria for an early diagnosis of anorexia nervosa. You have lost too much weight. You are too thin for your age and height." Meg hesitated for a moment and then replied, "You know, that is not possible. I have gotten two expert opinions that say I am not too thin. Thank you for your time, but I'll be leaving now."

Meg knew what she was doing and what she wanted. She lined up appointments with her interior designer, her colorist, her dermatologist, and several other experts. As she was making these appointments, she thought to herself, "That's so silly, that idea from the eating disorder clinic. I know I am fine in my weight. After all, Mrs. Lang and the nice UPS delivery person told me I am not too thin." Meg always went for expert advice when she needed help.

Comment: How many times have we seen patients who would never go to their stylist or dry cleaner for advice about an illness such as diabetes but think that anyone they know or meet who thinks their weight is fine is acceptable as an expert? Anorexic thinness in young women is almost always ego-syntonic. The cognitive distortion of filtering is alive and well: any opinion that does not agree with their perceptual distortion that they are just fine is filtered out, whether that opinion is from a parent, physician, or psychologist.

Sometimes, when I share the opinion, based on evaluation, that a young woman has early anorexia nervosa, and she says others think she is fine, I might reply, "Well, let's ask the plumber about your hair color, and the bakery owner about your interior design. How about it?" The reply is, "No, of course not. That's silly. I want experts to advise me." Our "normative cultural distress" is so common that a woman believes she is "normal" in weight only when she is more than 15% below the ideal body weight, not just the population average. We have to use motivational techniques to help women accept help about weight.

It's Hard to Say Goodbye

Kent and Barb were staring gloomily into their Diet Cokes. "I sure miss Ed," said Barb. "He was always there for us. When no one else understood, he did. When he was around I knew what to do with my stress."

"Yeah, it's a bummer," said Kent. "When I was a fat, pimply junior in high school, Ed came to my rescue, too."

After a few more minutes of reminiscing, Alissa and Twyla stopped by. "Hey, what are you guys so down about?"

Once Kent and Barb explained it to the two new arrivals, Alissa and Twyla nodded in agreement. "It's sure hard to find loyal friends these days," said Alissa. "And then when you lose one, the world is a lot scarier. Like, I'm going to a college across country this fall, and I don't know how I'll handle it." Twyla chimed in with, "Totally agree with you. I'm returning to professional dance school for the summer program. My treatment is over, but what will I do with all those mirrors?"

Brent joined the group. "OK, don't tell me. I know what you are talking about. You have been reading my mind. It's Ed. He's gone, left town, scooted, vamoosed. I'm so tempted to run after him, search the Internet. I know if I asked him to come back, he would. After all, he's not dead, just gone away. Every once in a while, I imagine him telling me to remember to follow his plan, especially when Mom and Dad get on my case, which is most of the time."

Laurissa had finished her group therapy notes and was walking past the group. "Today was a graduation, not a wake, and here you all are look-ing like your best friend has passed. I'd like you to get back on track and remember the real Ed. Sure, Ed was always there—always there in a bad way so you didn't have to deal with the agony and messiness of adoles-cence. Each of you were trapped by Ed's confident advice that if you lost enough weight, or bulked up enough muscle, everything in life would go your way. No, you are not losing a friend. You are losing a noose, a strangler vine that wouldn't let you keep growing emotionally. Yes, you felt good for the moment when you followed him, when you either starved yourself, or did a ginormous workout, or had that 4:30 afternoon binge.

"Remember, today's unhealthy solutions become tomorrow's problems, whether it's drugs, eating disorders, or self-cutting. Your emotions went into the deep freeze. Now you are having to deal with them—hooray for feeling emotions. Emotions are feelings, not commands. Remember the exercises we did to cultivate positive emotions. We meant not only to kick Ed in the butt, not only to pick weeds, but to grow roses.

"After a couple of weeks of vacation for me, we'll resume the group therapy for anyone who is in the area. Hey, dudes, I'm not scolding you. It's totally natural to miss someone who gave the illusion of help—it was a form of help, but very temporary, and with an enormous price tag. How about holding a passing-away service for Ed. Then we'll have a celebration for your new life, led by yourself, by your true feelings, by the knowledge you have worked so hard to obtain. It's normal to mourn for Ed, but only for a bit. It's normal to be a bit scared without his dictatorship. But you have yourself back on a healthy pattern of dealing with life, you have each other, you have your new buddies. It's time to say goodbye. Love you guys."

Comment: Eating disorders (Ed) are problem solvers, but even bigger problem givers. You would have to be a little bit nuts to say, "No, don't straighten my broken leg," or "Don't take out my inflamed appendix." But eating disorders are different, and that is one reason that parents, and the public in general, don't understand that they are not simply a voluntary habit. Once developed, eating disorders have a life of their own. They do actually make some feelings better for a while; they allow a person to avoid making some difficult decisions; they allow guys and gals to deflect hurt feelings from unkind comments; they give the illusion that there is an effective sense of control; that others will like them more. But then the price tag comes in: the developmental arrest, the medical complications, the self-isolation, the treadmill of relentless exercise.

Many, not all, of our patients go through a time when they have improved in their eating disordered behavior and are recognizing the true need of dealing with life's issues in healthy ways, but they are not yet solid. This is the time when it is so tempting to call Ed back into the picture.

Thermometers and Thermostats

"Oh, I am so sleek and thin. Sometimes, I have a silver center surrounded by glass like a glamorous piece of jewelry dangling from the ears of a celebrity. And you know what silver costs these days! Otherwise, my center is red and people can't stop looking at me. Red never goes out of style—like brightening up a boring, black cocktail dress with a red handbag and shoes, or Marilyn Monroe's lipstick. I am so fashionable, people check me out every day—a thermometer. They want me. They need me."

"I can't argue with you. You certainly are glamorous—long and thin. I'm pretty clunky myself, usually rectangular or square. Nothing fancy about being beige or dull gray. Lots of times, people try to hide me. I'm a wallflower compared to you. I may only get looked at a couple of times a year. Then, someone pushes a few buttons on me, goes away, and I continue to gather dust for another six months."

"I feel sorry for you, my clunky thermostat friend. Wish I could do something for you. Oops, hold on. My silver-colored center just shot up. The sun is shining brightly on the terrace, where fabulous people are having cocktails, and they all keep staring at me. Believe me, I get plenty of attention."

"For a thermostat, I'm feeling a little happier for a change. My owner, a bearded guy who eats lots of granola and rides his bike everywhere, came up to me the other day and changed a few of the dials. He said, 'You know, little thermostat, you saved me hundreds of bucks last winter.' I may not be glamorous, but I do important work."

"Well, you are still a clunky piece of metal that hardly ever gets noticed. You are not thin and sleek. You don't have a silver or red center that goes up and down. Oops, excuse me for a moment. I suddenly shrunk to this little itty bitty thing, and I'm feeling very cold. Ouch, I fell! My silver center is running out! I'm being swept up and put in the trash! Help me! Help me! Help . . ."

And then there was silence.

Meanwhile, the thermostat continued to do his job day after day, changing the temperature cycle, switching from air conditioning to heat, turning the furnace on and off. Not very glamorous, but much valued.

Comment: In an interview in the *New York Times*, Professor Cornel West (2011) is quoted as saying, "You've got to be a thermostat rather than a thermometer. A thermostat shapes the climate of opinion; a thermometer just reflects it." What a wonderful summary of the difference between thermometers and thermostats! I encourage patients to become thermostats, not thermometers. Most patients with anorexia nervosa act like thermometers: when the fashion climate, or their friends, or the movies say thinner is in, they follow the climate and slim. Hemlines up, hemlines down. And it's sad. So often, they look glamorous only when dressed up, but medically they are starved and bony. Of course, guys follow trends and can be thermometers too: "Bulk up those pecs; get that body fat down." In contrast, a person who is a thermostat sets the climate, doesn't follow it, or more accurately, doesn't follow it when it is unhealthy. The thermostat controls the temperature, while the thermometer simply follows the temperature set by the thermostat.

When the daughter of a friend of mine was eating a second hot dog during lunch with her dance team comrades, one said, "Ellie, you're going to get fat. That's your second hot dog. I wouldn't eat even one hot dog." Ellie calmly went on eating her second hot dog, and gently said, "You know, Liz, these hot dogs are surprisingly good. We work out hard and need to eat enough calories to maintain our strength for the dance team. I wonder if you might have an eating disorder, or the beginning of one. There's a friend of my dad who coordinates an eating disorder clinic. I'd be glad to give you his name. And, oh, I think I'll get that chocolate ice cream for dessert." Ellie was setting the climate, not following it.

When patients learn to be a thermostat, not a thermometer, they become empowered to examine cultural trends and then decide whether to follow them or not. More importantly, they let other people know (in a nonjudgmental way) what they think and why they do what they do. Kudos to Professor West for his summary of the difference between thermometers and thermostats. Goofy story, maybe. Important concept, yes.

The Girl in the Yellow Dress

Carla was an experienced Marine Corps sergeant who had seen service in Iraq and Afghanistan on three tours of duty. She was invited to the eating disorder evening group at the local community center to tell her story, because the group had helped her in the past. What a commanding presence she was: outfitted in desert camouflage gear, with broad shoulders but feminine in physique, with a squared-away appearance that engendered instant respect. On planes, passengers wanted to shake her hand and thank her. This is what she said at the meeting: "Guys, it's war out there, and war is hell, but someone has to protect our country, even if you don't agree with every policy. I want to tell you a story that keeps me up at night to this day, and when I do sleep, I have nightmares. The VA is doing its best to help, and it's coming along, but slowly."

"One day, we were in a small town in Afghanistan, being friendly with the locals to show them that we were on the side of peace. As we drove slowly through town, making stops to hand out diapers and vitamins to groups of young mothers and their children, we were on the look-out for IEDs—that's improvised explosive devices for you civvies. Toward the end of the town, I saw one of those damn IEDs on the side of the road—disguised as a tin can behind a clump of weeds. I knew my duty. I stopped the jeep and started to walk cautiously toward the IED to inspect it and see if we could either disable or move it, so it wouldn't do any harm. Can't believe what happened. A young girl, about 8 or 9, had been following our slowly moving jeep. She darted out ahead of me and picked up the IED. You know what happened. The blast shredded her body and threw me back against the jeep and concussed one of my buddies, and tore a hole in the face of another. When I came to my senses, I half-crawled over to what remained of the girl—only a few pieces of her yellow dress and a couple of shredded flowers she was trying to give me remained.

"That's only one of the traumatic events that happened in Afghanistan, but the worst. I can't get it out of my mind. If only I had been faster in getting to it. If only I had seen her and warned her away. If only. But "if onlys" don't count. This precious little girl was gone forever. I wake up at night in a sweat dreaming of the explosion and trying to warn the girl. Every time I hear a car backfire, I hit the concrete instinctively. I break down when I see little girls in yellow dresses. No, I'm not going back to my eating disorder and this PTSD will eventually get better. But that's what war does to you. I am accepting another tour of duty, partly because I believe that women belong in the armed forces, in every role. Any thoughts?"

After a few moments of silence, Leslie stood up and spoke with tears in her eyes. "What a story. But you know, Carla, it's war over here, too. I was raped at a party by someone I thought was a friend. I can't get it out of my mind either. I get the sweats at night and go right down to the refrigerator for a binge to settle down. I know it's not healthy, but these nightmares terrorize me. Sometimes I don't even remember that I had a binge, except for the bulge in my stomach in the morning. And all those reminders during a regular day that trigger my memories—not only memories—but it's like being right back there saying, 'No, no . . . ,' but he doesn't stop. My heart is racing. It's hard to breathe. Even if a friendly guy in my class taps my shoulder to ask a question, it freaks me out. And then I want to binge."

"Yeah," said Kyle. "I saw my cousin shoot himself in the head playing with a pistol he found in his dad's drawer. He thought it was empty. I can't go to any movies now that have guns. And those sweats you are talking about. That's me. When the flashback comes, my heart feels like it's coming out of my chest, it's beating so strongly. I feel hot and cold at the same time. I think that's what got me started with dieting and body building, and now I can't quit."

And so it went. Marie was sexually assaulted in her own bedroom by a cousin while their parents visited in the living room. It happened every time the families visited. She just couldn't tell her parents. They would never believe it. She decided that if she became so thin and bony that no one would be attracted to her, she would be safe; but she never felt safe, except in this group.

Everyone gave Carla a big hug at the end of the group. They all realized they were in this thing together—bad things, really bad things, happen in Iraq and Afghanistan, but also in the good old USA, and other places. The group members made a decision to be more open about what happened to each one of them in the past, and to text each other if they were having a flashback. War is hell wherever it happens.

Comment: Carla's story is a true story told to me by a patient. To this day, she can't forget the trauma and violence in Iraq and Afghanistan, but especially the tragedy of the little girl in the yellow dress. Whether trauma, sexual or other, is related to an increased chance of developing eating disorders is somewhat controversial. Now, after far too long, the armed services are getting honest about the high prevalence of PTSD in service personnel. At least one-third of patients with eating disorders whom I have treated have had traumatic experiences and then relive the experiences. These vary from bad memories to a daily reliving of the trauma, often triggered by innocuous stimuli. Most have night terrors, as well. For some of these patients, binge eating, dieting, or extreme exercise has become their "solution." The methods of treating PTSD are still evolving and generally improving. But certainly, no history and examination of a patient with an eating disorder are complete without a detailed, compassionate, gentle inquiry into a history of trauma—and no, it should not be done at the first meeting, but only when trust has been gained. Whether or not the trauma is directly related to the onset and maintenance of the eating disorder is not the point—identification and treatment of PTSD is a package deal in treating patients with eating disorders. There are no "Lone Rangers" when it comes to eating disorders—virtually all of them come as package deals, and these days, PTSD and trauma, whether overseas or stateside, are too often part of the picture.

Prescribing Psychotherapy*

Clinicians at times may be unsure about which method of psychotherapy is best for patients with eating disorders. Some clinicians may have training that emphasized only one method of therapy, such as evidence-based cognitive behavioral therapy or psychodynamic therapy. Teaching in medical schools and graduate schools even varies by geography.

A sequence of psychotherapeutic methods may be more helpful than any single method. I have found that a sequence of methods, as described below, meets the needs of most patients with eating disorders when a clinician has a long-term relationship with the patient. Health plan limitations are a reality, but whenever possible, a progressive sequence of psychotherapeutic methods adapted to the severity of the eating disorder supports the patient's return to psychological freedom from the eating disorder and ability to move on with the challenges of life.

Background

The history of psychiatry has been marked by tension between psychodynamic psychiatry and biological psychiatry. The former method has emphasized an understanding of the psychological meaning behind human behavior, whereas the latter has studied the biological substrate of normal and abnormal behavior and emphasized psychopharmacology. Psychodynamic theories and practice dominated psychiatric thinking in the United States until the 1960s, when more systematic methods of diagnosis, epidemiologic studies, and more effective methods of treatment began to cast doubt on some of the classic psychodynamic assumptions. Categories of diagnosis and treatment trials, rather than intrapsychic process issues, came to the forefront. As a result, psychiatry tended to adopt an either/or way of thinking, which led to artificial polarities that asked such questions as, "Is the condition treatable through psychotherapy or should medications and other psychical methods be used?"

Recent studies suggest several major changes are taking place in the field of psychiatry with respect to psychotherapy. Many psychiatric illnesses have been shown to respond best to a combination of psychological and

*Pages 349–65 are adapted from Arnold Andersen, "Prescribing Psychotherapy," in *Directions in Psychiatry*, vol. 9, lesson 17, F. F. Flach, ed., Hatherleigh Co., 1989. With permission of Hatherleigh Press.

psychopharmacologic methods, even though one modality may play the major role. More than one method of psychotherapy is now available, providing alternatives to the once-dominant technique of psychoanalytic psychotherapy. As a result, prescribing a sequence of psychotherapy methods to accommodate the patient's changing needs and capacity for psychotherapeutic work may prove most beneficial.

In place of the either/or polarized thinking between physical and psychological methods of treatment or a dogmatic insistence on one particular form of psychotherapy, the practicing psychiatrist now has the flexibility in prescribing psychotherapy much like the internist has in prescribing an antibiotic. Although it would be naive and premature to assume that psychotherapy prescription has the same empirical support as the rational prescription of an antibiotic, enough studies on psychotherapy research have been published to suggest the analogy is a useful one. Just as a physician must be able to answer certain questions before prescribing a medication, the psychiatrist should find answers to similar questions before beginning a course of psychotherapy. He or she must determine the goals to be attained with the method of treatment; review the evidence that the chosen method has a strong possibility of improving the specific condition of a particular patient; assess the risks involved; explore the available alternatives; and establish which aspect of the total condition psychotherapy can be expected to help. Finally, the psychiatrist must determine how psychotherapy can best be integrated with psychopharmacology for conditions in which pharmacology or other physical methods have been demonstrated to be effective so that each modality can work most effectively in partnership.

Definition of Psychotherapy

Jerome D. Frank (1982), a widely respected student of comparative psychotherapy systems, defines psychotherapy as follows:

> Psychotherapy is a planned, emotionally charged, confiding interaction between a trained, socially sanctioned healer and a sufferer. During this interaction the healer seeks to relieve the sufferer's distress through symbolic communications, primarily words but also sometimes bodily activities. The healer may or may not involve the patient's relatives and others in the healing rituals. Psychotherapy often includes helping the patient to accept and endure

suffering as an inevitable aspect of life that can be used as an opportunity for personal growth.

The two essential purposes of psychotherapy, in Frank's view, are to *restore morale and to help the patient solve specific life problems.*

The FDA Tests: Safety and Efficacy

If psychotherapy is to be prescribed in a manner somewhat analogous to prescribing medication, it may be worthwhile to ask first whether psychotherapy meets the US Food and Drug Administration's (FDA) basic tests for approving new medical treatments—safety and efficacy. Any treatment that has the potential for helping to heal has some potential for misuse. Freud himself said that the application of psychoanalysis to schizophrenia, for example, was a mistaken use of the art, but he went ahead and used psychoanalytic thinking to suggest an etiology for schizophrenia. Following the ancient medical dictum of *primum non nocere*, above all, do no harm, *psychotherapy, applied properly,* and following the ethical guidelines of the American Psychiatric Association, *can be said to be a safe, although not entirely risk-free, procedure. The efficacy of psychotherapy has been a more controversial issue.* The extreme views present in psychiatry suggest, on the one hand, that psychotherapy by a trained individual has no specific effectiveness beyond that which would be accomplished by any caring individual. The other extreme suggests psychotherapy is specifically curative for virtually any psychiatric disorder. The evidence suggests psychotherapy has a definite but variable benefit according to the disorder, being much more effective in bulimia nervosa and nonpsychotic depression than in schizophrenia or dementia. Anorexia nervosa has been more difficult to study because patients are often hospitalized and suffer from severe medical complications, but short of strictly randomly assigned studies of psychotherapeutically treated versus not treated methods (probably unethical), *the current preponderance of evidence supports the prescription of CBT, especially for anorexia nervosa.*

The basic test of whether a hypothesis is a scientific statement or a philosophic statement is achieved by determining if the proposed method can be experimentally tested so that the hypothesis can be either refuted or confirmed (Kuhn, 1970). Some statements regarding psychotherapy can be tested empirically, but others remain more related to philosophic issues. The prescription of a particular form of psychotherapy should ideally develop out of testable forms of treatment. Recent experimental work in the *psychotherapies* (probably a better word than *psychotherapy* as a single generic term) have examined the therapeutic effectiveness of specific forms of psychotherapy for well-defined disorders, using as controls either patients who received no active treatment or those given other modes of treatment, such as medication. Using those procedures for testing, we can say CBT, for example, appears to be as effective as tricyclic antidepressants or SSRIs in treating moderately depressed, nonpsychotic individuals (Simons et al., 1985). It is more effective than medication in treating bulimia nervosa. Monosymptomatic phobias, to use another example, respond routinely to systematic behavioral desensitization (Marks, 1969).

In place of the question, "Does psychotherapy work?" (which would be about as ambiguous as the question, "Do medicines work?"), practicing psychiatrists should be asked, "Does psychotherapeutic method A work for patients with disorder B, using operational definition C of practical application for improvement in their disorder?" This more scientific question not only fails to inhibit psychotherapy treatment but paves the way for progress in the field so that the psychiatrist can become increasingly more effective. A scientific mindset toward the traditional prescription of psychotherapy does not minimize the need for the art of psychotherapy or the need for sensitive relational skills.

Why has psychotherapy not been examined in a more scientific manner? For one thing, research in that area can be much more difficult than research conducted in the field of organic medical disease, where reductionist methods of biochemistry and neurophysiology have led to great advances. Some theoretical statements central to certain forms of psychotherapy are phrased in terms not testable by the scientific method. For example, two central tenets of psychoanalysis, the existence of the unconscious and the belief in psychic determinism (Brenner, 1955), are philosophic, not scientific, statements.

Second, therapists who sincerely and energetically treat individuals one by one in the outpatient setting, using traditional psychotherapy methods, are usually not trained in the experimental approach to hypothesis testing. In addition, they often feel that the improvement of an individual patient under their treatment validates their psychotherapeutic approach.

Other therapists may feel that a scientific approach will inhibit the art of psychotherapy or take the place of empathetic interpersonal relationships. Finally, many training programs teach a particular form of psychotherapy in a dogmatic manner without examining its grounds for credibility or its ability relative to other forms of psychotherapeutic treatment to alleviate psychiatric disorders. This critique of unexamined teaching applies to both biologically based and psychotherapeutically rigid programs. The book *Perspectives of Psychiatry* (McHugh and Slavney, 1983) describes how multiple methods of approaching mental life and human behavior, each with its own strengths and vulnerabilities, can be integrated and used in the diagnosis and treatment of patients with psychiatric illness.

Without implying that simple reductionist methods will ever suffice completely for testing psychotherapeutic paradigms, psychotherapeutic models can and should be tested by appropriate evidence-seeking methods, for a number of reasons. In this day of increasing scrutiny of treatment modalities by third-party payers and governmental sources, data are needed to show that the methods of treatment administered are indeed effective. Psychotherapy can be a long, expensive process and may appear to critical eyes to be an outmoded, high-cost treatment that can be replaced by more-easily-prescribed medications. Several evidence-based forms of psychotherapy have been demonstrated to be effective in a time-limited approach, typically 8–16 sessions. Resistance by psychiatrists to a more scientific approach toward psychotherapy may eventually lead to reduced levels of payment by medical insurance companies when effectiveness cannot be confirmed. The major reasons for a scientific approach to psychotherapy, however, are more fundamental: we want to know if what we are doing to help people is more effective than the mere passage of time or a general level of caring that could be given by a nontrained individual. We wish to continually improve in our practice, and that can be done only by using valid and reliable methods of scrutinizing our treatment approaches for evidence of effectiveness. We need to know that the methods we are using are indeed the best ones for a particular patient.

By using a more evidence-based approach to prescribing psychotherapy, there is no doubt that many psychiatric conditions that cause great suffering can and have been shown to improve substantially with psychotherapy, even if the process is lengthy and costly. Few third-party payers would object to long-term treatment of diabetes or recurring cancer. In short, the needs of both psychiatrists and their patients will be better met by the adoption of a scientific approach to psychotherapy without sacrificing the utterly essential qualifications of human respect and empathy in the process of patient care. The distinguished psychiatrist and philosopher Karl Jaspers (1963) spoke of the need for psychiatrists to have a dual-orientation approach to the patient. On the one hand, the psychiatrist must rigorously take a history and do a full mental status examination so that a clear, scientific definition of the psychopathology involved can be assessed. Only then can he or she enter into an empathic relationship with the patient, appreciating the nature of the existential suffering and offering understanding, hope, and a specific means of improvement. A scientific effort at evaluation of the various forms of psychotherapy in no way reduces the field of psychiatric treatment to a simplistic method or robs it of the richness and complexity of understanding and relieving human suffering.

Prescribing a Method of Psychotherapy

The methods of psychotherapy can be summarized by describing for each method several essential facts: the "key players," the basic idea underlying the method, the basic mode of application, the disorders for which each method has been shown to be suited, and some general comments regarding employment (table 17.1). The use of a single method of psychotherapy based on unexamined teaching that may be decades old is no longer appropriate for many general psychiatrists. In its place, a small group of sequential, complementary methods of psychotherapy, each having some shared as well as some unique features, needs to be learned so the appropriate method can be prescribed in order. If each proponent of each different kind of psychotherapy were mentioned, the list of individual names would quickly grow into hundreds. In practice, however, only a few major forms of psychotherapy are commonly chosen, and they can be categorized according to one of the following goals: to understand the nature of illness; to improve distressed moods; to change abnormal behaviors; to change painful, ineffective, or abnormal ways of thinking; to deal with existential issues of meaning and suffering; to improve dysfunctional family patterns; to make "meaningful connections" on the basis of insight and interpretation of transference; to deal with living in the here and now; to build a "toolbox" of lasting patterns of action and thinking that

Table 17.1. The methods of psychotherapy

Method	Key players	Central concept	Mode of application	Disorders/situations best treated	Comments
Behavioral therapy (BT)	Marks; Wolpe	Progressive desensitization along a hierarchy of increasing fears leads to less restricted, more normal behavior.	Teach method of relaxation; pair relaxation with a hierarchy of increasing fears until feared object, situation, or condition is tolerated.	Monosymptomatic phobias; panic attacks; inhibited sexual response; binge eating	Real-life (in vivo) or ideational (in vitro) methods both effective. Other examples include sensate focus therapy (sexual disorders) and response inhibition (bulimia nervosa).
Cognitive behavioral therapy (CBT)	Beck; Rush; Garner; Garfinkel; Fairburn	Painful moods, self-defeating behaviors, and abnormal eating behaviors result from overvalued or irrational beliefs ("grids") and automatic thoughts.	Identify irrational mental "grids"; challenge and refute irrational beliefs by evidence gathering; practice new appropriate and supportive ways of thinking and acting.	Mild to moderate nonpsychotic depression; binge-eating disorder; bulimia nervosa; obsessive-compulsive disorders; probably anorexia nervosa	Often paired with behavioral methods.
Dialectical behavioral therapy (DBT)	Linehan	Patterns of abnormal behaviors and thinking can be changed by increasing emotional and cognitive regulation.	Combines CBT with distress tolerance, acceptance, and mindfulness meditation.	Borderline personality disorder; suicidal ideation; substance abuse; mood disorders; some eating disorders	Reduces rate of rehospitalization and reduces suicidal gestures in year after treatment.

(*continued*)

Table 171. (continued)

Method	Key players	Central concept	Mode of application	Disorders/situations best treated	Comments
Existential psychotherapy	Frankl; Yallom	Issues of meaning, values, identity, suffering, and finiteness are central to authentic living.	Clarify values and identity; deal with fears of nothingness and the meaning of painful experiences.	(1) Use as a concluding method in a sequence of psychotherapies. (2) For existential issues rather than for severe major psychiatric disorders.	Has roots in philosophy and religion—may have agnostic or theistic forms. Overlaps fields of philosophy and religion.
Family therapy	Minuchin; Halley	An individual patient's symptoms are often an expression of underlying family dysfunction.	Identify maladaptive systems of family functioning, inappropriate norms, undercommunication, and lack of generational boundaries. Establish healthy, age-appropriate functioning.	The younger the patient, the more likely family therapy is necessary and useful for anorexia nervosa, as adjunct in schizophrenia and mood disorders, behavioral disorders of children, and distressed family states.	Multiple innovative techniques include reassignment of roles, "care lists," dramatization of family patterns, clarification of communications.
Interpersonal psychotherapy (IPT)	Klerman; Paykel; Sullivan; Weissman	Improvement in distressed relationships leads indirectly to improvement in the specific psychiatric disorder.	Time-limited (12–16 sessions); uses practical diagrams of relationships, directive; generally does not focus on the disorder itself.	Ambulatory patients with bulimia nervosa; postpartum depression; distressed family functioning	Rated as moderately effective, slightly slower than CBT, for bulimia nervosa; interrupts one leg of triangle of mood-thinking-behavioral interaction.

Mindfulness	Kabat-Zinn	Mindfulness is a feature of human consciousness, which a person can increasingly become aware of in the here and now.	Teach nonjudgmental acceptance and awareness of ongoing emotions and physical and mental sensations.	Anxiety disorders; stress reduction; grief; pain; depression	Derived from the nonreligious component of Buddhism; has preventive value.
Psychodynamic methods	Adler; Freud; Jung; Kernberg; Klein; Kohut	Confusing or painful feelings, behaviors, and relationships are linked in a causal way with crucial developmental experiences of both an intrapsychic and interpersonal nature.	Free associations, dream work, and interpretations of the transference of relationship lead to insightful understanding of personal development, working through of painful feelings or dysfunctional ways of thinking and behaving, and developing new patterns of living.	Insightful, motivated, distressed individuals with internal conflicts, situational stresses, unsatisfying relationships; some personality disorders; complex eating disorders	Newer forms include transactional analysis, object relations, and self-psychology schools. Short-term dynamic therapy described by Sifneos.

(continued)

Table 17.1. (continued)

Method	Key players	Central concept	Mode of application	Disorders/situations best treated	Comments
Psychoeducation	Donley; Tomlinson; Anderson; Garner; Garfinkel	Education about the nature and course of illness empowers the patient to deal with disorders in a healthy way.	Provide nonjudgmental information about the illness to the patient and family; clarify misinformation. Aims to create alliance with the treatment team.	Essential for all disorders in the diagnostic and treatment phases; the first step, and intrinsic to, continuing treatment where additional forms of psychotherapy are appropriate.	Basic but often underused; creates trust when given in warm, supportive manner.
Reality therapy	Glasser	Holding individuals accountable for responsible behavior leads to more improvement than insight-oriented methods for these individuals.	Confront patients with irresponsible behaviors by limit setting and positive reinforcement of healthy behavior. Emphasis is on here and now, not insight.	Antisocial behavior; histrionic behavior	Best documented form of psychotherapy for antisocial behavior.
Supportive psychotherapy	Bloch	Acute traumatic events or chronic stresses lead to emotional distress and loss of or regression of preexisting defense mechanisms.	Give reassurance and explanation; offer specific suggestions; restore morale; change the environment where necessary.	Overwhelming life circumstances; severe personality disorders; adjunctive treatment for major mental illness	Reintegration of preexisting defenses is the goal, not working through and "sealing over," not "uncovering" or developing more mature defenses.

Note: See the Suggested Readings for publications supporting studies of these psychotherapeutic methods.

continue after therapy is concluded; and to emphasize supportive empathetic care.

Many different psychotherapy methods share important features, such as development of a trusting interpersonal relationship, showing empathy, and timely responses or interpretations. Enough empirical work has been done, however, to suggest that—unless one's practice is limited to a specific type of patient—a sequential or concurrent combination of several psychotherapy techniques is probably best for most patients. It is crucial for the therapist, if concomitant methods are used, such as CBT and psychodynamic psychotherapy, to be aware of which method is at the forefront for each treatment session. The essential decisions regarding psychotherapy that need to be made include the following:

- Will psychotherapeutic methods be central or adjunctive for this disorder?
- What skills or experiences does the patient bring to the therapy situation that may make one method more appropriate than another? For example, a non-insightful patient with severe alexithymia may not benefit from an insight-oriented form of psychotherapy.
- Are there contraindications to a particular form of therapy? Any treatment that can help can also be used in a harmful manner.
- Does the practitioner have the skills necessary to implement the chosen form of psychotherapy?

Practicing psychiatrists may be prisoners of their own methods of training. There is a tendency to practice unreflectedly the kind of training that one has worked hard to learn in the past, often accentuated by a sense of personal benefit and psychological understanding obtained by the therapist during the training period. Being a prisoner of one's method of learning, however, does not serve the psychiatrist or the patient well. Openness to new evidence-based methods that leads to taking courses and workshops in additional evidence-based forms of psychotherapy is essential.

Psychotherapeutic Options

Some examples may be useful in illustrating the choice of a method of psychotherapy for a specific disorder in a patient. Incidentally, the term *patient*, which derives from the word for "suffering," is used here rather than *client*. Although the term *client* has been advocated recently to designate the sufferer and represents a worthy effort to see the suffering individual as the initiator of the therapeutic services, we feel the term is less suitable to the historical role of the physician, psychologist, or other mental health professional as a caregiver.

Mr. A has suffered an acute myocardial infarction at age 49. He is doing well medically in the intensive care unit but is complaining of depression. He has a compulsive personality and was raised in a family characterized by angry striving rather than supportive interaction and reasonable goals. The consultation-liaison psychiatrist identifies the need for some control on the patient's part during treatment and asks the medical staff to allow Mr. A to independently take a single small dose of an antianxiety agent from a bedside single-dose supply when he feels very anxious. He is given control of time-limited small IV doses of morphine when he has cardiac pain. He is given precise and comforting psychoeducation concerning the mild nature of his infarction, the absence of need for myocardial revascularization, and the probability of a return to work and marital relations in 6 weeks. He is given nonblaming information regarding his type A driven personality and a specific referral to a mindfulness group following discharge. His therapy has been designed to be supportive, informative, and directive, attempting to integrate his existing defenses and suggesting nonblaming ways to diminish his compulsive lifestyle, which may predispose him to increased risk for future cardiac symptoms. He is taught a method of relaxation that he finds lowers his blood pressure.

Ms. B suffers from panic disorder that has made her fearful of continuing her volunteer work in the community. Fearing new attacks, she has begun to experience anticipatory anxiety, and she has also developed secondary depressive symptoms. The outpatient psychiatrist she has chosen prescribes behavioral desensitization integrated with cognitive behavioral methods of psychotherapy to alleviate the panic attacks and to diminish the resulting anticipatory anxiety and avoidance behavior. Using educational material by Claire Weeks (1969), the psychiatrist explains to the patient a plan to engage a psychotherapy assistant in the beginning of treatment to help the patient walk through situations like those that triggered panic attacks in the past, such as a movie theater, driving over a long bridge, and shopping in a crowded department store. The patient learns to become an observer of the panic attack, watching it crescendo and then diminish, experiencing lower and lower peak anxiety with each successful "walking through" of a panic attack. The patient's beliefs that she is dying or going crazy are identified and cognitively refuted using evidence for and against her cognitive distortion. A support group is recommended.

Ms. C has grown up in a family marked by three generations of alcoholism and has been the object of both physical and verbal abuse. She has developed a self-defeating pattern of trying to please everyone around her. Through 2 years of twice-weekly dynamic psychotherapy, she has effectively reconstructed her developmental pattern whereby she grew up switching generational roles to become a parent to her parent, anticipating her father's violent rages, having learned to say and do whatever was necessary to inhibit his rages. Her anger toward her ineffective mother who has enabled her father's alcoholism becomes apparent to her for the first time as she learns not to be frightened of angry feelings. She learns not to take responsibility for her parents' behaviors or to blame herself for their behaviors; she becomes appropriately assertive. Through dynamic therapy, she frees herself of her sense of fatalism about following the path of her mother by being a woman who is destined to choose an alcoholic husband.

D is a 16-year-old antisocial young man who had repeatedly been brought before the courts for a number of minor offenses, including stealing. More recently, his offenses have become more serious and include armed robbery and cocaine abuse. Through his family's efforts, he has been placed in a closed unit for disordered adolescents. In that setting, he attempts to blame his parents and his environment for his behavior. His psychotherapist, prescribing reality therapy (Glasser, 1965), asks him to focus on his own irresponsible and illegal behavior—not accepting excuses for it. He is confronted with his lack of remorse, with his law breaking, and with a probable future involving long jail sentences. Only after limits on his behavior are consistently enforced for several months on a closed unit does he develop some depression and—for the first time—a sense of personal suffering and a bond with his therapist. He is granted short supervised passes with specific tasks to accomplish only when his behavior on the unit becomes responsible. He is told to "cut the b.s." when he tries to blame his parents for his behavior. He is eventually promoted to the position of chair of the daily unit group meetings and begins to take remedial school courses to obtain his GED.

Ms. E is a 24-year-old woman with paranoid schizophrenia who has suffered many relapses despite adequate doses of neuroleptic medication.

Her family lives in an intense emotional atmosphere characterized by hostility and unclear communications. Through family therapy as an adjunct to her medication, the family's emotional tone becomes less intense, more calm, and more appropriate, and individual family members learn to express their feelings through words. Because of the interest shown toward them and their struggle with the chronic illness of their daughter, the parents begin to feel less overwhelmed and are able to quietly discuss issues, lowering the tense atmosphere in the family. In the year following family therapy, the patient greatly reduces the number of repeat hospital admissions she needs, and her haloperidol (Haldol) dose is lowered to half the previous dose.

Choosing a Sequence of Psychotherapy Methods for Eating Disorders

Not only can one particular form of psychotherapy be more appropriate for a particular disorder in a given individual. but a sequence of psychotherapy methods can often be the most useful prescription for a patient's needs. The following are some examples.

Ms. A, a 19-year-old woman with a 7-year history of anorexia nervosa, bulimic subtype, enters a hospital for treatment of her eating disorder. Because her weight is very low, her mental concentration is poor, and she feels cold, the initial prescription is one for supportive and psychoeducational psychotherapy aimed at restoring her morale and instilling a sense of hope for the future along with knowledge about her illness. Psychotherapy is given in short daily sessions for the first 2 weeks. Once medical stabilization has taken place and nutritional rehabilitation is under way, an 8-week program in CBT is begun. Emphasis in psychotherapy shifts to cognitive behavioral work, identifying the patient's many irrational beliefs about the overvaluation of thinness and her fear that normal eating will make her fat. She learns to challenge and refute the abnormal patterns of thinking, trying for the first time to see the environment as it really is, and showing a willingness to accept praise when given rather than listening only to criticism. When she is transitioned to partial psychiatric hospital (day program) after attaining 85% of healthy body weight, and showing some skill in beginning CBT methods, the emphasis on CBT continues more intensively in the partial hospital. For the first 6 months of outpatient psychotherapy, CBT is continued, with the emphasis gradually shifting from CBT alone to a beginning focus on psychodynamic psychotherapy, helping the patient recognize the connections between her own life experiences and the function her eating disorder serves. She recognizes that becoming extremely thin when she was 13 was a way to keep her parents from separating. It also allowed her to gain attention that had been disproportionately given to her extroverted older sister. Later, when her parents' marital relationship improved and that purpose was no longer necessary to keeping her eating disorder, she began to recognize that her thinness additionally allowed her to avoid her fears of sexual development and possible advances from young men. She comes to understand that her eating disorder is also based on a phobic avoidance of developing a personal identity. She identifies her early childhood lack of internalization of a stable, nurturing object due to the impoverished relationship with her mother, who was frequently hospitalized for mental illness.

During the last 6 months of an 18-month outpatient psychotherapy experience, the emphasis gradually shifts to existential psychotherapy, helping Ms. A make sense of her suffering, but with a return to either CBT reinforcement or a dynamic interpretation of the transference relationship when either is appropriate. The patient is then able to express her rage at years of wasted time and to reexamine her inherited family values, no longer afraid to change what she believes in. She develops a commitment to help others to avoid her experience of an eating disorder and to live each day to the fullest without regret for the past or fear of the future. She finds the story of Viktor Frankl (1962) helpful in allowing her to get beyond her self-imprisonment of anorexia nervosa.

Dr. C, a 35-year-old physician on the faculty of a university, presents with bipolar II mood disorder and muscle dysmorphic disorder, sometimes called "reverse anorexia nervosa." During the early phase of mood stabilization with lithium and an antidepressant, the psychotherapeutic emphasis is on supportive and psychoeducational psychotherapy to give him hope for eventual improvement beyond each mood shift and to understand both of his disorders, while respecting his intellect and desire for knowledge of research studies. Through cognitive and dynamic therapy, he stops feeling guilty and self-blaming during depressive episodes, which have been accompanied by thoughts of suicide; he begins to be able to say, "It, the illness, is here again," not that "I am my illness." He can say with conviction that "I feel sad, but I know that I am a good person." He begins to identify and change triggers of his mood shifts, including working late at night in the laboratory, continuing verbal fights on holidays with his parents, and feelings of inadequacy in dating only women who are needy. During the CBT phase of his therapy, he is able to change his overvalued belief in the necessity of large muscularity and very low body fat. He agrees to cover the mirrors in his house except for a small section to let him see to brush his hair and brush his teeth, as a way to stop his mirror gazing and self-criticism for thinking he is puny. Through psychodynamic psychotherapy, he recognizes his anger at his mother's psychological unavailability during his youth because of her mood disorder, which made her frequently ill and in need of him to act as a supportive parent. He understands why he has feared women who are like his aunt who smothered him with unending hugs. Through his psychodynamic and existential phases of psychotherapy, he attempts to moderate his overvalued ambition of becoming board-certified in three specialties in order to prove his worth to himself; he becomes less concerned about international fame for his research and starts placing greater value on developing caring relationships with women who are not needy or predatory. He finds that daily prescribed exercise helps regulate his mood. He gradually comes to view himself as fit and attractive, not tiny and unattractive.

In summary, choosing a method of psychotherapy is an important, and can be a rational, decision in patient care. Sufficient research is now available to choose a particular form of psychotherapy or a sequence of psychotherapy methods that are appropriate for a given patient. The psychiatrist's psychotherapeutic techniques need to be examined and updated when the methods used are overly restrictive or inadequate for the patient's needs. By keeping in mind the general guidelines of Dr. Frank (1982)—psychotherapy always has two main purposes: restoring morale and helping to solve problems—the clinician's choice of psychotherapy technique or techniques may determine the effectiveness of the intervention. Transcending all the particular methods of psychotherapy is respect for the patient as a unique individual, empathy for his or her suffering, and an attempt to match the patient's particular disorder with the most effective therapy available. At times, psychotherapy will provide the major, or sole, emphasis in treatment, but at other times it serves a vital adjunctive role. For eating disorders, evidence-based psychotherapy, especially CBT, but also IPT and DPT, are essential. Further, especially for eating disorders, psychotherapy is for many patients best prescribed in a sequential manner. There is no psychiatric disorder for which psychotherapy is not an essential part of comprehensive treatment. Any psychiatric disorder, whether resulting from stressful events, from a vulnerable temperament, or from distressed relationships, or when it springs from well-documented genetic or biochemical causes, always creates human suffering (even an elated manic episode takes its toll), dysfunctional patterns of thinking and behaving, and eventually an altered sense of personal identity and worth. Choosing an effective method of psychotherapy or a sequence of psychotherapy methods based on the most scientific studies available and following the guiding principles of ethical treatment will allow psychiatry to continue to deal with the broad range of mental disorders that affect human beings.

Summary

The treatment of eating disorders most often involves a combination of medical and psychotherapeutic methods. For the very ill patient, such as an individual with anorexia nervosa and a BMI of 10–12, the initial treatment is primarily medical for several weeks. For a patient struggling with bulimia nervosa who is at normal weight and has normal electrolytes and normal findings on medical evaluation, the treatment may be primarily psychotherapeutic from the beginning. Most patients may need a combination of medical and psychotherapeutic interventions, with a changing ratio of these two components as treatment progresses. Treatment also varies, of course, with age and with psychological mindedness—and unfortunately, with health plans' allowable length of stay. Psychoeducation from the very beginning of treatment, even for highly medically compromised patients, prepares the way for psychotherapy that can identify and change underlying cognitive distortions. Once a patient is medically stable (if initially treated in the intensive care unit) and able to progress in an inpatient psychiatric unit or a residential care program, the practice of writing a letter to the illness as friend and foe begins to establish a psychotherapeutic interaction based on the individualizing features of these letters. The clinician can then plan a sequence of personalized psychotherapeutic methods, based both on the eating disorder diagnosis and on the comorbid features. For example, for a patient diagnosed with bulimia nervosa who also meets the criteria for borderline personality disorder with past self-harm attempts, in the second phase of the sequence—evidence-based manualized psychotherapy—the clinician may choose dialectical behavioral therapy rather than cognitive behavioral therapy, although these two methods are increasingly being blended. For younger patients especially, and in groups, stories often communicate concepts that more technical terms do not. Beyond words, however, stories offer visualization and employ different parts of the brain, utilizing the strengths of even very ill patients.

SUGGESTED READINGS
The following are additional illustrative publications supporting studies of the psychotherapeutic methods listed in table 17.1, with an emphasis on practical application (including workbooks). The emphasis is on seminal original publications.

GENERAL OVERVIEW OF PSYCHOTHERAPIES
Gabbard, Glen O., Judith S. Beck, and Jeremy Holmes. *Oxford Textbook of Psychotherapy*. Oxford: Oxford University Press, 2007.

BEHAVIORAL THERAPY
O'Leary, K. Daniel, and G. Terence Wilson. *Behavior Therapy: Application and Outcome*. Englewood Cliffs, NJ: Prentice-Hall, 1975, pp. 7–12.

COGNITIVE BEHAVIORAL THERAPY
Fairburn, Christopher G, Zafra Cooper, and Roz Shafran. Cognitive behaviour therapy for eating disorders: A "transdiagnostic" theory and treatment. *Behavior Research and Therapy* 41(5):509–28, 2003.

DEPRESSION
Greenberger, Dennis, and Christine Padesky. *Mind Over Mood*. New York: Guilford Press, 1995.

DIALECTICAL BEHAVIORAL THERAPY
Linehan, Marsha M. *Cognitive Behavioral Treatment of Borderline Personality Disorder*. New York: Guilford Press, 1993.
Linehan, Marsha M. *DBT Skills Training Manual*, 2nd ed. New York: Guilford Press, 2014.

EATING DISORDERS
Grilo, Carlos M., and James E. Mitchell, eds. *The Treatment of Eating Disorders: A Clinical Handbook*. New York: Guilford Press. 2010.

EXISTENTIAL PSYCHOTHERAPY
Yalom, Irvin D. *Existential Psychotherapy*. New York: Basic Books, 1980.

FAMILY THERAPY

Madanes, Cloé, Alan S. Gurman, and David P. Kniskern, eds. *Handbook of Family Therapy*, vol. 2. Philadelphia: Brunner/Mazel, 1991, pp. 396–416.

INTERPERSONAL PSYCHOTHERAPY

Weissman, Myrna, John Markowitz, and Gerald Klerman. *Comprehensive Guide to Interpersonal Psychotherapy*. New York: Basic Books, 2000.

MINDFULNESS

Kabat-Zinn, Jon. *Full Catastrophe Living*. New York: Bantam Doubleday/Dell Publishing Group, 1990.

PSYCHODYNAMIC PSYCHOTHERAPY

Gabbard, Glen O. *Long-Term Psychodynamic Psychotherapy*. Arlington, VA: American Psychiatric Association Publishing, 2010.

PSYCHOEDUCATION

Garner, David. Psychoeducational principles in treatment. In: David Garner and Paul Garfinkel, eds. *Handbook of Treatment for Eating Disorders*. 1997, pp. 145–73.

REALITY THERAPY

Glasser, William. *Stations of the Mind: New Directions for Reality Therapy*. New York: Harper & Row, 1981.

SUPPORTIVE PSYCHOTHERAPY

Winston, Arnold, Richard N. Rosenthal, and Henry Pinsker. *Introduction to Supportive Psychotherapy*. Washington, DC: American Psychiatric Publishing, 2004.

REFERENCES

Brenner C. 1955. Two fundamental hypotheses. In: *An Elementary Textbook of Psychoanalysis*. New York: Doubleday and Company.

Frank JD. 1982. Therapeutic components shared by all psychotherapies. In: Harvey JH and Parks MM, eds. *Psychotherapy Research and Behavior Change*. Washington, DC: American Psychological Association.

Frankl VE. 1962. *Man's Search for Meaning*. New York: Simon & Schuster.

Glasser W. 1965. *Reality Therapy: A New Approach to Psychiatry*. New York: Harper.

Iacono D, Markesbery WR, Gross M, et al. 2009. Clinically silent AD, neuronal hypertrophy, and linguistic skills in early life. *Neurology* 73:665–73.

Jaspers K. 1963. *General Psychopathology*. Chicago: University of Chicago Press.

Kabat-Zinn J. 1990. *Full Catastrophe Living*. New York: Bantam Doubleday/Dell Publishing Group.

Kuhn TS. 1970. *The Structure of Scientific Revolutions*. Chicago: University of Chicago Press.

Marks IM. 1969. *Fears and Phobias*. London: William Heinemann Medical Books.

McHugh PR and Slavney PR. 1983. *The Perspectives of Psychiatry*. Baltimore: Johns Hopkins University Press.

Rodin J, Silberstein L, and Striegel-Moore. 1985. Women and weight: A normative discontent. In: Sonderegger TT, ed. *Psychiatry and Gender.* Lincoln: University of Nebraska Press, pp. 267–307.

Serpell L and Treasure J. 2002. Bulimia nervosa: Friend or foe? The pros and cons of bulimia nervosa. *International Journal of Eating Disorders* 32:164–70.

Serpell LJ, Treasure J, Teasdale J, and Sullivan V. 1999. Anorexia nervosa: Friend or foe? *International Journal of Eating Disorders* 25:177–86.

Simons AD, Lustman PJ, Wetzel RD, and Murphy GE. 1985. Predicting response to cognitive therapy of depression: The role of learned resourcefulness. *Cognitive Therapy and Research* 9(1):79–89.

Weeks C. 1969. *Hope and Help for Your Nerves.* New York: Bantam Books.

West, C. 2011. *New York Times,* Sunday Magazine, July 24, p. 11.

Contributors

Ovidio Bermudez, MD, is the Chief Clinical Officer and Medical Director of Child & Adolescent at Eating Recovery Center, Denver.

Carrie Brown, MD, is an attending physician on ACUTE at Denver Health and an Assistant Professor of Medicine at the University of Colorado School of Medicine.

Craig Johnson, PhD, is the Chief Science Officer of Eating Recovery Center and Clinical Professor of Psychiatry at the University of Oklahoma College of Medicine.

Mori Krantz, MD, is the cardiologist for ACUTE at Denver Health and a Professor of Medicine at the University of Colorado School of Medicine.

Russell Marx, MD, is an attending psychiatrist at Eating Recovery Center, Denver, and the Chief Science Officer for NEDA.

Margherita Mascolo, MD, is the Medical Director of ACUTE at Denver Health and an Associate Professor of Medicine at the University of Colorado School of Medicine.

Jennifer McBride, MD, is an attending primary care physician at Eating Recovery Center, Denver.

Anne Marie O'Melia, MS, MD, is the Medical Director of Eating Recovery Center, Denver, for Adult Services, Lowry campus, and Medical Director of Eating Recovery Center, Ohio.

Cynthia Pikus, PhD, is the Senior Clinical Director for Adult Services at Eating Recovery Center, Denver.

Katherine Sachs, MD, is an attending physician on ACUTE at Denver Health and an Assistant Professor of Medicine at the University of Colorado School of Medicine.

Kristine Walsh, MD, MPH, is an attending primary care physician at Eating Recovery Center, Denver.

Kenneth Weiner, MD, is the Founder and Chief Executive Office of Eating Recovery Center, Denver, and an Associate Professor of Psychiatry at the University of Colorado School of Medicine.

Patricia Westmoreland, MD, is an attending psychiatrist at Eating Recovery Center, Denver.

Index